NurseThink® for Students

Conceptual Clinical Cases

Next Gen Clinical Judgment:
From Fundamentals to NCLEX®

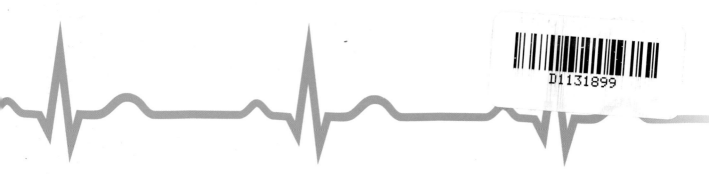

Tim J. Bristol

PhD, RN, CNE, ANEF, FAAN

Karin J. Sherrill

RN, MSN, CNE, ANEF, FAADN

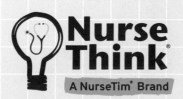

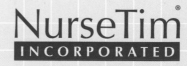

Follow Us On Social Media 🅵 🅾 @NurseThink / NurseThink.com / Help@NurseThink.com

Executive Editor: Tim Bristol
General Manager: Mitch Fisk
Project Coordinator: Rebecca Synoground
Design Account Director: Cory Dammann
Design, Layout, & Production: Shayla Johnson
Marketing Manager: Kelly Christian
Video Production Assistant: Hans Bristol
Photography: © Shutterstock

Published by NurseTim, Inc., P.O. Box 86, Waconia, MN 55387

This book is designed for use as a supplement to learning and clinical judgment. This resource should not be used as a replacement for the care that can be provided by medical professionals. Neither the authors, contributors, or publisher assume any responsibility for injury or damage to persons or property resulting from the interpretation and application of information contained within this resource.

The authors developed this content based on current research and available information at the time of publication. Due to the constantly changing nature of the medical knowledge base, the procedures and best practices contained herein should be evaluated by the reader on an ongoing basis to ensure content legitimacy within this field of study. NCLEX®, NCLEX-RN®, and NCLEX-PN® are federally registered trademarks and service marks of the National Council of State Boards of Nursing, Inc. This publication and subsequent publications are not endorsed by the National Council of State Boards of Nursing, Inc.

Additional copies of this publication are available at www.NurseThink.com.

ISBN: 978-0-9987347-7-4

Printed in the United States of America

First Edition

Table of Contents

Table of Contents

SECTION 4

Care of the Multi-Concept Client

Index

Focused Index for Go To Clinical Cases

About the Authors

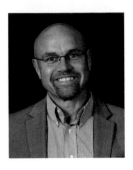

Dr. Tim Bristol is a nurse educator from Minneapolis, Minnesota. He has taught students at all levels to include LPN, ADN, BSN, MSN, and PhD. Through NCLEX® reviews and coaching, NurseTim® brings clinical judgment to life for students and faculty at all levels. He works with programs and organizations internationally on everything from student remediation and retention to exams and curricular success. He helps ensure that clinical is the focus of everything that happens in nursing education. He also enjoys working internationally and leads many service learning trips each year with his wife and four children. Over the past 12 years, he has led over 600 travelers abroad focusing on community development and nursing.

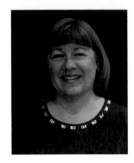

Karin J. Sherrill is a Nurse Educator with a passion for faculty development, test item writing, active teaching strategies, and the integration of the clinical judgment model in nursing education. She has taught ADN and BSN students locally and internationally for almost three decades. Karin has worked closely with publishing and technology companies, as well as testing and professional organizations to advance student success and nursing education. She loves to develop ways to escalate the level of thinking and decision making of the future bedside nurse. Karin's favorite classroom saying is "If your brain doesn't hurt, I haven't done my job."

Letter From the Authors

Every minute that you study should feel as if you are standing next to the client, whether it's in their home, in their hospital room, in their community, or at their school. By studying this way, you are learning in the same way that you will apply new information as a professional nurse. It is about developing a habit of collecting clinical cues, analyzing the information, and prioritizing the actions. The clients in this book will help you study as if you are the nurse providing the care – it creates realism. You will learn by helping each person in this book navigate a very difficult, but realistic health related experience. We hope you will address each of these clients with the seriousness and professionalism that they deserve. They are real. From our experience, you will save time studying by developing these key habits of NurseThink® and Clinical Judgment. Making it real will allow you to become the thinking nurse you are striving to be.

- Karin & Tim

Reviewers and Contributors

Mary Boyce, MSN, RN, CCRN, CNE
Nursing Faculty
Mesa Community College
Mesa, AZ

Anne Brett, PhD, RN
Faculty
College of Doctoral Studies at University of Phoenix
Consultation Manager, NurseTim Inc.
Germantown, WI

Kristofer Bristol, BSN, RN
Registered Nurse
University of Minnesota Medical Center
Minneapolis, MN

Clare Buck
Nursing Student
Clemson University
Clemson, SC

Roni Collazo, PhD, RN
Division Chair
Estrella Mountain Community College
Avondale, AZ

Elise Dando, MSN, RN
Registered Nurse
Mayo Clinic Hospital
Phoenix, AZ

Susan Feinstein, MSN, RN, CNS-BC
Nursing Faculty
Cochran School of Nursing
Yonkers, NY

Jennifer S. Graber, EdD, PMHNP-BC
Assistant Professor
University of Delaware
Newark, DE

Mark C. Hand, PhD, RN, CNE
Department Chair BSN Nursing
East Carolina University
Greenville, NC

Maria Harmann, MSN, RN
Nursing Faculty
GateWay Community College
Phoenix, AZ

Judith W. Herrman, PhD, RN, ANEF, FAAN
Professor Emerita
University of Delaware, School of Nursing
Newark, DE

Barbara Horning, ASN, RN
Registered Nurse
Good Samaritan Society
Waconia, MN

Paige J. Lodien
Nursing Student
Crown College
St. Bonifacius, MN

Linda Merritt, PhD, RNC-NIC, CNE
Assistant Professor
Texas Woman's University
Dallas, TX

Melissa Moser, MSN, RN, CNEcl
Assistant Professor of Nursing
Lake Region State College
Devils Lake, ND

Jason Mott, PhD, RN, CNE
Assistant Professor
University of Wisconsin
Oshkosh, WI

Darcy A. Nelson, PhD, RN, HN-BC
Nursing Faculty
Ridgewater College
Hutchinson, MN

Nicole C. Orent, MSN, RN, CNE
Nursing Faculty
Scottsdale Community College
Scottsdale, AZ

L. Jane Rosati, EdD, MSN, RN, ANEF
Professor
Daytona State College
Daytona Beach, FL

Kathryn Shaffer, EdD, MSN, RN, CNE
Assistant Professor
Thomas Jefferson University, College of Nursing
Philadelphia, PA

Bryan M. Sherrill, BS, BA, EIT
Graduate Student
Columbia University
New York, NY

Winsome Stephenson, PhD, MSN, RN, CNE
Nurse Educator
NurseTim, Inc.
Waconia, MN

Stephanie W. Terry, Ph.D., RN, CNE
Nurse Educator
NurseTim, Inc.
Waconia, MN

Melissa Williams, MSN-Ed, RN, CPN
Nursing Faculty
Glendale Community College
Glendale, AZ

Introduction

Scan QR Code to access the
10-Minute-Mentor 🔘
NurseThink.com/casestudy-book

The NurseThink®
Way of Thinking

The NurseThink® Way of Thinking uses a **conceptual approach** to apply **Next Gen Clinical Judgment**. The strategies of **Prioritization Power** and **THIN Thinking** allow the student to develop a systematic way of improving clinical judgment in the classroom, lab, simulation, and clinical.

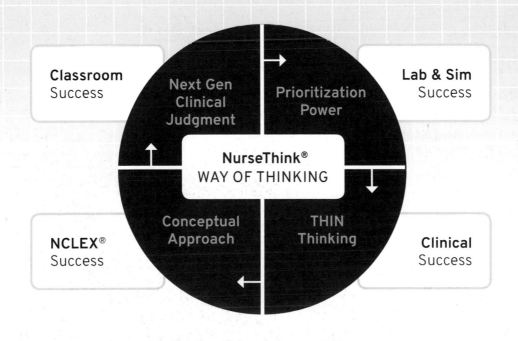

Classroom
Success

Next Gen
Clinical
Judgment

Prioritization
Power

Lab & Sim
Success

NurseThink®
WAY OF THINKING

NCLEX®
Success

Conceptual
Approach

THIN
Thinking

Clinical
Success

NurseThink® Conceptual Approach

A **conceptual approach** to learning helps to save time studying. Using the process of compare and contrast, a student can learn at a higher level than with just memorization. For example, reviewing the concept of oxygenation can be addressed consistently in a variety of conditions (known as exemplars). Whether a client is experiencing an oxygenation problem from pneumonia, pulmonary edema, or a pulmonary embolus, the nurse's actions to address the oxygenation deficit are similar. For this reason, it is important for the nurse to recognize problems of oxygenation and intervene safely, regardless of the underlying cause or illness. The habits formed by the NurseThink® conceptual approach will develop clinical judgment that guides the nurse towards the best action.

NurseThink® Next Gen Clinical Judgment

NurseThink® Next Gen Clinical Judgment originates from evidence and best practices in nursing education. The focus of Next Gen Learning is to apply clinical judgment, also known as the doing that happens after critical thinking and clinical decision making. Next Gen Learning includes the recognition of clinical cues that alert the nurse to formulate and prioritize a hypothesis about which actions need to be taken. Once the action is taken, the nurse needs to determine if it was effective and re-evaluate the hypothesis if necessary.

> **Apply Next Gen Clinical Judgment when you see this symbol.**

NurseThink® Prioritization Power

Prioritization Power is the strategy used when identifying a client's highest priority needs. The Prioritization Power activities may include: priority assessments, priority labs or diagnostics findings, priority complications, priority interventions, priority medications, priority concerns, and/or priority client education or discharge concerns. When completing the Prioritization Power items consider, "What should the nurse do 1st, 2nd, and 3rd?" or "Which lab should the nurse obtain 1st, 2nd, or 3rd?" Know that the correct answer to a test item will be in the top three priorities – guaranteed!

> **Apply Prioritization Power when you see this symbol.**

NurseThink® THIN Thinking

THIN Thinking is a unique strategy by NurseThink®. **THIN** Thinking allows for efficient processing of information that will benefit the student when taking multiple choice and alternative exams questions. This method ensures higher-order mental processing, rather than memorization. Often, students select an answer based on recognition of material and answer by association. This strategy encourages the student to read the question and focus on the intent of what the item is asking. Next, the student will apply the **THIN** mnemonic to guide the decision towards the highest priority answer. This strategy is especially valuable when confused by a question or stuck between two answers.

> **Apply THIN Thinking when you see this symbol.**

To implement THIN Thinking, consider this process:

T: TOP THREE

What are the three highest needs, concepts, questions, components, or elements noted in this question? Ask yourself: What is this question addressing? What are the top three needs?" This is where to apply **Prioritization Power!** Use these prioritization strategies to best determine the Top Three.

> **Maslow's Hierarchy of Needs:** This is a theory that places basic physiological needs as a higher priority than psychological needs. A greater challenge occurs when comparing the priority of safety to physiological needs. For example, if a client is not breathing, that is the priority. But, if the client is not breathing from a car accident and the car is on fire, moving the client to a safe environment should occur before addressing the fact that they are not breathing (making safety a higher priority).

> **ABCs:** This is everyone's favorite. Is there a time when circulation is a higher priority than airway or breathing? Yes. Consider a client with diabetic ketoacidosis and a respiratory rate of 28 breaths per minute. Although alarming, this is a good thing because it indicates that they are attempting to compensate for the metabolic acidosis from the ketosis state. In this case, airway and breathing are not a problem. Move on to circulation.

> **Actual versus Potential:** In most cases, an actual problem will take precedence over a potential problem unless the potential problem presents a greater risk to safety than the actual problem. For example, while an alert client may have an actual problem of vomiting, a client who is nauseated while in c-spine precautions is a higher priority because of the concerns for airway safety.

> **Acute versus Chronic:** Given a choice between acute and chronic, an acute situation will almost always be the higher priority. A good example of this would be a client with COPD. While their disease is being maintained with medications and oxygen, they are considered chronic. When there is evidence of respiratory distress or exacerbations of the symptoms (respiratory rate, ABGs, pulse ox, etc.) the client becomes acute by showing a change in their baseline condition.

> **Least Invasive First:** It is important for the nurse to consider less invasive options before increasing the client's risk of injury with an invasive option. For example, standing a male client at the bedside every two hours to use a urinal is a better option than applying adult diapers. Applying adult diapers is a better option than applying a condom catheter. Applying a condom catheter is a better option than placing a Foley catheter.

> **Safe Practice:** This is always a priority. Safety concerns may include evaluation of the risk for falls, prevention of injury when performing a skill, reduction of risk for hospital acquired infections (HAI), and more.

H: HELP QUICK!

What can the nurse do quickly to relieve the problem? What strategies can the nurse perform immediately while waiting for another intervention or healthcare professional? What interventions may be implemented urgently? Will it help to elevate the head of the bed? What if oxygen is applied? Will the dizziness be improved if the client sits down? How can the nurse act now to help the client? These are the types of questions that the nurse should be asking to help the client as quickly as possible.

I: IDENTIFY RISK TO SAFETY

What are the top safety concerns of the client? The National Council Licensure Examination (NCLEX®) is an exam about safety—many questions are going to address client safety or discuss a threat to client safety. Because of this, it is important to consider the highest concerns for safety experienced by the client. Safety concerns may include evaluation of the risk for falls, prevention of injury, reduction of risk for hospital acquired infections (HAI), and more.

N: NURSING PROCESS

Many questions represent a step of the nursing process. Although it is possible for a test question to refer to any step of the nursing process, the NCLEX® exam is focused on nursing actions. Assessment, Implementation, and Evaluation of care are often the focus of test items. Reflect on "what action should the nurse take next?" knowing that an action can be an assessment, intervention, or evaluation. When determining a priority action, ask yourself, "have I fully assessed what I need in order to safely perform this intervention?" For example, a client with surgical pain of 8 out of 10 needs pain medicine (intervention). A higher priority would be to assess the vital signs to confirm that the medication can be safely delivered without injury to the client.

The Value of Studying with Unfolding Clinical Cases

Never has a nursing school graduate said "my nursing program had too much clinical time!" The more common comment by students is "I wish we had more time in clinical." Most students recognize the value of clinical learning, especially when it is engaging and focused. That is the value of clinical case studies. Many professional disciplines, including nursing, medicine, teaching, and law, all use case studies as a means of teaching and learning. Clinical cases are effective in assisting nursing students to develop critical judgment and enhance problem solving skills while facilitating learning through unfolding scenarios that mimic realistic clinical situations. The process of applying knowledge and concepts in a clinical setting or working with case studies assists students in moving beyond memorization of facts and recall of information into thinking like a nurse and develops an ability to transfer knowledge in similar situations.

The clinical cases in this book will unfold requiring each case to be completed in a systematic, beginning-to-end, order. That means that each case needs to be completed using NurseThink® and Next Gen Clinical Judgment. Much like clients in the health care system, it is important to look comprehensively at the healthcare journey to put the pieces together. When a nurse addresses only a single snapshot in time, holistic care cannot be achieved.

Terms Used Throughout the Clinical Cases

These are terms and abbreviations that are used on the NCLEX® exam and will be used throughout the clinical cases.

> **UAP: Unlicensed assistive personnel** is the term for any healthcare provider who does not have a license, including nurse's aides, assistants, or techs.

> **HCP: Healthcare Provider** include all professionals with prescriptive privileges, including physicians, nurse anesthetists, physician assistants, nurse practitioners, and nurse midwives.

> **Prescriptions:** The term used for any "orders" from the HCP, not just medication related options. For example, a provider can "prescribe" physical therapy or a low sodium diet.

Key

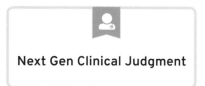

Next Gen Clinical Judgment

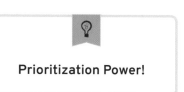

Prioritization Power!

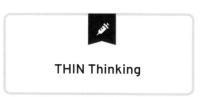

THIN Thinking

Next Gen Clinical Judgment

Examples of Using Prioritization Power and THIN Thinking

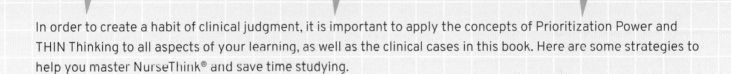

In order to create a habit of clinical judgment, it is important to apply the concepts of Prioritization Power and THIN Thinking to all aspects of your learning, as well as the clinical cases in this book. Here are some strategies to help you master NurseThink® and save time studying.

Prioritization Power with Study Time

Reading

1. Read a section of the textbook (no more than 1-2 pages)

2. Summarize the material in 2-4 sentences. Consider speaking it out loud, recording it, and/or writing it in a notebook.

3. Use Prioritization Power to choose the Top 3 of what was read.

   a. Pathophysiology findings

   b. Assessment findings

   c. Lab findings

   d. Interventions

   e. Medications

   f. Potential problems or complications

   g. Education/Discharge needs

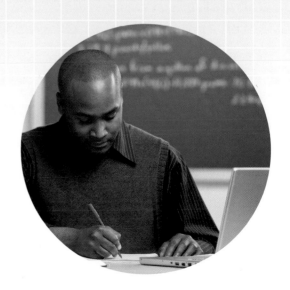

Study Group Learning

1. Bring the Prioritization Power summaries and compare/contrast with your study buddies. This will help you save so much time studying.

2. Complete a Clinical Case in this book and compare/contrast with your study buddies.

3. Challenge your group by asking "what if" for each illness/condition/concept. For example – "What if the client became dizzy, what would I do 1st, 2nd, and 3rd?"

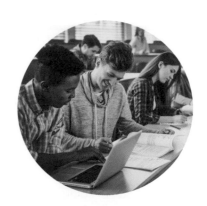

In Class (explore the NurseThink® NoteBook at NurseThink.com)

Organize your Notes into Next Gen Learning by creating a new template. Take your notes in class, then use Prioritization Power after class (within 24 hours) while the information is fresh. Study for the exam from your Prioritization Power Summaries in the right-hand column.

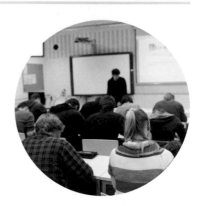

CHRONIC KIDNEY DISEASE	
Notes	**Prioritization Power**
> Maintain fluid and electrolyte balance (K, Na, Ca, Phos) > Dialysis catheter, bruit (hear) & thrill (feel) > Hold meds before dialysis – but not insulin > Weak bones from lack of Vitamin D (Ca) – risk for fractures > Hypertension (HTN), edema from excess fluid > Anemia (lack of erythropoietin (EPO))	**Priority Assessments** 1. Fluid status (lungs, edema, blood pressure (BP)) 2. Electrolytes (K, Na, Ca, Phos) 3. Dialysis Catheter (bruit & thrill) **Priority Labs** 1. Potassium (dysrhythmias) 2. Hemoglobin (anemia – lack of erythropoietin) 3. ABGs (metabolic alkalosis) **Priority Interventions** 1. Daily weights, I/O (fluid status) 2. Lung sounds (crackles) 3. Protect fistula (no tight clothing, no BPs, no IVs) **Priority Complications** 1. Heart failure (HF), Pulmonary Edema (crackles, short of breath (SOB) first) 2. Dysrhythmias (irregular pulse felt) 3. Tissue hypoxia (anemia) **Priority Discharge Goals** 1. Weigh self each day 2. Report shortness of breath 3. Follow renal diet

THIN Thinking with Go To Clinical Cases

As discussed in Chapter 1, THIN Thinking uses an acronym to help strategize the priorities in client care. Here is a quick review.

T: TOP THREE — This is where to apply Prioritization Power! Consider these prioritization options:

> Maslow's Hierarchy of Needs
> ABCs
> Actual versus Potential
> Acute versus Chronic
> Least Invasive First
> Safe Practice

H: HELP QUICK! — What can the nurse do quickly to relieve the problem?

I: IDENTIFY RISK TO SAFETY — What are the top safety concerns of the client?

N: NURSING PROCESS — Many questions represent a step of the nursing process.

Prioritization Power and THIN Thinking with Testing

Try this approach to apply thinking to test items and improve your performance.

1. Read the question more than once. Read JUST the question, NOT the answer choices.
2. Use **Prioritization Power** – Generate all alternatives, then choose the Top 3 Priorities.
3. NOW read the answer choices
4. Taking Actions – (Apply **THIN Thinking**)
5. Evaluating Options – Re-read the question – does the answer make the most sense?

Study Time Examples

EXAMPLE ⓵

Q: The nurse is caring for a client with liver failure who is having a percutaneous liver biopsy. The assessment findings include a heart rate of 115 beats per minute, a respiration of 24 breaths, and a blood pressure of 82/50 (60) mmHg. The client is lethargic and difficult to arouse. Which action should the nurse perform first?

Apply Prioritization Power!

1. **Read JUST the Question – Not the Answers**

2. **Prioritization Power!**
   You have enough assessment information – need to act (The Top 3 Priorities are in italic).

   > *Assess biopsy site for hemorrhage.*
   > Hold pressure at biopsy site if there is bleeding.
   > *Oxygen for change of level of consciousness (LOC) from decreased perfusion.*
   > *Positioning with head of bed down to improve perfusion.*
   > IV fluids to improve perfusion.

3. **NOW Read Answer Options**

   1. Type and cross for 2 units of PRBCs.
   2. Apply oxygen at /nasal cannula.
   3. Apply pressure to the biopsy site.
   4. Place the head of bed flat.

4. **Apply THIN Thinking - H**
   Help Quick — Need to act, there is enough information given that further assessment is not the top priority.

   1. Lower head of bed (NurseThink® Strategy: Least Invasive First)
   2. Apply O$_2$ (NurseThink® Strategy: ABCs)
   3. Assess site (NurseThink® Strategy: Nursing Process)

5. **Evaluate Options**
   Reevaluate vital signs (VS) in 2-3 minutes to determine if interventions were adequate. If not, continue prioritizing care.

Scan QR code to see the correct answers.
Nursethink.com/book-register/casestudy-book

EXAMPLE (2)

Q: The nurse is caring for a client experiencing an acute asthma event. The client is dyspneic with a respiratory rate of 34. The breath sounds are diminished throughout all lung fields. What should be the nurse's next action?

Apply Prioritization Power!

1. **Read JUST the Question – Not the Answers**

2. **Prioritization Power!**

   You have enough assessment information – need to act. Top 3 priorities in italic.

   > *Raise head of the bed*
   > Encourage relaxation, decrease anxiety
   > *Assess pulse oximeter reading – apply O_2 if needed*
   > *Deliver bronchodilator*
   > Determine what precipitated this event

3. **NOW Read Answer Options**

   1. Encourage the client to use the incentive spirometer, cough and deep breath.
   2. Administer albuterol via nebulizer as prescribed.
   3. Request an arterial blood gas be drawn as prescribed.
   4. Assess oxygen saturation reading.

4. **Apply THIN Thinking - H**

   Help Quick – Need to act, there is enough information given that further assessment is not the top priority.

   1. Raise the head of bed (NurseThink® Strategy: Least invasive first)
   2. Assess pulse oximeter reading (NurseThink® Strategy: Nursing Process)
   3. Deliver albuterol (NurseThink® Strategy: Help Quick!)

5. **Evaluate Options**

   Reassess oxygen saturation if O_2 is applied and reassess lung sounds with albuterol delivery.

Scan QR code to see the correct answers.
Nursethink.com/book-register/casestudy-book

Now – try this full question, applying the same steps as examples 1 and 2.

Q: **The nurse is caring for a client with acute kidney injury secondary to septic shock. An IV of 0.9% NaCl is running at 125 mL/hr. Assessment shows crackles in the lungs, distended neck veins, and 1+ pitting edema in the feet. What should be the nurse's next action?**

1. Determine if a diuretic has been ordered.
2. Assess the blood pressure.
3. Evaluate the oxygen saturation reading.
4. Stop the IV infusion.

Apply Prioritization Power!

1. Read JUST the Question – Not the Answers

2. Prioritization Power!

3. NOW Read Answer Options

4. Apply THIN Thinking

5. Evaluate Options

Stem, Answers, and Rationale

Stem: What should be the nurses next action? (The best response is noted by the ◉ symbol.)

1. Determine if a diuretic has been ordered. *This is an intervention.*

2. Assess the blood pressure. *ABCs – Oxygenation assessment comes first.*

3. ◉ Evaluate the oxygen saturation reading. *Further assessment is needed to determine if hypoxia is present.*

4. Stop the IV infusion. *This is an intervention.*

THIN Thinking: Nursing Process – Further respiratory assessment is needed and is a priority over interventions. ABCs places airway before circulation. **NCLEX®**: Physiological Adaptation. **QSEN**: Patient-centered care.

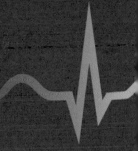

SECTION 2

Concept Overview

Unfolding Concepts I

Sexuality / Circulation / Protection / Homeostasis / Respiration / Nutrition / Hormonal Regulation

Many of the concepts in Chapters 3 and 4 are commonly seen in clients and help with Next Gen Clinical Judgment. The goal of this section is to review and refresh on topics that will appear in the Go to Clinical Cases throughout the book. Be sure to follow the QR code on each page to access additional resources to help save time studying.

The Unfolding Concepts in Chapter 3 are physiological in nature. Each map provides the definition of the concept, the priority assessment or cues, and lab findings. Related concepts are listed to deliver additional guidance when caring for clients. Additionally, normal and abnormal findings are reviewed.

To best understand this material, it is important to apply the concepts as a nurse would. Be sure to explore the online resources for assistance and coaching in NurseThink®.

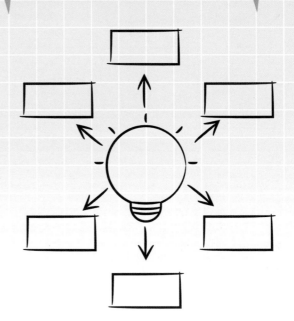

Clinical Hint: Use these Unfolding Concept Maps with every Go To Clinical Case (Patient Assignment) in the book. This will develop your Clinical Judgment Muscles!

Reproduction

Definition

The process by which humans produce a new life.

Requirements for Normal Reproduction

> Sexual Maturity
> Functional Reproductive System
> Functional Endocrine System
> Access to Partner/Sperm/Ova

Priority Assessment or Cues

> Maternal Health, Nutrition, Weight & Lifestyle Behaviors
> Current Medications
> Gravidity, Term Births, Preterm Births, Abortions/ Miscarriages, Living Children (GTPAL)
> Menstrual Cycle Regularity
> Nausea/Vomiting/Hydration Status
> Blood Pressure, Edema
> Fetal Heart Tones and Movement
> Uterine Contractions, Spotting, Membrane Rupture
> Cervical Dilation

Priority Labs

Sexually Transmitted Infections Screenings, Human chorionic gonadotropin (hCG). Rh Factor, CBC, Hormone Levels

Effective Reproduction

> Fertilization
> Implantation
> Maintenance of Pregnancy
> Healthy Delivery
> Healthy Term Neonate

Ineffective Reproduction

> Infertility
> Fetal Demise
> High Risk Pregnancy
> Fetal Loss
> Miscarriage
> Maternal Fetal Complications
> Male Infertility

Related Concepts

> Sexuality
> Nutrition
> Metabolism
> Comfort
> Coping
> Mood and Affect
> Grief

**Additional related concepts may be considered based on the client's situation.*

Sexuality

Definition

The factors allow a person to experience and express them self as a sexual being. Facilitates a person's gender identity.

Influences of Sexuality Perception

> Sexual Attitudes & Behaviors
> Adequacy of Hormones
> Adequacy of Sexual Physiology
> Acceptance of Self

Priority Assessment or Cues

> Physical Assessment of Sex Organs
> Physical, Sexual, & Psychological Health Status
> Sexual Relationships
> Sexual Desire, Connection, Consent, & Choice
> Sexual Self-Concept

Priority Labs

Cultures for Sexually Transmitted Infections (STI), Hormone Levels

Normal Sexuality

> Positive Attitudes & Behaviors
> Well-Being
> Healthy Association with Others
> Free of Pain and Discomfort

Altered Sexuality

> Altered Libido
> Depression
> Adolescent Pregnancy
> Erectile Dysfunction
> Gender Identity Confusion
> Sexually Transmitted Infection

Related Concepts

> Safety
> Comfort
> Coping
> Immunity
> Reproduction
> Interpersonal Relationships
> Anxiety
> Communication

**Additional related concepts may be considered based on the client's situation.

Perfusion

Scan the QR Code to access *Go To Clinical Cases* that correlate with the Unfolding Concepts.

NurseThink.com/casestudy-book

Definition

The ability for the body to move blood through the vascular system to deliver nutrients and oxygen to the cells, while removing cellular waste.

Requirements for Normal Perfusion

> Functioning Cardiopulmonary System Including Vascular Tone and Adequate Pump
> Adequate Fluid Volume in the Vascular Space
> Free from Blockages Including Clots and Atherosclerosis

Priority Assessment or Cues

> Blood Pressure (Mean Arterial Pressure-MAP)
> Pulses - Capillary Refill
> Level of Consciousness (LOC)
> Bowel Sounds
> Urine Output
> Pain
> Skin color
> Temperature

Priority Labs

Hgb/Hct, RBC, Protein/Albumin, BUN/Creatinine, Cardiac & Liver Enzymes, Change to Brain Natriuretic Peptide (BNP)

Adequate Perfusion

> Alert/Oriented
> MAP > 65 mmHg
> Urine Output > 30 mL/hr
> Pulses WNL
> Warm to Touch
> Tissue Color WNL

Inadequate Perfusion

> Light-headed or Confused
> Sensation Loss
> Decreased Organ Function
> Ischemic Pain
> Cell & Tissue Necrosis

Related Concepts

> Clotting
> Comfort
> Oxygenation
> Digestion/Elimination
> Mobility/Sensory
> Tissue Integrity
> Reproduction
> Fluid and Electrolytes Balance
> Inflammation
> Intracranial Regulation

**Additional related concepts may be considered based on the client's situation.*

Clotting

Definition

The process by which blood will convert from a liquid to a semisolid state to stop bleeding. May include either a excess or inability to form a clot.

Requirements for Normal Coagulation

> Integrity of the Tissues and Vessels
> Functioning Bone Marrow & Liver for Hemostasis
> Free of Bleeding Disorders and Hypercoagulability States
> Free of Venous Stasis

Priority Assessment or Cues – Excess Clotting (Venous/Arterial)

> Mentation
> Pulses - Capillary Refill
> Tissue Color and Temperature
> Breathing Pattern - Oxygen saturation
> Pain

Priority Assessment or Cues – Lack of Clotting (Bleeding)

> Assessments of Perfusion (See Perfusion Concept Map)
> Stool Color

Priority Labs Excess Clotting

D-Dimer, Platelets, Coagulation Panel (INR, PT, PTT)

Priority Labs for Lack of Clotting

Platelets, Hct/Hgb, Coagulation Panel (INR, PT, PTT)

Normal Coagulation

> Warm to Touch
> Pulses WNL
> Activity Tolerance

Excess Clotting

> Decreased Circulation
> Hypoxia
> Pain
> Limited Movement
> Organ Failure

Lack of Clotting

> Hemorrhage
> Hypo/Hyperthermia

Related Concepts

> Oxygenation
> Mobility
> Comfort
> Immunity
> Perfusion
> Intracranial Regulation

**Additional related concepts may be considered based on the client's situation.*

Immunity, Inflammation, Infection

Definition

The ability for a body to protect and defend itself from disease and illness using an active or passive process.

Requirements for Normal Immunity and Defense

> Intact Non-Specific Defenses or Barriers
> Functional Lymphatic System
> Optimal Innate Immune Response
> Functional Inflammatory Response
> Appropriate Adaptive (Acquired) Immune Response Both Active and Passive

Priority Assessment or Cues – Infection and Inflammation

> Temperature, Blood Pressure, Respiratory Rate
> Signs of Redness, Swelling, Drainage, Pain
> Color of Tissue and Body Fluids
> Skin – Warmth, Rash, and Swelling
> Lymph Nodes
> Immunization History

Priority Labs

White Blood Cells and Differential, Bacterial and Viral Cultures, C-reactive protein (CRP), Allergy Testing, Antibody Levels

Adequate Immunity

> Alert/Oriented
> Afebrile
> MAP > 65 mmHg
> Tissue Color WNL
> Body Fluids WNL
> Skin WNL
> Lymph Nodes WNL
> Wound Healing

Inadequate Immunity

> Hyper/Hypothermia
> Signs of Sepsis
> Discoloration of Tissue and Body Fluids
> Skin Warmth, Rash
> Enlarged Lymph Nodes
> Cancer
> Inability to Fight Infection
> Chronic Inflammation

Related Concepts

> Comfort
> Mobility
> Tissue Integrity
> Coping
> Nutrition
> Cellular Regulation
> Functional Ability
> Thermoregulation

**Additional related concepts may be considered based on the client's situation.

Acid-Base Balance

Scan the QR Code to access *Go To Clinical Cases* that correlate with the Unfolding Concepts.

NurseThink.com/casestudy-book

Definition

The process of regulating the pH, bicarbonate, and carbon dioxide concentration of body fluids and gasses.

Requirements for Normal Acid-Base Balance

> Normal Respiratory and Renal Functioning
> Normal Digestion Functioning
> Absence of Vomiting or Diarrhea with Balanced Nutrition
> Krebs Cycle
> Normal Anion Gap
> Oxyhemoglobin Disassociation Curve

Priority Assessment or Cues

> Respiratory Rate
> Level of Consciousness
> Dysrhythmias
> Tetany, Paresthesias, Seizures
> Gastrointestinal Output
> Urine Output
> Ingestions of Acidic/Alkaline Medication

Priority Labs

Arterial Blood Gas, Anion Gap, Electrolytes

Normal Acid-Base Balance

> Respirations 16-20 bpm (adult)
> Lack of Excessive Gastrointestinal Output
> Kidney Function WNL

Abnormal Acid-Base Balance

> Bradypnea/Tachypnea
> Kussmaul Respirations
> Vomiting and/or Diarrhea
> Excess Nasogastric Secretions
> Level of Consciousness (LOC)
> Tetany, Tingling of Extremities
> Seizures
> Dysrhythmias

Related Concepts

> Fluid and Electrolyte Balance
> Perfusion
> Gas Exchange
> Elimination
> Nutrition

**Additional related concepts may be considered based on the client's situation.

CONCEPT: HOMEOSTASIS

Fluid Balance

Scan the QR Code to access *Go To Clinical Cases* that correlate with the Unfolding Concepts.

NurseThink.com/casestudy-book

Definition
The regulation of fluid volume within the body. Controlled by fluctuations of osmolality, plasma concentration, and electrolytes.

Requirements for Normal Fluid Balance
> Fluid & Electrolyte Intake and Absorption
> Normal Functioning of Renin-Angiotensin-Aldosterone System
> Sufficient Cardiac Output
> Normal Functioning of Adrenal, and Pituitary Glands
> Regulation of Body Fluid Compartments with Osmosis, Diffusion, & Active Transport

Priority Assessment or Cues
> Temperature, Heart Rate and Rhythm, Respiratory Rate
> Level of Consciousness & Seizures
> Lung and Heart Sounds
> Urine and Body Fluid Output
> Edema, Jugular Vein, Liver Palpation
> Muscle Strength and Abnormal Movement
> Skin Turgor, Mucous Membranes
> Weight & Intake/Output
> Central Venous Pressure (CVP)

Priority Labs
Electrolytes, Serum & Urine Osmolality, BUN, Creatinine & Ratio, Brain Natriuretic Peptide (BNP)

Normal Fluid Balance
> Vital Signs (VS)
> Alert/Oriented
> Lung and Heart Sounds WNL
> Equal Intake and Output
> Strength & Movement WNL
> Skin Turgor and Mucous Membranes WNL
> No Weight Gain or Loss
> CVP 2 - 6 mmHg

Abnormal Fluid Balance
> Tachycardia, Tachypnea
> Irregular Heart Rhythm & Dysrhythmias
> Confusion, Disorientation
> Weakness and Seizures
> Unequal Intake and Output

Fluid Volume Excess
> Hypertension
> Crackles in Lungs, Short of Breath
> Inadequate Urine and/or Body Fluid Output
> Jugular Vein Distension, Elevated CVP
> Edema, Weight Gain

Fluid Volume Deficit
> Febrile, Hypotension
> Skin Tenting, Dry Mucous Membranes
> Weight Loss
> Inadequate Urine
> Decreased CVP

Related Concepts
> Nutrition
> Tissue Integrity
> Perfusion
> Gas Exchange
> Elimination
> Cognition

**Additional related concepts may be considered based on the client's situation.*

Electrolyte Balance

Scan the QR Code to access *Go To Clinical Cases* that correlate with the Unfolding Concepts.

NurseThink.com/casestudy-book

Definition

The process of regulating plasma concentrations of electrolytes.

Requirements for Electrolyte Balance

> Electrolyte Intake and Absorption
> Normal Functioning of Aldosterone System
> Normal Functioning of Adrenal, Parathyroid, and Pituitary Glands
> Regulation of Acid-Base Balance

Priority Assessment or Cues

> Heart Rate and Rhythm
> Level of Consciousness & Seizures
> Urine and Body Fluid Output
> Muscle Strength and Abnormal Movement
> Weight & Intake/Output

Priority Labs

Electrolytes, Serum & Urine Osmolality, BUN, Creatinine & Ratio, Brain Natriuretic Peptide (BNP)

Normal Electrolyte Balance

> VS WNL
> Alert/Oriented
> Equal Intake and Output
> Strength & Movement WNL
> No Weight Gain or Loss

Abnormal Electrolyte Balance

> Tachycardia, Irregular Heart Rhythm & Dysrhythmias
> Confusion, Disorientation
> Weakness, Twitching, Seizures, Coma
> Inadequate or excessive urine and/or Body Fluid Output
> Weight Gain or Loss

Related Concepts

> Acid-Base Balance
> Nutrition
> Gas Exchange
> Elimination
> Cognition

**Additional related concepts may be considered based on the client's situation.*

Oxygenation/ Gas Exchange

Scan the QR Code to access *Go To Clinical Cases* that correlate with the Unfolding Concepts.

NurseThink.com/casestudy-book

Definition

The transportation of oxygen to the cells and carbon dioxide from the cells.

Requirements for Normal Oxygenation/Gas Exchange

> Adequate Functioning of the Respiratory System with the Ability to Inhale and Exhale with Intact Lung Elasticity and Lung Expansion

> Adequate Perfusion for the Exchange of Gas

> Adequate Neurologic Function

> Efficient Cellular Metabolism Including Hemoglobin

Priority Assessment or Cues

> Respiratory Rate, Depth, Effort
> Oxygen saturation
> Level of Consciousness
> Skin Color
> Capillary Refill
> Use of accessory muscles
> Positioning
> Nasal flaring

Priority Labs

Hemoglobin, Arterial Blood Gasses

Adequate Oxygenation/Gas Exchange

> Alert/Oriented
> Eupnea
> Oxygen saturation >94%
> Arterial pH 7.35-7.45
> Skin Color WNL
> Capillary Refill WNL
> Adequate Hemoglobin

Inadequate Oxygenation/Gas Exchange

> Altered Mental Status
> Respiratory Distress
> Respiratory Failure
> Hypoxemia
> Anoxia

Related Concepts

> Perfusion
> Clotting
> Mobility
> Acid-Base Balance
> Nutrition

**Additional related concepts may be considered based on the client's situation.*

Cellular Regulation

Scan the QR Code to access *Go To Clinical Cases* that correlate with the Unfolding Concepts.

NurseThink.com/casestudy-book

Definition
The process by which cells replicate, proliferate, and grow.

Requirements for Normal Cellular Regulation
> Normal DNA and Manufacturing of Proteins
> Healthy Life-Style: Balance of Sleep, Exercise, & Nutrition
> Normal Weight
> No Exposure to Known Carcinogens

Priority Assessment or Cues
> Lifestyle
> Family History
> Exposure to Carcinogens
> Temperature
> Pain, Level of Activity
> Focused Assessment of Body System Abnormality (Cough, Lump, Bowel Change, etc.)
> Weight

Priority Labs
CBC, Tumor Markers, Prostate-Specific Antigen (PSA), Genetic Markers, Organ Specific Labs

Normal Cellular Regulation
> Lack of Abnormal Symptoms, Growths, or other Health Concerns
> Stable Weight

Abnormal Cellular Regulation
> Pain
> Fever, Fatigue
> Abnormal Bleeding
> Cough
> Skin Growths
> Lumps or Mass (Benign or Malignant)
> Change in Bowel Pattern
> Reoccurring Illness/ Infections
> Weight Loss or Gain

Related Concepts
> Tissue Integrity
> Comfort
> Coping
> Grief
> Immunity
> Interpersonal Relationships
> Nutrition/Elimination

**Additional related concepts may be considered based on the client's situation.*

Intracranial Regulation

Scan the QR Code to access *Go To Clinical Cases* that correlate with the Unfolding Concepts.

NurseThink.com/casestudy-book

Definition

The processes which impact intracranial compensation and adaptation to change.

Requirements for Normal Intracranial Regulation

> Adequate Function of Neurons and Neurotransmitters
> Adequate Perfusion of Blood, Oxygen, and Glucose
> Adequate Autoregulation
> Cerebral Spinal Fluid Production and Reabsorption

Priority Assessment or Cues

> Level of Consciousness, Orientation, Cognition
> Pupillary Reaction
> Cranial Nerves
> Movement and Sensation
> Seizures
> Temperature, Pulse Pressure, Respiratory Rate/Rhythm

Priority Labs

Glucose, Sodium, ABGs, Serum Osmolality

Normal Intracranial Regulation

> Alert/Oriented
> PERRLA
> Cranial Nerves Intact
> Moves all Extremities Equally with Full Sensation
> Lack of Seizures
> Vital Signs (VS)

Abnormal Intracranial Regulation

> Disoriented and/or Obtunded
> Abnormal Cranial Nerves
> Lack of Movement or Sensation
> Seizure Activity
> Hyper/Hypothermia
> Widening Pulse Pressure
> Abnormal Respiratory Pattern
> Increased Intracranial Pressure
> Unequal or unreactive pupils

Related Concepts

> Sensory Perception
> Cognition
> Mobility
> Gas Exchange
> Perfusion
> Functional Ability

**Additional related concepts may be considered based on the client's situation.

Thermoregulation

Scan the QR Code to access *Go To Clinical Cases* that correlate with the Unfolding Concepts.

NurseThink.com/casestudy-book

Definition

The process of maintaining core body temperature within an optimal physiological range.

Requirements for Normal Thermoregulation

> Normal Hypothalamus Functioning
> Chemical Thermogenesis
> Normal Sweat Gland and Skeletal Muscle Functioning
> Sufficient Blood Flow
> Brown Fat in the Newborn
> Normal Thyroid Regulation

Priority Assessment or Cues

> Temperature
> Environmental Temperature Assessment
> Hydration Status
> Infection
> Tissue Perfusion

Priority Labs

CBC, Sodium, Lactic Acid, Cultures and Sensitivity

Normal Thermoregulation Balance

> Normothermia
> Around 37°C/98.6°F
> Adaptation to Environmental Temperature Change

Abnormal Thermoregulation Balance

> Hypothermia < 36°C OR 95°F
> Severe Hyperthermia > 40°C OR 104°F (adult)
> Tach/Bradypnea
> Tach/Bradycardia
> Dehydration, Hyponatremia
> Tissue Ischemia & Necrosis

Related Concepts

> Fluid & Electrolyte Balance
> Metabolism
> Perfusion
> Tissue Integrity
> Intracranial Regulation
> Immunity, Infection, Inflammation

**Additional related concepts may be considered based on the client's situation.*

Nutrition and Digestion

Definition

The process by which the body ingests, absorbs, transports, uses, and eliminates nutrients.

Requirements for Normal Nutrition & Digestion

> Functioning Gastrointestinal Tract and Associated Organs
> Adequate Ingestion of Nutrients and Water

Priority Assessment or Cues

> Food History/Diary
> Allergies to Foods
> Height, Weight, BMI, Growth Patterns
> Muscle Tone, Strength, Agility, Reflexes
> Cognitive & Mood
> Level of Energy
> Bowel Sounds
> Bowel Patterns

Priority Labs

Albumin/Protein, Hgb/Hct, Electrolytes

Adequate Nutrition & Digestion

> Calorie and Dietary Intake Adequate
> Height, Weight, Body Mass Index (BMI), Growth WNL
> Adequate Muscle Movement and Strength
> Alert, Cooperative
> Adequate Energy to Complete Activities of Daily Living (ADLs)
> Bowel Sounds WNL
> Stools WNL

Inadequate Nutrition & Digestion

> Insufficient Calorie or Nutritional Intake
> Abnormal BMI, Growth for Age
> Weak, Tired, Lethargic
> Muscle Wasting
> Hypo/Hyperactive Bowel Sounds
> Abnormal Bowel Pattern or Appearance

Related Concepts

> Metabolism
> Cognition
> Interpersonal Relationships
> Fluid & Electrolyte Balance
> Thermoregulation
> Development
> Clotting

**Additional related concepts may be considered based on the client's situation.*

Elimination

Scan the QR Code to access *Go To Clinical Cases* that correlate with the Unfolding Concepts.

NurseThink.com/casestudy-book

Definition

The excretion of waste products from the kidneys and intestines.

Requirements for Normal Elimination

> Normal Bowel and Bladder Ability to Expel Contents
> Peristalsis
> Adequate Hydration and Food Intake

Priority Assessment or Cues

> Bowel Sounds, Abdominal Assessment
> Bowel and Bladder Toilet Habits (Continence, Urgency, Frequency, etc.)
> Urine Output, Color, Clarity
> Feces Color, Consistency, Frequency
> Use of Bowel Aids
> Nutritional Assessment (Quantity, Fiber, Liquids, etc.)
> Activity Level
> Medications
> Fecal or Urinary Diversions
> Hemorrhoids

Priority Labs

Urine Specific Gravity, Amylase, Lipase, WBC, Electrolytes, BUN, Creatinine, Creatinine Clearance, Urinalysis, Urine/Stool Culture

Normal Elimination

> Free of Bowel and Bladder Habit Change
> Urine and Stool WNL
> Adequate Nutrition and Fluid Intake
> Regular Physical Activity
> Functioning Urinary/Fecal Diversions

Abnormal Elimination – Bowel

> Hypo/Hyperactive Bowel Sounds
> Flat or Distended Abdomen
> Diarrhea, Incontinence, Constipation, Impaction, Obstruction
> Bowel Aid Dependency
> Abnormal Color or Consistency of Feces
> Inadequate Nutrition
> Skin Excoriation and Breakdown
> Hemorrhoids

Abnormal Elimination - Bladder

> Urinary Retention
> Dilute or Concentrated Urine
> Incontinence, Urgency
> Skin Excoriation and Breakdown

Related Concepts

> Nutrition
> Coping
> Metabolism
> Mobility
> Cognition
> Fluid and Electrolyte Balance
> Tissue Integrity

**Additional related concepts may be considered based on the client's situation.

Metabolism

Scan the QR Code to access *Go To Clinical Cases* that correlate with the Unfolding Concepts.

NurseThink.com/casestudy-book

Definition

The processes of biochemical reactions occurring in the cells to produce energy, repair, and facilitate growth of cells in order to maintain life.

Requirements for Normal Metabolism

> Ingestion of Nutrients
> Cells and Organs to Synthesize and Secrete Hormones
> Hormone Target Cells
> Organ Perfusion

Priority Assessment or Cues

> Fluid and Electrolyte Assessment
> Weight, Height, Body Mass Index (BMI), Growth Chart
> Heart Rate, Blood Pressure, Temperature
> Muscle Strength

Priority Labs

Glucose, Thyroid Stimulating Hormone (TSH), T3, T4, T7, Calcium, Sodium, Cortisol, Adrenocorticotropic hormone (ACTH), Hemoglobin A1C

Normal Metabolism

> Heart Rate, Blood Pressure, Temperature WNL
> Height, Weight, BMI, Growth WNL
> Adequate Muscle Movement and Strength
> Adequate Energy to Complete ADLs
> Euglycemia
> Equal Intake/Output

Abnormal Metabolism

> Tachy/Bradycardia Hyper/Hypothermia
> Hyper/Hypotensive
> BMI Normal for Age and Sex (Around 18.5 to 25)
> Week, Tired, Lethargic
> Muscle Wasting
> Anxiety, Restlessness, Abnormal Sleep Patterns
> Ascites and/or Edema
> Hyper/Hypoglycemia
> Abnormal Hormone Levels

Related Concepts

> Nutrition
> Mobility
> Coping
> Perfusion
> Reproduction
> Fluid and Electrolyte Balance

**Additional related concepts may be considered based on the client's situation.*

CHAPTER

4

Unfolding Concepts II

Movement, Sensory, Nerve Conduction / Comfort / Adaptation / Emotion / Cognition

The Unfolding Concepts in Chapter 4 are psychosocial in nature. Each map provides the definition of the concept, the priority assessment or cues, and lab findings. Related concepts are listed to deliver additional guidance when applying specific client cases. Additionally, common normal and abnormal findings are reviewed.

To best understand this material, it is important to apply these concepts as if directly caring for a client. Be sure to visit the website by scanning the QR code to further explore the concepts.

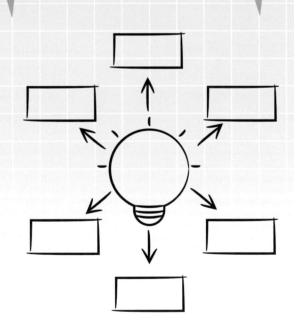

Clinical Hint: Use these Unfolding Concept Maps with every Go To Clinical Case (Patient Assignment) in the book. This will develop your Clinical Judgment Muscles!

CONCEPT: MOVEMENT, SENSORY,
NERVE CONDUCTION

Mobility

Scan the QR Code to access *Go To Clinical Cases*
that correlate with the Unfolding Concepts.

NurseThink.com/casestudy-book

Definition
The ability for the body to move as desired.

Requirements for Normal Mobility
> Adequate Energy
> Muscle Strength and Skeletal Stability
> Joint Function
> Neuromuscular Coordination
> Physical Development

Priority Assessment or Cues
> Age Limitations for Movement
> Gross and Fine Movements & Coordination
> Strength and Synchronized Efforts
> Blood Pressure
> Edema, Swelling, and Skin Breakdown
> Respiratory Pattern and Effort
> Dietary Intake – Bowel Patterns
> Risk for Falls
> Pain
> Medications

Priority Labs
Albumin/Total Protein, Hgb/Hct, Calcium, Potassium, Erythrocyte Sedimentation Rate (ESR)

Normal Mobility
> Heart Rate, Blood Pressure (BP), Respiratory Rate. WNL
> Adequate Muscle Movement and Strength
> Adequate Energy
> Physically Independent
> Controlled Weight

Impaired Mobility
> Orthostatic Hypotension
> Dizziness
> Obesity
> Muscle Wasting
> Week, Tired, Lethargic
> Musculoskeletal Injury
> Neuromuscular Impairment Muscle atrophy, Joint Crepitus
> Pain
> Dyspnea with Exertion
> Swelling of Extremities
> Contractures
> Skin Breakdown

Related Concepts
> Tissue Integrity
> Nutrition
> Elimination
> Perfusion
> Functional Ability
> Comfort
> Intracranial Regulation
> Gas Exchange

**Additional related concepts may be considered based on the client's situation.*

Sensory

Scan the QR Code to access **Go To Clinical Cases** that correlate with the Unfolding Concepts.

NurseThink.com/casestudy-book

Definition

A person's ability to receive, process and translate stimulus into a purposeful and meaningful response.

Requirements for Normal Reproduction

> External Stimuli
> Intact Neural System
> Intact and Functioning, Visual, Taste, Auditory, and Integumentary Senses

Priority Assessment or Cues

> Cranial Nerves
> Hearing and Visual Acuity
> Sensation to Touch
> Sensation of Taste – Food Preferences
> Ability to Smell
> Medications

Priority Labs

None

Normal Sensory Perception

> Hearing Range of 0 dB to 25 dB (adults)
> Visual Acuity 20/20
> Intact Skin Sensation – Distinguishes between Sharp/Blunt and Hot/Cold
> Taste includes Sweet, Salt, Sour, Bitter
> Smelling Intact

Abnormal Sensory Perception

> Unable to Detect dB Ranges (Difficulty Communicating)
> Visually Impaired (Accidents)
> Lack of Sensation of Touch (Thermal Injuries)
> Neuropathy
> Distorted Taste (Lack of Appetite)
> Distorted Smell (Consumes Spoiled Food)
> Perception Impairment

Related Concepts

> Safety
> Comfort
> Nutrition
> Mobility
> Communication
> Human Development
> Intracranial Regulation
> Interpersonal Relationships

**Additional related concepts may be considered based on the client's situation.

CONCEPT: COMFORT

Comfort

Scan the QR Code to access *Go To Clinical Cases* that correlate with the Unfolding Concepts.

NurseThink.com/casestudy-book

Definition

A state of physical and emotional tranquility.

Requirements for Normal Comfort

> Effective circulatory system
> Able to discern from comfort to discomfort
> Without noxious stimuli
> Intact neurological/sensory system
> Ability for emotional well-being

Priority Assessment or Cues

> Vital Signs
> Pain Scale
> Body Posture and Movement
> Functional Ability
> Communication and Interactions
> Mood and Affect
> Medications & Alternative Methods Used

Priority Labs

Erythrocyte Sedimentation Rate (ESR), C-Reactive Protein (CRP), Drug levels

Acceptable Comfort

> Heart Rate (HR), Blood Pressure (BP), Respiratory Rate (RR) WNL
> Pain Within Acceptable Limits (Client Determined)
> Movement to Perform Activities of Daily Living (ADLs)
> Communicates and Interacts Freely

Impaired Comfort

> Increased HR, BP, RR
> Pain at Unacceptable Limit
> Impaired Movement
> Unable to Perform ADLs
> Withdrawn, Socially Isolated, Depressed

Related Concepts

> Mobility
> Sensory Perception
> Mood and Affect
> Functional Ability

**Additional related concepts may be considered based on the client's situation.

Coping

Scan the QR Code to access *Go To Clinical Cases* that correlate with the Unfolding Concepts.

NurseThink.com/casestudy-book

Definition

AA fluctuating process that requires cognitive thoughts and behavioral actions to adapt to changing situations that are difficult.

Influences for Coping

> Individual Perceptions
> Life Experiences
> Availability of Adequate Resources and Support Systems

Priority Assessment or Cues

> Affect & Behavior
> Verbal and Non-Verbal Communication
> Activities of Daily Living (ADLs) and Independent ADLs
> Available Resources and Support Systems
> Physiological Responses to Stress (HR, BP, etc.)

Priority Labs

Glucose, Drug Screen

Resilience

> Healthy Lifestyle Choices
> Self-Care Adherence
> Identification of Stressors
> Appropriate Communication
> Use of Resources
> Physiological Responses WNL
> Successful Relationships
> Regimen Compliance

Maladaptive Behavior

> Substance Abuse/ Addiction
> Violence
> Eating disorders
> Post-Traumatic Stress Disorder
> Obsessive-Compulsive Disorder
> Suicide
> Lack of Self Care
> Unsuccessful Relationships
> Denial
> Risk taking

Related Concepts

> Functional Ability
> Family Dynamics
> Perfusion
> Mood & Affect
> Rest
> Immunity
> Sexuality
> Cognition
> Development
> Culture/Spirituality

**Additional related concepts may be considered based on the client's situation.*

Mood and Affect

Scan the QR Code to access *Go To Clinical Cases* that correlate with the Unfolding Concepts.

NurseThink.com/casestudy-book

Definition

An emotional state and how it is expressed.

Influences for Mood and Affect

> Cognitive Development that is Consistent with Developmental Age
> Neurological Balance of Neurotransmitters
> Balance of Hormones
> Individual Experiences

Priority Assessment or Cues

> Mental State
> Activities of Daily Living (ADLs)
> Ability to Provide Insight and Reasoning
> Responses in Expression and Gestures
> Mood, Thought, Eating Disorders
> Stress Level and Ability to Cope
> Medications

Priority Labs

Toxicology Screens and hormone levels

Normal Mood and Affect

> Positive Relationships
> Healthy Sleep and Eating Patterns
> Problem Solving Abilities
> Productive in Society

Abnormal Mood and Affect

> Abnormal Sleep Patterns
> Addictions
> Violence/Agitation
> Sadness, Suicidal
> Impaired Health
> Isolation

Related Concepts

> Nutrition
> Safety
> Grief
> Cognition
> Coping
> Functioning Ability
> Sensory Perception
> Interpersonal Relationships
> Sleep

**Additional related concepts may be considered based on the client's situation.

Grief

Scan the QR Code to access *Go To Clinical Cases* that correlate with the Unfolding Concepts.

NurseThink.com/casestudy-book

Definition

The reaction to either real or perceived loss and the way it impacts psychosocial and physical well-being.

Influences for Grief

> Actual Loss
> Perceived Loss
> Anticipatory Loss
> Personal experiences

Priority Assessment or Cues

> Acknowledgement of Loss
> Emotional Response to Grief
> Stages of Grief
> Support Systems

Priority Labs

N/A

Adaptative Grief

> Acknowledgement of Loss and Emotions
> Appropriate Use of Available Resources and Support Systems
> Acceptance and Rebuilding
> Memorialization of Loss
> Resolution

Maladaptive Grief

> Denial
> Prolonged Mourning
> Mental or Emotional Immobilization
> Physical Symptoms or Illness

Related Concepts

> Human Development
> Safety
> Immunity
> Comfort
> Diversity
> Coping
> End of Life
> Interpersonal Relationships

**Additional related concepts may be considered based on the client's situation.*

Cognitive Functioning

Scan the QR Code to access *Go To Clinical Cases* that correlate with the Unfolding Concepts.

NurseThink.com/casestudy-book

Definition

A process by which an individual understands, learns, stores, retrieves, and utilizes new information.

Influences for Cognitive Functioning

> Appropriate Growth and Development
> Adequate Cerebral Oxygenation, Tissue Perfusion and Nutrition
> Intact Neurological and Metabolic Function
> Opportunities for Growth Through Education

Priority Assessment or Cues

> Blood Pressure (BP), Mean Arterial Pressure (MAP), Pulse Oximeter, Respiratory Rate (RR)
> Level of Consciousness
> Cognitive & Intelligence Level
> Ability to Send and Receive Information
> Communication – Language Barriers
> Ability to Learn, Understand, and Remember
> Use of Mind Altering Substances

Priority Labs

ABGs, Hgb/Hct, Glucose, Electrolytes, Ammonia, Toxicology Screens

Normal Cognitive Functioning

> BP (MAP), Oxygenation, RR WNL
> Treatment Compliance
> Lifestyle Management
> Clear Communication

Abnormal Cognitive Functioning

> Frequent Injuries
> Institutionalized Dependence
> Unsuccessful Relationships
> Poor Health Outcomes
> Inability to process stimuli
> Inability to perform ADL's

Related Concepts

> Intracranial Regulation
> Acid-Base Balance
> Perfusion
> Nutrition
> Safety
> Human Development
> Functional Ability
> Sensory Perception
> Metabolism
> Sleep

**Additional related concepts may be considered based on the client's situation.*

Clinical Cases & Exemplars

Sexuality

Reproduction / Sexuality

According to the World Health Organization (WHO), "Sexual health is a state of physical, mental and social well-being in relation to sexuality. It requires a positive and respectful approach to sexuality and sexual relationships, as well as the possibility of having pleasurable and safe sexual experiences, free of coercion, discrimination, and violence." (www.who.int) Although this definition is accurate in describing intimacy, it is not all-encompassing. Sexuality also includes perceptions of sex, sexual acts, gender identity, and sexual orientation, all of which can impact a person's sexual health.

Reproduction requires a fine balance on the health and illness continuum. Reproductive health spans from childhood to middle-adulthood in most people, and although it is mostly a natural, healthy process, some people experience difficulty and illness. Consider the physical, emotional, and social impact of sexually transmitted infections, difficulties of fertility, and cancers of sexual organs. Each of these has a damaging and lasting impact on one's ability to be sexually healthy.

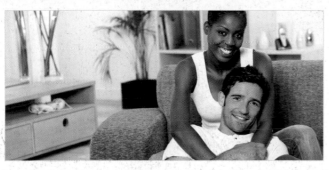

Next Gen Clinical Judgment:

> How are sexuality beliefs and practices different among various cultures, religions, and generations?

> What impact does reproductive health have on sexuality?

> What impact does sexuality have on reproductive health?

> How are reproductive and sexual health different between men and women?

Case 1: Infertility, Conception, and Complications

Related Concepts: Circulation, Nutrition, Adaptation
Threaded Topics: Grief, Loss, Violence, Communication,
Family Dynamics

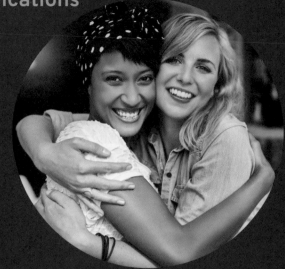

Anna Frey-Walters is a 30-year-old client who arrives at the clinic today with her wife of two years, Carol. Anna states that they want to conceive and have a child together. They have decided that Anna will carry their baby, Carol will be the egg donor, and a chosen male friend will be the sperm donor. Anna and Carol report that they are both healthy, run five miles a day together, and do not take any medications or vitamins.

Both Anna and Carol report having multiple partners before they met. They have never been tested for sexually transmitted infections. Carol reports that she had some heterosexual relationships in the past that were sexual. They are unsure of their friend's medical history and are hesitant to ask him, afraid that he'll change his mind about being the sperm donor.

---

1. **NurseThink® Prioritization Power!**

   Evaluate the information in the case above and pick the **Top 3 Priority** concerns or cues.

   1. _____

   2. _____

   3. _____

---

2. **Based on the priority concerns, which action(s) should the nurse anticipate? Select all that apply.**

   1. Both women being placed on folic acid 400 mcg, daily by mouth.
   2. A discussion about the importance of knowing their friend's health history.
   3. Performance of a pelvic exam on Anna to rule out sexually transmitted infections.
   4. Obtaining blood work on Carol to rule out sexually transmitted infections.
   5. Exploring why they want to have children.

The male friend willingly shares his health history information and no concerns arise. Anna and Carol return to the clinic today to begin fertility testing for Anna. The provider draws some baseline labs.

Nurse Think
HEALTHCARE SYSTEM

Name: Anna Frey-Walters
Health Care Provider: Martina Hines, FNP
Code Status: Full code

Age: 30 years
Allergies: NKDA

LABORATORY REPORT

Lab	Normal	May 8		
WBC	4,000-10,000 μ/L	6.2		
Hemoglobin	12 -17.0 g/dL	**11.0 L**		
Hematocrit (%)	36 - 51%	**35 L**		
RBC	4.2 – 5.9 cells/L	**3.9 L**		
Platelets	150,000 to 350,000 μL	192,000		
Calcium	9 – 10.5 mg/dL	**8.9 L**		
Chloride	98 - 106 mEq/L	99		
Magnesium	1.5 - 2.4 mEq/L	2.4		
Phosphorus	3.0 - 4.5 mg/dL	4.3		
Potassium	3.5 - 5.0 mEq/L	**3.4 L**		
Sodium	136 - 145 mEq/L	145		
Glucose, fasting	70 100 mg/dL	79		
BUN	8 – 20 mg/dL	**36 H**		
Creatinine	0.7-1.3 mg/dL	0.9		
Total Protein	6 - 7.8 g/dL	6.8		
Albumin	3.5 - 5.0 g/dL	3.7		
CPK	30 - 170 U/L	57		
LDH	60 - 100 U/L	95		
AST	0 - 35 U/L	28		
ALT	0 - 35 U/L	29		
GGT	9 - 48 U/L	38		
Total Bilirubin	0.3 - 1.2 mg/dL	0.9		

3. After reviewing the lab report, which question(s) should the nurse ask? Select all that apply.

1. "Do you ever feel cold or weak?"
2. "What color are your stools?"
3. "How much water do you drink each day?"
4. "How much protein do you consume each day?"
5. "How much dairy do you consume each day?"

> **Clinical Hint:** Signs of anemia include: fatigue, loss of energy, tachycardia, shortness of breath, headache, lack of mental focus, dizziness, pale skin, leg cramps, and insomnia.

The nurse learns that Anna chooses to maintain a strict vegan diet. She ran five miles today before coming to the clinic.

4. Which suggestions should the nurse give? Select all that apply.

1. It is unsafe for Anna to conceive.
2. Anna requires vitamin supplements with calcium and iron.
3. She should consume more water.
4. Additional testing is needed.
5. She should go off of her vegan diet during pregnancy.

5. The nurses in the office have never cared for a lesbian couple and feel the need to learn how to meet Anna and Carol's needs better. How should the nurses obtain more information?

1. Ask Carol and Anna to share with the nurse what they feel is appropriate.
2. Ask someone from the lesbian community to provide an in-service to the staff.
3. Perform a literature search on the care of the lesbian client and couple.
4. Ask a friend who is in a same-sex relationship what can be done to help this couple.

6. The health care provider prescribes a hysterosalpingography for Anna. What should the nurse teach Anna about this procedure? Select all that apply.

1. The procedure is performed after the follicular phase of the menstrual cycle.
2. Anna may experience moderate to severe cramping, along with shoulder pain, during the procedure.
3. Radiopaque dye is injected through the cervix, entering the uterus, and fallopian tube, allowing for visualization of abnormalities.
4. Anna will be given a nonsteroidal anti-inflammatory immediately prior to the procedure.
5. After the procedure, Anna needs to report severe cramping, bleeding, fever or malodorous discharge.

7. The fertility tests are completed, and no abnormalities are detected. Carol is placed on gonadotropin 75 units, subcutaneously, once a day for five days, starting on cycle day 3. How can the nurse suggest that Anna be more involved?

1. Instruct Anna in how to administer the daily injections.
2. Have Anna pick up the prescription from the pharmacy.
3. Instruct Anna of the side effects to monitor.
4. Instruct Anna how to draw up the medication.

> **Next Gen Clinical Judgment:**
> Visit the Office of Women's Health at
> www.womenshealth.gov/a-z-topics/infertility
>
>
>
> Review 3 areas that you did not know that would be beneficial for Anna and Carol to know. Record them here and teach them to a classmate.
>
> _____
>
> _____
>
> _____

8. **Carol calls the clinic a few days later and reports that she is experiencing swelling of her hands, feet, and is short of breath. What action should the nurse take?**

   1. Administer the human chorionic gonadotropin (hCG) to stimulate Carol's ovaries.
   2. Postpone the infertility treatment until the next cycle.
   3. Prep Carol for oocyte retrieval.
   4. Instruct Carol to increase her fluids.

9. **Carol and Anna are disappointed that they have to wait for a for another cycle before they can complete in vitro fertilization (IVF). What action is most appropriate for the nurse to take?**

   1. Inform them that they should consider other options because pregnancy is too dangerous.
   2. State that God's plan is for them not to have children.
   3. Allow them to express their feelings and provide a supportive atmosphere.
   4. Suggest that maybe Anna should be the donor and Carol the carrier.

10. **The next cycle goes well, and Carol is ready for the human chorionic gonadotropin (hCG) injection to be administered. What information should the nurse provide to Carol about this medication?**

    1. Carol must refrain from intercourse after receiving this medication.
    2. The injection is given subcutaneously by the nurse 7 to 9 days after her last injection of gonadotropin.
    3. Egg retrieval will be performed in approximately 24 to 36 hours after she receives the medication.
    4. The injection will be given intramuscularly by the nurse three days after her last injection of gonadotropin.

11. **The medication is successful, and the health care provider retrieves 10 eggs. Five days later, Anna comes to the clinic for embryo transfer. Which action(s) should the nurse take before the procedure. Select all that apply.**

    1. Verify that informed consent has been obtained.
    2. Confirm that the client has had nothing by mouth.
    3. Confirm with the physician how many embryos will be transferred.
    4. Conduct a timeout and document the time out.
    5. Obtain baseline vital signs.

    Next Gen Clinical Judgment: Infertility practices are frequently points for ethical dilemmas from zygote disposal to selective reduction. Perform a web search and read 3 journal articles about the ethics of infertility.

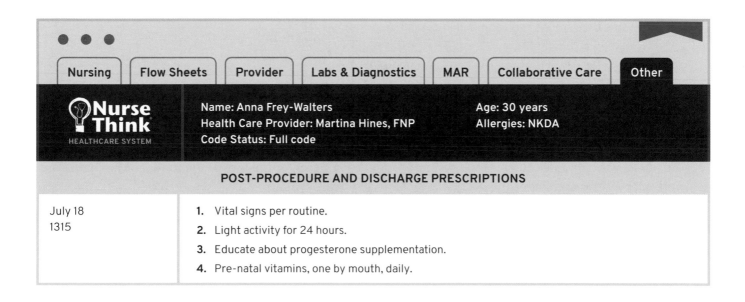

| Nursing | Flow Sheets | Provider | Labs & Diagnostics | MAR | Collaborative Care | Other |

NurseThink HEALTHCARE SYSTEM

Name: Anna Frey-Walters
Health Care Provider: Martina Hines, FNP
Code Status: Full code

Age: 30 years
Allergies: NKDA

POST-PROCEDURE AND DISCHARGE PRESCRIPTIONS

July 18 1315	1. Vital signs per routine.
	2. Light activity for 24 hours.
	3. Educate about progesterone supplementation.
	4. Pre-natal vitamins, one by mouth, daily.

12. **Explain the rationale for each of the instructions after the procedure.**

    1. Vital signs per routine._____

    2. Light activity for 24 hours._____

    3. Educate about progesterone supplementation._____

    4. Pre-natal vitamins, one by mouth, daily. _____

13. **A pregnancy test 14 days later confirms that Anna is pregnant. At six weeks gestation, Carol and Anna come to the clinic for an ultrasound. What is the most appropriate way for the nurse to address them?**

    1. Carol as the father of the baby and Anna as the mother.
    2. Carol as the significant other and Anna as the mother.
    3. Carol as the other mother and Anna as the mother.
    4. Carol by her first name and Anna as the mother.

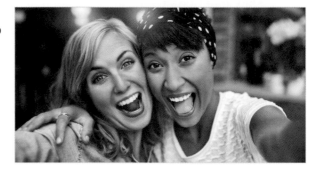

14. **Carol and Anna ask what Anna can be eating to ensure she is getting the right nutrients for her and their baby. Plan an appropriate meal for her based on Choose My Plate.**

    _____

    _____

    _____

    Scan the QR code on your phone to find more information. →

    www.choosemyplate.gov/moms-pregnancy-breastfeeding

15. **At 16 weeks gestation, Carol and Anna return to the clinic for a check-up and ultrasound. The uterus has not increased in size, and the health care provider determines there has been a missed miscarriage. A dilation and curettage (D&C) procedure is scheduled and performed. Which discharge instruction(s) should the nurse provide to Anna? Select all that apply.**

    1. Report heavy or bright red vaginal bleeding.
    2. Have someone remain with her for the first three hours.
    3. Report any fever, chills, or foul-smelling discharge.
    4. Delay pregnancy for at least 2 months.
    5. Take the antibiotics until she feels better.
    6. Eat food high in iron and protein.

16. **The nurse wants to offer support and comfort to Anna and Carol for the loss of the pregnancy. What is the most appropriate statement the nurse can make to them at this time?**

    1. "It may be for the best since sometimes there is something wrong with the fetus."
    2. "There is always next time since you have more embryos."
    3. "You can start adoption procedures because that often helps."
    4. "I am so sorry for your loss; this must be very difficult."

17. **Which nursing intervention(s) is/are most likely to offer comfort to Anna and Carol? Select all that apply.**

    1. Telling Anna, she may have done something to cause this.
    2. Encourage Anna and Carol to talk about their feelings.
    3. Suggest that Carol be the carrier and Anna donate the eggs for the next cycle.
    4. Sit and listen to their concerns.
    5. Recommend a referral to a support group.
    6. Provide a follow-up call after discharge to check on them.

18. **A week later, Anna comes into the clinic saturating a pad with blood every hour. Methylergonovine 0.2 mg intramuscular (IM) is prescribed. Before giving the medicine, the nurse notes the blood pressure is 145/95 (112 mmHg). The nurse holds the medication and contacts the provider. Complete an SBAR communication to the health care provider.**

    S – _____

    B – _____

    A – _____

    R – _____

    Clinical Hint:
    S - Situation
    B - Background
    A - Assessment
    R - Recommendation

19. **After several months, Anna and Carol undergo another round of in vitro fertilization. Anna is now 32 weeks pregnant and comes into the clinic for a visit with some bruises on her arms and abdomen. Anna confides in the nurse that Carol occasionally hits her. What is the nurse's best response?**

    1. "I am glad you have shared this with me. No one has the right to hit you."
    2. "Thank you for telling me; I'll place it in your chart, now let's assess you and the baby."
    3. "Good to know but I am sure Carol is just feeling stressed, don't you agree?"
    4. "Has this happened to you in other relationships?"

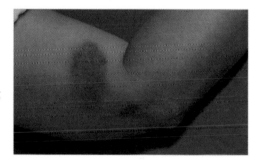

20. **THIN Thinking Time!**

    What actions should the nurse take in response to this reported abuse? Apply **THIN Thinking.**

    T – _____

    H – _____

    I – _____

    N – _____

    T - Top 3
    H - Help Quick
    I - Identify Risk to Safety
    N - Nursing Process

    Scan to access the
    10-Minute-Mentor →
    on THIN Thinking.

    NurseThink.com/THINThinking

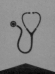
Case 2: Pregnancy with Delivery

Related Concepts: Comfort, Thermoregulation, Circulation, Hormonal
Threaded Topics: Diabetes Management, Medication Safety, Nutrition, Communication, Wellness

Olivia Hernandez is a 28-year-old who gave birth to a 4800-gram infant three years ago at 36 weeks gestation. Her daughter spent a week in the Neonatal Intensive Care Unit with unstable blood glucose levels, breathing, and feeding problems. She is currently 28 weeks pregnant with her second child. She is 5 ft 3 inches tall, and her pre-pregnancy weight was 170 pounds. She has an O+ blood type, is human immunodeficiency virus (HIV) negative, rubella immune, and is venereal disease research laboratory test (VDRL) non-reactive. She is married to Juan, her husband of six years. Both Olivia's mother and grandmother have type 2 diabetes.

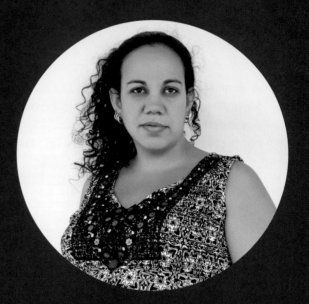

Olivia comes to the health care provider for a prenatal visit and glucose challenge test. The provider notes that she had gained 8 pounds since her last appointment two weeks ago. Olivia says she fasted the night before coming to the clinic, and typically eats a diet of rice, beans, tortillas, and some meat, prepared by her mother and grandmother.

---

1. **NurseThink® Prioritization Power!**
   Evaluate the information in the case above and determine the **Top 3 Priority** concerns or cues.

   1. _____

   2. _____

   3. _____

---

2. **Based on the priority concerns, which action(s) should the nurse perform? Select all that apply.**

   1. Complete a glucose challenge test.
   2. Obtain a blood pressure.
   3. Complete a 3-hour oral glucose challenge test.
   4. Obtain a finger sample blood glucose level.
   5. Complete a 24-hour food recall.

3. **The nurse is administering the glucose challenge test. Which instruction(s) should be given to Olivia? Select all that apply.**
   1. Serum blood sample will be drawn in 1, 2, and 3-hour intervals.
   2. Client will be provided 100 grams of oral glucose.
   3. Client will be provided 50 grams of oral glucose.
   4. Serum blood sample will be drawn after 1 hour has passed.
   5. Based on the results additional testing may be needed.
   6. Client will not need to fast when the screen is done.

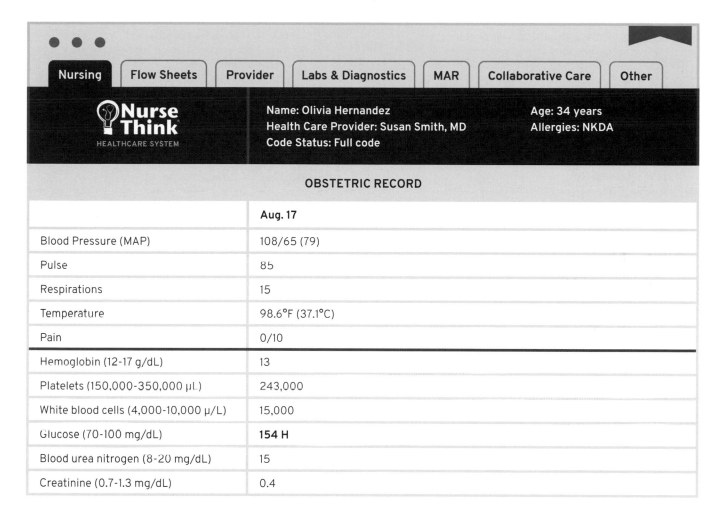

| | Nursing | Flow Sheets | Provider | Labs & Diagnostics | MAR | Collaborative Care | Other |

NurseThink HEALTHCARE SYSTEM

Name: Olivia Hernandez
Health Care Provider: Susan Smith, MD
Code Status: Full code

Age: 34 years
Allergies: NKDA

OBSTETRIC RECORD

	Aug. 17
Blood Pressure (MAP)	108/65 (79)
Pulse	85
Respirations	15
Temperature	98.6°F (37.1°C)
Pain	0/10
Hemoglobin (12-17 g/dL)	13
Platelets (150,000-350,000 µL)	243,000
White blood cells (4,000-10,000 µ/L)	15,000
Glucose (70-100 mg/dL)	**154 H**
Blood urea nitrogen (8-20 mg/dL)	15
Creatinine (0.7-1.3 mg/dL)	0.4

4. **Based on the information in the electronic record, what action should the nurse take next?**
   1. Instruct Olivia that her test indicates she has gestational diabetes.
   2. Educate Olivia on a gestational diabetic diet.
   3. Instruct Olivia that the test was negative and no further testing is needed.
   4. Inform Olivia that it is likely that additional tests are indicated on another day.

5. **Olivia asks the nurse about the 3-hour glucose challenge test. What information should the nurse provide Olivia? Select all that apply.**

   1. She will need to fast the night before and during the test.
   2. Blood will be drawn at the start of the test, and at 1, 2, and 3 hours.
   3. She may have a cup of coffee the morning of the test.
   4. She will drink a 100 grams oral glucose solution after the first blood draw.
   5. Olivia will drink a 50 grams oral glucose solution after the second blood draw.

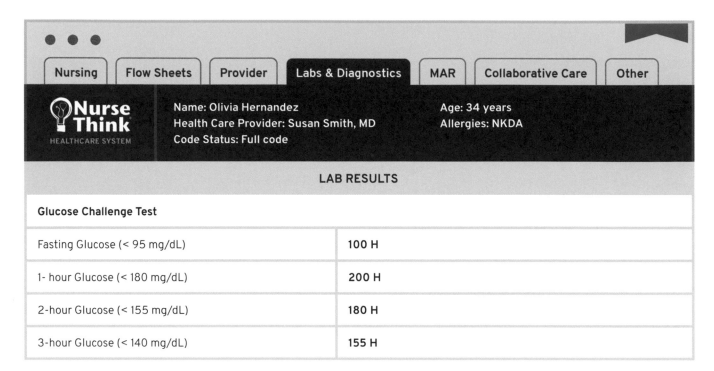

| Nursing | Flow Sheets | Provider | Labs & Diagnostics | MAR | Collaborative Care | Other |

NurseThink HEALTHCARE SYSTEM

Name: Olivia Hernandez
Health Care Provider: Susan Smith, MD
Code Status: Full code

Age: 34 years
Allergies: NKDA

LAB RESULTS

Glucose Challenge Test	
Fasting Glucose (< 95 mg/dL)	100 H
1- hour Glucose (< 180 mg/dL)	200 H
2-hour Glucose (< 155 mg/dL)	180 H
3-hour Glucose (< 140 mg/dL)	155 H

6. **Explain the rationale for each of these post-procedure prescriptions.**

   1. Dietary Instructions._____
   2. Moderate exercise program._____
   3. Instructions for self-monitoring of blood glucose._____
   4. Daily dietary log and record all blood glucose levels. Bring these to the next appointment.

   _____

7. **Olivia meets with the diabetes nurse educator about her diet before leaving the clinic. She identifies that her preference is a plant-based diet, preferring beans and grains to meat. She is counseled using the Latin American Diet Food Pyramid. Plan an appropriate meal for her based on her preferences and the Latin American Diet Food Pyramid.**

   _____

   _____

   _____

   Scan the QR code on your phone to find more information. →

   oldwayspt.org/traditional-diets/latin-american-diet

Olivia returns to the clinic four weeks later for her prenatal visit with her food and blood glucose diary. She says she is having a hard time following the diet because her mother and grandmother insist on cooking for her and continue cooking food that is high in fat, salt, and sugar. Her blood glucose levels are persistently greater than 95 mg/dL fasting, and 2-hours post-meal levels are consistently higher than 120 mg/dL.

8. **The provider places Olivia on lispro injections. Explain the rationale for each of these insulin instructions.**
    1. Reason for the medication._____
    2. Administration 5-10 minutes before meals._____
    3. Need to eat immediately after injection._____
    4. Instructions for Olivia's husband about insulin administration and symptoms of hypoglycemia.

    _____

9. **NurseThink® Prioritization Power!**
    Evaluate the information in the case provided and pick the **Top 3 Priority** education needs about insulin administration.

    1. _____
    2. _____
    3. _____

10. **The provider orders a nonstress test to assess fetal status. What should the nurse expect to find if the results are normal?**
    1. Two accelerations of fetal heart rate (FHR) within 20 minutes that are least 15 beats per minute above the baseline rate and last for a minimum of 15 seconds each.
    2. Three contractions that last at least 40 seconds within 10 minutes without the presence of late or significant variable decelerations.
    3. The absence of two fetal heart rate acceleration within 20 minutes.
    4. Three uterine contractions within a 10-minute period with late fetal heart decelerations.

11. **To prepare for the nonstress test, which action(s) should the nurse take? Select all that apply.**
    1. Place client in a side-lying position.
    2. Record vital signs.
    3. Apply electronic fetal monitor.
    4. Record baseline FHR and monitor for 20-30 minutes.
    5. Instruct Olivia to mark the paper with each perceived fetal movement.
    6. Stimulate uterine contractions until three contractions occur within 10 minutes.

Olivia experiences no further complications with her pregnancy. She is able to maintain her glucose levels within an acceptable range with insulin therapy. At 40 weeks gestation, she goes into labor and reports to triage in the labor and delivery department.

12. **Which prescription(s) should the admitting nurse anticipate from the health care provider? Select all that apply.**
    1. Monitor blood glucose levels every 1 to 2 hours.
    2. Administer IV fluid of D10W at 125 mL/hr.
    3. Monitor fetal heart rate patterns throughout labor.
    4. Monitor urinary output closely.
    5. Assess maternal vital signs every 2 hours.

13. **Olivia is connected to a fetal monitor, and early decelerations are noted. What action should the nurse take first?**
    1. Continue to monitor the client.
    2. Change maternal position to side-lying.
    3. Increase the rate of maintenance IV fluid.
    4. Administer oxygen at 8 to 10 L/minute.

14. **THIN Thinking Time!**

    Olivia's labor is progressing, her membranes rupture, with clear amniotic fluid and an epidural catheter is placed. Use **THIN Thinking** to prioritize her care during an epidural block.

    T - Top 3
    H - Help Quick
    I - Identify Risk to Safety
    N - Nursing Process

    T – _____

    H – _____

    I – _____

    N – _____

    Scan to access the 10-Minute-Mentor → *on THIN Thinking.*

    NurseThink.com/THINThinking

15. **Six hours later, Olivia successfully delivers a baby girl, vaginally. The infant is crying and is vigorous. What action should the nurse take first?**
    1. Place the infant on the mother's chest.
    2. Dry and stimulate the infant.
    3. Obtain vital signs of the infant.
    4. Obtain measurements of the infant.

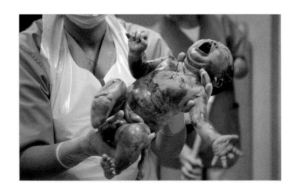

Olivia's baby's Apgar Scores are 8 at 1 minute of age and 9 at 5 minutes of age and the infant weighs 8 lbs. 5 oz. The initial blood glucose level of the infant is 52 mg/dL. She successfully breastfeeds for 15 minutes. After the feeding, the infant's blood glucose is 72 mg/dL. Four hours have passed, and Olivia and her baby girl are ready to be transferred to the mother/baby unit. Olivia's blood glucose has remained stable.

16. **Prepare the SBAR handoff report for the accepting nurse?**

S - _____

B - _____

A - _____

R - _____

Clinical Hint:
S - Situation
B - Background
A - Assessment
R - Recommendation

17. **NurseThink® Prioritization Power!**

Based on the SBAR report, what are postpartum nurse's **Top 3 Concerns**?

1. _____

2. _____

3. _____

18. **Upon assessment, the nurse notices the uterus is flaccid and displaced to the right. What action should the nurse take first?**

1. Check bladder status and encourage voiding.
2. Notify the health care provider.
3. Place an indwelling urinary catheter.
4. Perform fundal massage.

19. **Olivia is successfully breastfeeding her infant but is concerned about her baby getting enough fluids. She says, "My mother says I should be giving her water and formula." What is the nurse's best response?**

1. "Let me consult with the lactation specialist and see what can be done."
2. "Your infant will receive all the nutrition and water she needs from your breastmilk."
3. "I will bring you some water and formula for the baby."
4. "This is an old wives' tale, and you need to tell your mother that it's not true."

20. **Olivia experiences no further complications and is breastfeeding her daughter without difficulties. The nurse provides discharge teaching to Olivia. For each potential post-delivery complication, write the symptoms Olivia should report to her health care provider.**

Condition	Symptoms to Report
Infection	
Uterine subinvolution	
Signs of deep vein thrombosis	
Signs of postpartum depression	

Conceptual Debriefing & Case Reflection

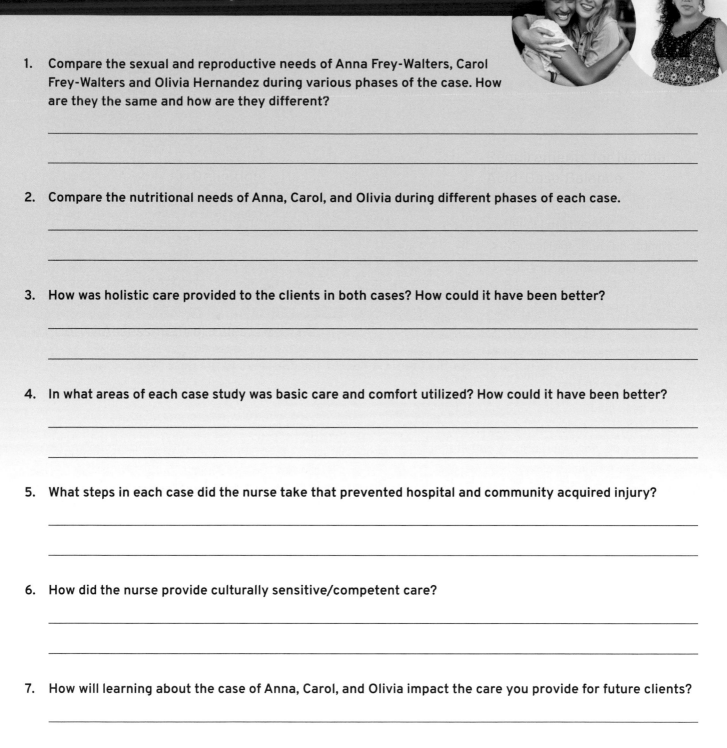

1. Compare the sexual and reproductive needs of Anna Frey-Walters, Carol Frey-Walters and Olivia Hernandez during various phases of the case. How are they the same and how are they different?

    _____

    _____

2. Compare the nutritional needs of Anna, Carol, and Olivia during different phases of each case.

    _____

    _____

3. How was holistic care provided to the clients in both cases? How could it have been better?

    _____

    _____

4. In what areas of each case study was basic care and comfort utilized? How could it have been better?

    _____

    _____

5. What steps in each case did the nurse take that prevented hospital and community acquired injury?

    _____

    _____

6. How did the nurse provide culturally sensitive/competent care?

    _____

    _____

7. How will learning about the case of Anna, Carol, and Olivia impact the care you provide for future clients?

    _____

    _____

Fundamental Quiz

1. A client is recently hospitalized for depression. He states that he does not feel like he has normal sexual feelings for his age. How should the nurse respond?

   1. "Normal feelings are only defined by you. Please tell me what you are feeling."
   2. "Your sexual feelings often change as you mature. I am sure that they will change."
   3. "It sounds as if you are confused. Please tell me what you are confused about."
   4. "It is not uncommon to have sexual feelings that are difficult to understand."

2. A married lesbian couple comes to the office to begin prenatal care. Which nursing response demonstrates bias?

   1. The nurse asks the couple: "Which one of you is the mother?"
   2. The nurse documents that the client is single.
   3. The nurse asks the client: "How was conception achieved?"
   4. The nurse asks the significant other "Are you excited about this pregnancy?"

3. A 13-year-old and her parent come to the clinic for an annual pediatric examination. The parent informs the nurse that the daughter started her period last year. What is the appropriate nursing response?

   1. The nurse asks the client if she has any questions about preventing pregnancy.
   2. The nurse counsels the client about the consequences of sexually transmitted infections.
   3. The nurse documents that the age of menarche as twelve years.
   4. The nurse records that the age of menopause for the client is thirteen.

4. A sexually active young adult comes to the clinic for lesions on the head of the penis. It is determined that he has genital herpes. Which educational statements is/are a priority before discharge? Select all that apply.

   1. You must wear a condom when you have an outbreak to prevent the spread of the virus.
   2. If you have only one partner, there will not be spread of the virus.
   3. Spread can occur when using a condom since the virus may be in a location not covered by the condom.
   4. Herpes can be cured with the use of daily medication.
   5. Having herpes increases your risk of getting human immunodeficiency virus (HIV).

5. The nurse asks the client to provide a 'teach-back' when demonstrating the proper way to perform a breast self-examination when she states "I could not possibly feel my breasts like that." How should the nurse respond?

   1. "I don't understand what the problem is, can you tell me more?"
   2. "What are your concerns?"
   3. "Would it be easier if your husband does it?"
   4. "It's really easy, let me show you again."

Advanced Quiz

6. A client returns to the room with continuous bladder irrigation after prostate removal. The client is taking ice chips and has an I.V. infusing at 100 mL/hour. The catheter is draining light pink urine. After 3 hours, the nurse notes that the urine output is red and has dropped to 15 mL and 10 mL for the last 2 consecutive hours. What should be the nurse's next action?

   1. Increase the fluid rate of the bladder irrigation.
   2. Assess the bladder using a bladder scanner.
   3. Increase the IV fluid rate.
   4. Assess the BUN, creatinine and potassium levels.

7. The nurse is caring for a pregnant client at 32 weeks gestation with an 8-year history of insulin-dependent diabetes. She comes to the clinic stating "I'm having low back pain, and there is some drainage in my underwear. I'm terrified and shaking." What should be the nurse's first action?

   1. Obtain a fingerstick glucose reading.
   2. Collect a urine specimen.
   3. Assess fetal heart sounds.
   4. Determine if there is a bloody show.

8. A client at 38-weeks gestation is admitted to triage with bright red vaginal bleeding. No contractions are reported, but she says that she has some 'abdominal cramping.' Vital signs are heart rate 100 beats per minute, blood pressure 108/67 (87 mmHg), and respirations 16 breaths per minute. Fetal heart rate is 120 beats per minute. What should the nurse do next?

   1. Determine if cervical dilation is present.
   2. Further, assess the abdominal cramping.
   3. Place an indwelling catheter and determine the urinary output.
   4. Observe the quantity of vaginal bleeding.

9. The nurse is caring for a client in active labor and begins to see late decelerations on the fetal heart monitor. Upon entering the room, the nurse observes this image. What should be the nurses next action?

   1. Place the client in a right lateral position.
   2. Notify the practitioner and prepare for surgery.
   3. Place O_2 at 8 liters by non-rebreather mask.
   4. Reassure the parents that everything is all right.

10. The grandmother of a stillborn infant tells the nurse she wants to see and hold the child. What is the nurse's best response?

    1. "I'll check with the provider first to see if it is all right."
    2. "Let me dress him first, and I'll bring him to you."
    3. "I don't think it's good for you to see him."
    4. "It will be better if I bring you a photo of him."

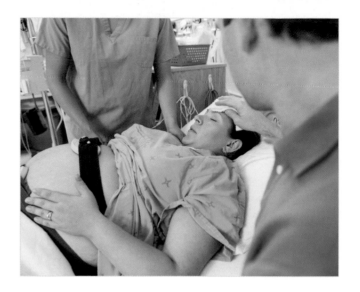

TESTS FOR PREGNANCY				
	Prenatal Tests Throughout	**First Trimester Months: 1-3**	**Second Trimester Months 4-6**	**Third Trimester Months 7-9**
Blood pressure	Screen for early signs of preeclampsia			
Urine Analysis	Screen for infection, preeclampsia, or diabetes			
Blood Tests	Screen for infections (syphilis, hepatitis B, and HIV) blood type (Rh factor), and anemia		QUAD screen: alpha-fetoprotein (AFP), estriol, human chorionic gonadotropin (hCG), and inhibit A); Glucose screening at 6-7 months	
Cervical Fluid				Group B Strep
Ultrasound	Gestational age		Growth and birth defects	
Carrier Genetic Screening		Cystic Fibrosis (CF), spinal muscular atrophy (SMA), thalassemia's, and hemoglobinopathies		
Cell-free Fetal DNA Testing (maternal serum sample)		After 9 weeks Down syndrome		
Chorionic Villus Sampling (placenta sample)		10-13 weeks Genetic conditions		
Amniocentesis (amniotic fluid)			Genetic and birth defects	Infant lung maturity and infections

Circulation

Perfusion / Clotting

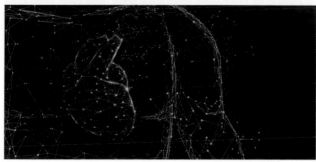

Circulation is the movement of blood through the body and is dependent on the strength and function of a beating heart. Perfusion, although often used interchangeably with circulation, refers to the passage of oxygenated blood through the capillaries to the tissues and cells of the body. In order to have adequate perfusion, both circulation (blood movement) and respiration (the ability to receive oxygen into the blood) are required. Without both of these components, perfusion will be insufficient in meeting the oxygen needs of the body.

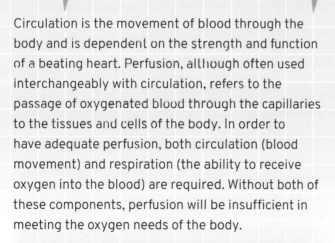

Clotting is a normal process within the body for most people. When the process of clotting is not functioning as expected, negative outcomes occur, including tissue necrosis from a blockage of blood flow or hemorrhage from the inability to form clots.

Next Gen Clinical Judgment:

If a client has poor circulation from a weak heart, what assessment changes can be observed?

> If there are excessive clots in the body, what changes will be seen in the peripheral circulation?

> What assessment differences will there be for a client with decreased perfusion from poor heart function compared to one with excessive clotting?

> How can the nurse determine if there is decreased perfusion to internal organs?

> Which serum labs are impacted by poor circulation or perfusion?

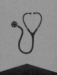
Case 1: Impaired Coronary Perfusion and Chest Pain

Related Concepts: Comfort, Adaptation: Coping & Stress
Threaded Topics: Health Promotion & Teaching, Clinical
Calculations, Legal Issues, Communication

Kandice Sheridan is a 49-year-old female in the emergency department for "achiness" in the elbows that is atypical and worsening over the last three days. She states that the feeling awakens her at night. Ms. Sheridan has felt more short of breath with activity lately and has been under a lot of stress at work. She is planning a trip overseas in a few days and wants to confirm there is nothing significantly wrong before leaving the country.

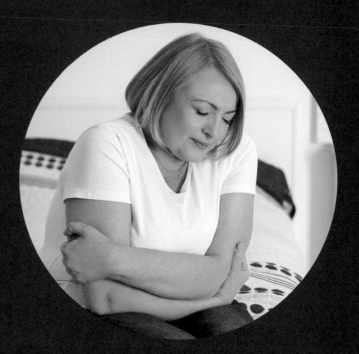

1. **The nurse is beginning the initial assessment. In what priority order should these actions be performed?**

    Answers: _____, _____, _____, _____, _____.

    1. PQRST pain assessment.
    2. Vital sign assessment.
    3. Health history and medication use.
    4. Place in a hospital gown.
    5. Assessment of contributing symptoms.

    Clinical Hint:
    P - Provocation/Palliation
    Q - Quality
    R - Radiation/Relief
    S - Severity/Symptoms
    T - Timing

    Clinical Hint: Mean Arterial Pressure (MAP) is a calculation that measures the blood perfusion to organs. A MAP < 65 mmHg indicates that there is inadequate perfusion. Ex: 145/88 (107). The MAP is 107.

Nursing	Flow Sheets	Provider	Labs & Diagnostics	MAR	Collaborative Care	Other

Nurse Think
HEALTHCARE SYSTEM

Name: Kandice Sheridan
Health Care Provider: M. Dixon M.D.
Code Status: Full Code

Age: 49 years
Allergies: NKDA

NURSING NOTE

June 1 0730	49-year-old female admitted with atypical pain in the elbows. Afebrile, RR 18, HR 88, BP 145/88 (107), sats 97% on room air (RA). Denies chest pain and shortness of breath at this time. Says her arms feel "heavy" and elbows feel "achy." Describes achiness as "less than during the night last night." Denies nausea or other discomforts. Skin moist to touch. History includes iron deficiency anemia, C-sections x 2, and appendectomy. Family history consists of a father with an acute myocardial infarction (AMI) at age 56.

2. NurseThink® Prioritization Power!

Evaluate the information within the Nursing Notes from the emergency department and pick the **Top 3 Priority** assessment findings.

1. _____

2. _____

3. _____

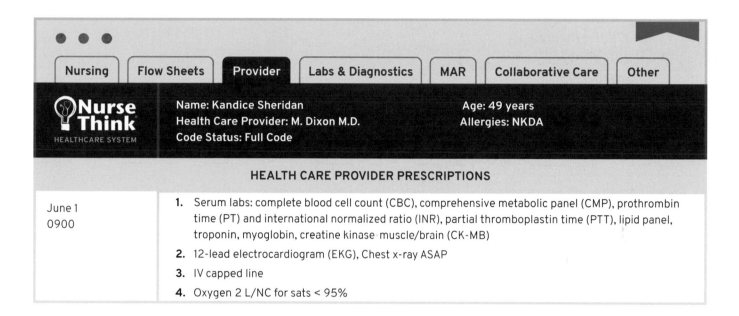

| Nursing | Flow Sheets | Provider | Labs & Diagnostics | MAR | Collaborative Care | Other |

Nurse Think HEALTHCARE SYSTEM

Name: Kandice Sheridan
Health Care Provider: M. Dixon M.D.
Code Status: Full Code

Age: 49 years
Allergies: NKDA

HEALTH CARE PROVIDER PRESCRIPTIONS

June 1 0900	1. Serum labs: complete blood cell count (CBC), comprehensive metabolic panel (CMP), prothrombin time (PT) and international normalized ratio (INR), partial thromboplastin time (PTT), lipid panel, troponin, myoglobin, creatine kinase muscle/brain (CK-MB)
	2. 12-lead electrocardiogram (EKG), Chest x-ray ASAP
	3. IV capped line
	4. Oxygen 2 L/NC for sats < 95%

3. After reviewing the orders, which action should the nurse take first?

1. Request serum lab draw.
2. Obtain 12-lead EKG.
3. Place IV capped line.
4. Apply O_2 at 2 L/nasal cannula.

4. In preparation for the IV insertion, the nurse should place a _____ gauge capped IV line.

5. Which observation(s) should the nurse make in the review of the 12-lead EKG? Select all that apply.

1. The client has tachycardia.
2. There is ST segment elevation in V leads.
3. The client has premature ventricular contractions (PVCs).
4. There is artifact on the tracing.
5. The tracing is normal.

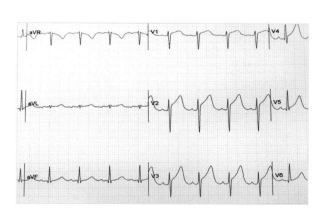

6. **After reviewing the EKG, what should be the nurse's next action?**

   1. Apply continuous EKG monitor.
   2. Check to see if the serum lab report is back.
   3. Notify the healthcare provider.
   4. Apply the ordered oxygen.

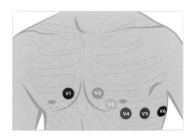

Nurse Think
HEALTHCARE SYSTEM

Name: Kandice Sheridan
Health Care Provider: M. Dixon M.D.
Code Status: Full Code

Age: 49 years
Allergies: NKDA

LABORATORY REPORT

Lab	Normal	1000		
WBC	4,000 - 10,000 µL	5,000		
Hemoglobin	12.0 - 17.0 g/dL	**11.1 L**		
Hematocrit	36.0 - 51.0%	39		
RBC	4.2 - 5.9 cells/L	**3.90 L**		
Platelets	150,000 - 350,000 µL	245,000		
Calcium	9 - 10.5 g/dL	9		
Chloride	98 - 106 mEq/L	98		
Magnesium	1.5 - 2.4 mEq/L	2.0		
Phosphorus	3.0 - 4.5 mg/dL	3.1		
Potassium	3.5 - 5.0 mEq/L	**3.3 L**		
Sodium	136 - 145 mEq/L	139		
Glucose	70 - 100 mg/dL	**110 H**		
BUN	8 - 20 mg/dL	20		
Creatinine	0.7 - 1.3 mg/dL	1.0		
Creatine Kinase (CPK)	30 - 170 U/L	**378 H**		
CPK-MB	3 - 5%	**6% H**		
Lactic Dehydrogenase (LDH)	60 - 100 U/L	**150 H**		
Aminotransferase, Aspartate (AST)	0 - 35 U/L	30		
Aminotransferase, Alanine (ALT)	0 - 35 U/L	33		
GGT	9 - 48 U/L	34		
T. Bilirubin	1.2 mg/dL	0.9		
Cholesterol	< 200 mg/dL	**254 H**		
Triglycerides	< 150 mg/dL	**298 H**		
Troponin I	< 0.5ng/mL	**0.10 H**		
Troponin T	< 10 ng/mL	**12 H**		
Myoglobin	< 170 ng/mL	168		
PT	11 - 12.5 seconds	11.5		
INR	0.8 - 1.1	0.8		
aPTT	25 - 35 seconds	32		

7. **NurseThink® Prioritization Power!**

   Evaluate the information on the lab report and pick the **Top 3 Priority** lab findings.

   1. _____

   2. _____

   3. _____

8. **THIN Thinking Time!**

   Reflect on the events that have occurred since Kandice Sheridan came to the emergency department and apply **THIN Thinking**.

   T – _____

   H – _____

   I – _____

   N – _____

   T - Top 3
   H - Help Quick
   I - Identify Risk to Safety
   N - Nursing Process

   Scan to access the 10-Minute-Mentor on THIN Thinking. →

   NurseThink.com/THINThinking

9. The nurse gathers the lab report and begins to prepare an SBAR conversation for the HCP. Complete each section of the communication form.

   S – _____

   B – _____

   A – _____

   R – _____

   Clinical Hint:
   S - Situation
   B - Background
   A - Assessment
   R - Recommendation

10. The nurse obtains several STAT verbal prescriptions from the HCP for a client experiencing an acute myocardial infarction. In what order should the nurse complete these actions?

    Answers: _____, _____, _____, _____, _____.

    1. Nitroglycerin (NTG) 0.4 mg SL x 3 PRN for pain.
    2. Consult Dr. Nemus, Cardiologist.
    3. Obtain blood pressure and heart rate.
    4. Read back the verbal orders.
    5. Morphine 2-4 mg IV PRN for pain unrelieved by NTG.

    Clinical Hint: Remember **MONA**?
    M - Morphine
    O - Oxygen
    N - Nitroglycerin
    A - Aspirin

11. After administering 4 mg of morphine sulfate IV for chest pain, the nurse discovers that the consent for an emergent coronary angiogram was not signed. The assessment shows that the client is alert, oriented and pain-free. What should the nurse do next?

    1. Obtain a signature before the morphine peaks in the bloodstream.
    2. Notify the cardiologist and cancel the procedure.
    3. Determine if a power of attorney is available.
    4. Ask the client's teenage son, who is at the bedside, to sign the consent.

12. The nurse teaches the client about expectations of the emergent coronary angiogram and reviews what the cardiologist told her about the possibility of open-heart surgery if the stent placement is unsuccessful. The client begins to cry saying that her father died after open-heart surgery. How should the nurse respond?

   1. "I'm sure you are frightened, this is a scary thing to go through."
   2. "Do you want me to get the cardiologist back in here to answer your questions?"
   3. "It's okay, your cardiologist is excellent; he's one of the best."
   4. "Would you like it if I called the chaplain?"

Hand-Off Report

Kandice Sheridan is a 49-year-old returning from the cardiac cath lab after an anterior wall ST-Elevation Myocardial Infarction (STEMI). The cardiologist was able to place a stent in her proximal left anterior descending (LAD) artery. She also has a 40% lesion in her circumflex and a 30% lesion in her right coronary artery (RCA) which do not require intervention at this time. She has a sheath in her right femoral artery. There is no bleeding at the groin site, and her pedal pulses are 3-4+ bilaterally. Her skin is warm to touch. Her vital signs are stable. The nurses review the prescriptions together.

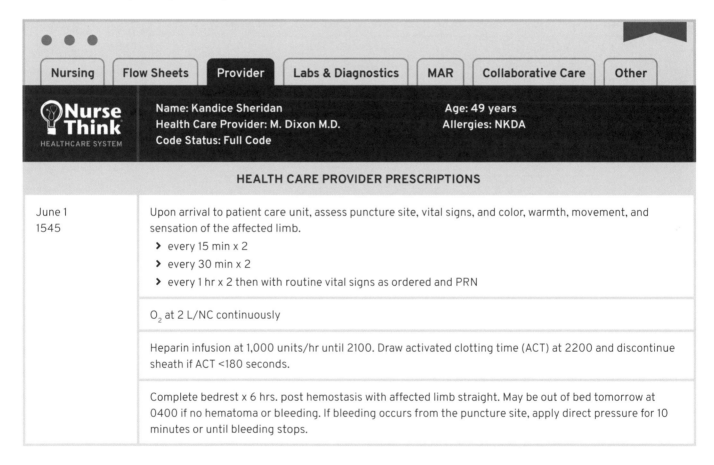

| Nursing | Flow Sheets | **Provider** | Labs & Diagnostics | MAR | Collaborative Care | Other |

NurseThink — HEALTHCARE SYSTEM

Name: Kandice Sheridan
Health Care Provider: M. Dixon M.D.
Code Status: Full Code

Age: 49 years
Allergies: NKDA

HEALTH CARE PROVIDER PRESCRIPTIONS

June 1 1545	Upon arrival to patient care unit, assess puncture site, vital signs, and color, warmth, movement, and sensation of the affected limb. > every 15 min x 2 > every 30 min x 2 > every 1 hr x 2 then with routine vital signs as ordered and PRN
	O₂ at 2 L/NC continuously
	Heparin infusion at 1,000 units/hr until 2100. Draw activated clotting time (ACT) at 2200 and discontinue sheath if ACT <180 seconds.
	Complete bedrest x 6 hrs. post hemostasis with affected limb straight. May be out of bed tomorrow at 0400 if no hematoma or bleeding. If bleeding occurs from the puncture site, apply direct pressure for 10 minutes or until bleeding stops.

13. The client returns from a cardiac catheterization procedure with a right groin sheath in place. What should the nurse include in the priority assessment of this client? Select all that apply.

   1. Blood pressure.
   2. Temperature.
   3. Right groin assessment.
   4. Lung sounds.
   5. Cardiac monitor.

Clinical Hint: After a procedure that involved the large vessels of the groin, the distal pulse assessment should include the popliteal, dorsalis pedis, and posterior tibialis arteries.

14. A client has 25,000 units of heparin in 500 mL NS infusing at 1,000 unit per hour via a 20 gauge IV in the left hand. At what rate should the pump be set?

    1. 10 mL/hr.
    2. 20 mL/hr.
    3. 25 mL/hr.
    4. 50 mL/hr.

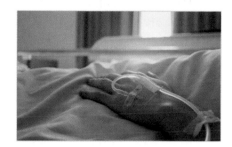

| Nursing | Flow Sheets | Provider | Labs & Diagnostics | MAR | Collaborative Care | Other |

NurseThink HEALTHCARE SYSTEM

Name: Kandice Sheridan
Health Care Provider: M. Dixon M.D.
Code Status: Full Code

Age: 49 years
Allergies: NKDA

VITAL SIGN RECORD

Time	BP (MAP)	HR	RR	Sats
1545	110/64 (79)	88	19	97% 2 L/NC
1601	105/62 (76)	97	20	98% 2 L/NC
1622	100/59 (73)	108	20	98% 2 L/NC

15. The nurse obtains the first three sets of vital signs. What should the nurse do next?

    1. Have the unlicensed assistive personal complete the remaining set of vital signs.
    2. Assess for bleeding at the sheath site.
    3. Re-evaluate the vital signs in 15 minutes.
    4. Notify the health care provider of the client's status.

The client is dehydrated and vital signs are stabilized after the intravenous fluid is administered. The sheaths are pulled at 2245 without complications.

16. While administering the ordered medications, Kandice asks why each of these medications are needed. Describe how the nurse should instruct her for each of these medications.

    1. Clopidogrel 75 mg daily, by mouth. _____

    2. Aspirin 81 mg daily, by mouth. _____

    3. Metoprolol 50 mg daily, by mouth. _____

    4. Atorvastatin 80 mg daily, by mouth. _____

17. Kandice asks what she can do to help decrease the risk for having another heart attack in the future. What should the nurse instruct? Select all that apply.

    1. Eat a diet low in cholesterol and saturated fats.
    2. Minimize carbohydrate intake.
    3. Walk 30 minutes 5 days a week.
    4. Increase dietary intake of fruit.
    5. Monitor serum lipid levels.

18. As the nurse enters Kandice's room on the morning of discharge, she finds her crying. When asked what is wrong, she states, "I'm so afraid I'll pass my bad genes to my children, and they'll have heart disease also." How should the nurse respond?

    1. "I don't think that will be an issue since your spouse has a good heart."
    2. "I'm sure you are afraid for them, maybe they'll be luckier than you."
    3. "They can make some lifestyle changes now, so their chances of heart disease are less."
    4. "With proper medication, they will have less chances of heart disease."

---

19. **NurseThink® Prioritization Power!**

    Evaluate the care of this client and pick the **Top 3 Priority** discharge needs.

    1. _____

    2. _____

    3. _____

---

20. Kandice returns to the office two weeks later appearing withdrawn and sad. The nurse asks how things are going and she states, "It's such an adjustment, I don't know if I can do it." What suggestions should the nurse make to the client?

    1. Request an antidepressant from the cardiologist.
    2. Participate in a cardiac support group.
    3. Encourage her spouse to be more supportive.
    4. Suggest she takes more time off of work.

Clinical Hint: Heart disease demands a lifetime of compliance with lifestyle change. Providing community support and resources for the client after discharge will improve the chances of long-term success.

Because heart disease is often familial it is important for the nurse to address concern for the blood relatives of the client. Prevention education is critical to slowing the cycle of disease and illness.

Next Gen Clinical Judgment: List all possible symptoms that can indicate impaired circulatory event. Consider the cues of each body system when it is experiencing a decrease in perfusion.

_____

_____

_____

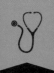
Case 2: Decreased Perfusion from Hypertension and Heart Failure

Related Concepts: Oxygenation, Mobility, Acid-base Balance
Threaded Topics : Legal Issues, Error Identification,
Communication, Teamwork, Patient Education, Medication
Safety

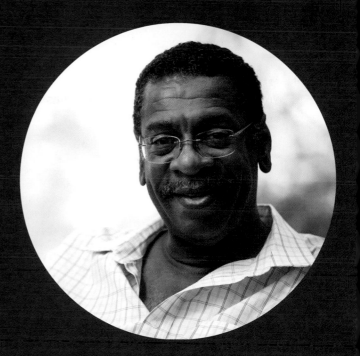

William Jones is a 69-year-old man with a 25-year history of hypertension. He was discharged from the Veteran's Hospital last week after a 2-day stay for hypertensive crisis. The home care nurse is making an initial visit to his home today. Mr. Jones greets the nurse at the door. He is tall with a large build. He walks with a limp and is mildly short of breath. His home is small but neat and well kept. There are no stairs or throw-rugs. He has a small dog, barking as the nurse enters. The smell of food cooking comes from the kitchen.

1. **The nurse performs an environmental assessment. Why would each observation listed be a potential concern and area for further assessment by the nurse? List the action that the nurse should take.**

    Large build_____

    Walks with a limp _____

    Mildly short of breath _____

    Small dog _____

    Smell of food _____

After completing the initial admission paperwork and physical assessment of Mr. Jones, the nurse documents the findings in the electronic record using a tablet computer.

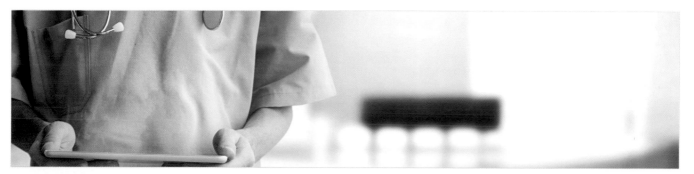

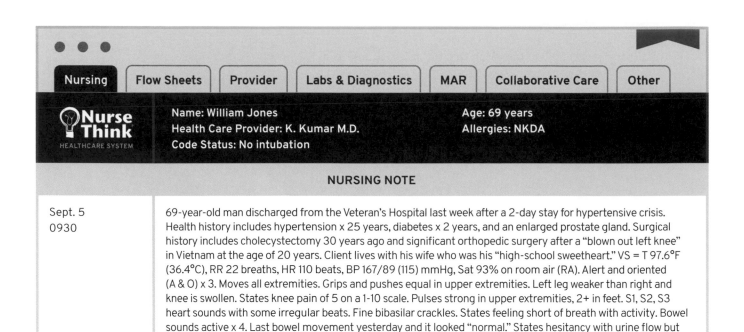

Nursing | Flow Sheets | Provider | Labs & Diagnostics | MAR | Collaborative Care | Other

Nurse Think
HEALTHCARE SYSTEM

Name: William Jones
Health Care Provider: K. Kumar M.D.
Code Status: No intubation

Age: 69 years
Allergies: NKDA

NURSING NOTE

Sept. 5 0930	69-year-old man discharged from the Veteran's Hospital last week after a 2-day stay for hypertensive crisis. Health history includes hypertension x 25 years, diabetes x 2 years, and an enlarged prostate gland. Surgical history includes cholecystectomy 30 years ago and significant orthopedic surgery after a "blown out left knee" in Vietnam at the age of 20 years. Client lives with his wife who was his "high-school sweetheart." VS = T 97.6°F (36.4°C), RR 22 breaths, HR 110 beats, BP 167/89 (115) mmHg, Sat 93% on room air (RA). Alert and oriented (A & O) x 3. Moves all extremities. Grips and pushes equal in upper extremities. Left leg weaker than right and knee is swollen. States knee pain of 5 on a 1-10 scale. Pulses strong in upper extremities, 2+ in feet. S1, S2, S3 heart sounds with some irregular beats. Fine bibasilar crackles. States feeling short of breath with activity. Bowel sounds active x 4. Last bowel movement yesterday and it looked "normal." States hesitancy with urine flow but denies burning. Up to void 1-2 times each night. Client states morning blood glucose was 178, and he checks it daily. Ht. 6'1" Wt. 263 pounds. BMI 34.7.

2. **NurseThink® Prioritization Power!**

   Evaluate the information within the admission note and pick the **Top 3 Priority** assessment concerns.

   1. _____

   2. _____

   3. _____

Next, the nurse reviews the client's medication list.

MY MEDICATIONS

Lisinopril 40 mg once a day by mouth

Atenolol 50 mg once a day by mouth

Metformin 1000 mg twice a day by mouth

Tamsulosin 0.4 mg once a day by mouth

Celecoxib 200 mg twice a day by mouth as needed

Clinical Hint: Always compare the actual medication bottles to a written/typed list that the client provides. Dosages may have changed and the list may be outdated.

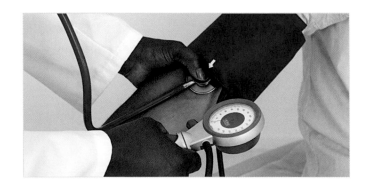

Next Gen Clinical Judgment: For each of these medications, review the drug category and priority teaching point.

3. After further inquiry, it is discovered that no morning medications have been taken. Which medications should the nurse suggest Mr. Jones take now? Select all that apply.

   1. Lisinopril.
   2. Atenolol.
   3. Metformin.
   4. Tamsulosin.
   5. Celecoxib.

   Read what the American Heart Association says about blood pressure management and hypertensive Crisis. →

   www.heart.org

   Explain why you chose each medication as a priority.

   _____

   _____

   _____

4. The nurse completes a Fall Risk Assessment for Mr. Jones. His score is 13 (at-risk is >10). Which intervention(s) would be most appropriate? Select all that apply.

   1. Ask him to find a new home for his dog.
   2. Request a physical therapy referral.
   3. Request an occupational therapy referral.
   4. Get a brace for his knee.
   5. Suggest grab bars in the bathroom.
   6. Place a red "Fall Risk" band on his wrist.

   Clinical Hint: Early fall risk assessment and interventions can save lives. The death rate from unintentional falls for adults aged 65 or more years has been increasing an average of 4.9% per year, according to the Centers for Disease Control and Prevention.

5. The nurse reviews Mr. Jones advanced directives. The forms indicate that he is agreeable to everything except being on life support. He has identified his wife as his Power of Attorney. How should the nurse interpret these preferences? Select all that apply.

   1. His wife is the proxy and will make his health care decisions.
   2. No intubation, should he stop breathing.
   3. Perform defibrillation if his heart stops.
   4. Provide nutritional support if he is in a vegetative state.
   5. Perform CPR if he is found unconscious and not breathing.

6. **NurseThink® Prioritization Power!**
   What additional concerns did the nurse not address on this visit?

   _____

   _____

   _____

   _____

7. One week later, Mr. Jones calls the home care nurse saying that he feels very short of breath since he awoke three hours ago and is having a hard time breathing. What actions should the nurse take next?

   1. Change the plan for the day and make a visit to Mr. Jones.
   2. Ask him to check his blood pressure and call you back.
   3. Have him take an extra antihypertensive medication and lay down.
   4. Tell him to hang up the phone and call an ambulance.

Mr. Jones chooses to have his wife drive him to the emergency department, where he is admitted. The nurse makes these notes in the electronic health record.

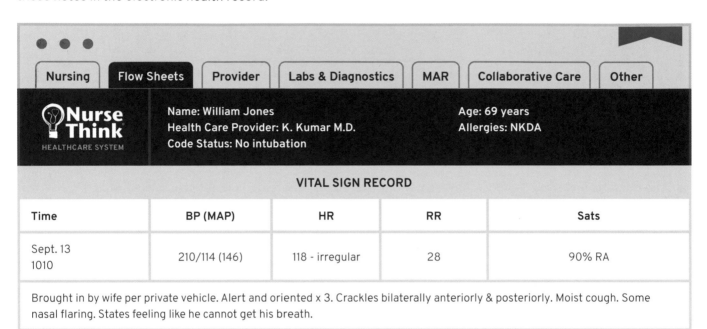

| Nursing | Flow Sheets | Provider | Labs & Diagnostics | MAR | Collaborative Care | Other |

Nurse Think HEALTHCARE SYSTEM

Name: William Jones
Health Care Provider: K. Kumar M.D.
Code Status: No intubation

Age: 69 years
Allergies: NKDA

VITAL SIGN RECORD

Time	BP (MAP)	HR	RR	Sats
Sept. 13 1010	210/114 (146)	118 - irregular	28	90% RA

Brought in by wife per private vehicle. Alert and oriented x 3. Crackles bilaterally anteriorly & posteriorly. Moist cough. Some nasal flaring. States feeling like he cannot get his breath.

8. **NurseThink® Prioritization Power!**

   Evaluate the information within the emergency department note and pick the **Top 3 Priority** actions.

   1. _____

   2. _____

   3. _____

9. The nurse discusses the situation with the emergency department provider. Which prescription(s) should the nurse question? Select all that apply.

   1. IV 0.9% sodium chloride at 100 mL/hr.
   2. Delivery of sodium nitroprusside intravenously.
   3. Portable chest x-ray.
   4. Furosemide 5 mg intravenously.
   5. Oxygen at 15 L by non-rebreather mask.
   6. Arterial blood gas.

   > **Clinical Hint:** A prescription can be a medication, therapy, or anything ordered by the health care provider.

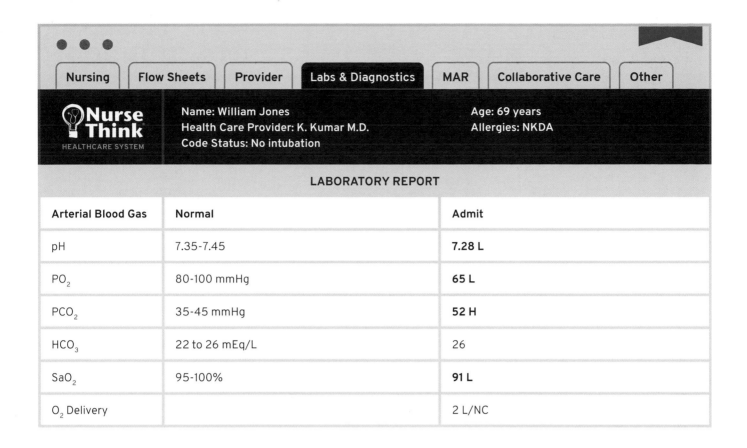

LABORATORY REPORT

Name: William Jones
Health Care Provider: K. Kumar M.D.
Code Status: No intubation

Age: 69 years
Allergies: NKDA

Arterial Blood Gas	Normal	Admit
pH	7.35-7.45	7.28 L
PO$_2$	80-100 mmHg	65 L
PCO$_2$	35-45 mmHg	52 H
HCO$_3$	22 to 26 mEq/L	26
SaO$_2$	95-100%	91 L
O$_2$ Delivery		2 L/NC

10. **The nurse receives the arterial blood gas results above. What conclusions should the nurse make about the client's situation?**
    1. In metabolic acidosis and has impaired renal function.
    2. In respiratory acidosis and needs more oxygen.
    3. Needs more oxygen and to breathe into a paper bag.
    4. Needs a bronchodilator and intubation.

    Clinical Hint: It is not important to "name" the blood gas but rather determine the best action the nurse should take in response to the lab report, based on the situation.

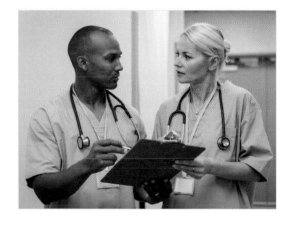

Handoff Report to ICU:

Mr. Jones is a 69-year-old with a history of hypertension, diabetes mellitus (DM) type II, and knee pain from a war injury. He came to the emergency department (E.D.) via private vehicle this morning after feeling severely short of breath. Upon admission to the E.D., he was found to be severely hypertensive and short of breath. His blood gases showed respiratory acidosis with hypoxemia, and his chest x-ray confirmed he is in acute cardiogenic heart failure. He's on 4 L/NC, and his saturations are at 93%. We gave him the "now" dose of furosemide 40 mg of IV about 10 minutes ago and started him on sodium nitroprusside intravenously at 0.1 mcg/kg/minute 15 minutes ago, and his last blood pressure was 211/115 (147) mmHg, heart rate is 120 in a sinus tachycardia, with rare premature ventricular contraction (PVC), respirations are 24 breaths per minute. His wife is in the intensive care unit (ICU) waiting room.

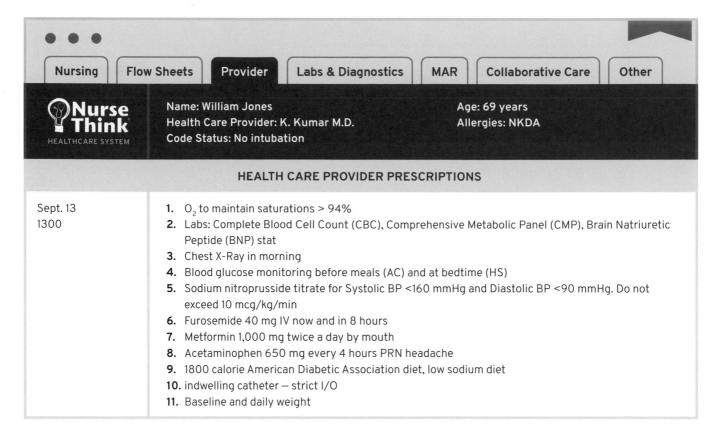

HEALTH CARE PROVIDER PRESCRIPTIONS

Sept. 13 1300	1. O₂ to maintain saturations > 94%

1. O_2 to maintain saturations > 94%
2. Labs: Complete Blood Cell Count (CBC), Comprehensive Metabolic Panel (CMP), Brain Natriuretic Peptide (BNP) stat
3. Chest X-Ray in morning
4. Blood glucose monitoring before meals (AC) and at bedtime (HS)
5. Sodium nitroprusside titrate for Systolic BP <160 mmHg and Diastolic BP <90 mmHg. Do not exceed 10 mcg/kg/min
6. Furosemide 40 mg IV now and in 8 hours
7. Metformin 1,000 mg twice a day by mouth
8. Acetaminophen 650 mg every 4 hours PRN headache
9. 1800 calorie American Diabetic Association diet, low sodium diet
10. indwelling catheter – strict I/O
11. Baseline and daily weight

Over the next couple of hours, the intensive care unit (ICU) nurse cares for Mr. Jones and documents the care in the electronic health record (EHR). Review the sequence of events listed below.

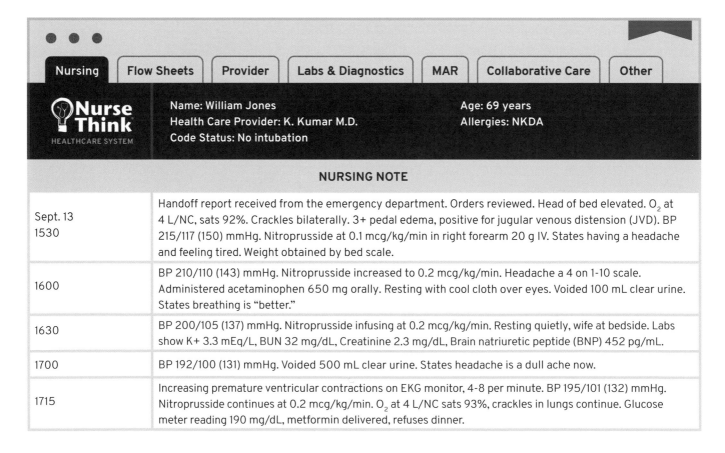

NURSING NOTE

Sept. 13 1530	Handoff report received from the emergency department. Orders reviewed. Head of bed elevated. O₂ at 4 L/NC, sats 92%. Crackles bilaterally. 3+ pedal edema, positive for jugular venous distension (JVD). BP 215/117 (150) mmHg. Nitroprusside at 0.1 mcg/kg/min in right forearm 20 g IV. States having a headache and feeling tired. Weight obtained by bed scale.
1600	BP 210/110 (143) mmHg. Nitroprusside increased to 0.2 mcg/kg/min. Headache a 4 on 1-10 scale. Administered acetaminophen 650 mg orally. Resting with cool cloth over eyes. Voided 100 mL clear urine. States breathing is "better."
1630	BP 200/105 (137) mmHg. Nitroprusside infusing at 0.2 mcg/kg/min. Resting quietly, wife at bedside. Labs show K+ 3.3 mEq/L, BUN 32 mg/dL, Creatinine 2.3 mg/dL, Brain natriuretic peptide (BNP) 452 pg/mL.
1700	BP 192/100 (131) mmHg. Voided 500 mL clear urine. States headache is a dull ache now.
1715	Increasing premature ventricular contractions on EKG monitor, 4-8 per minute. BP 195/101 (132) mmHg. Nitroprusside continues at 0.2 mcg/kg/min. O₂ at 4 L/NC sats 93%, crackles in lungs continue. Glucose meter reading 190 mg/dL, metformin delivered, refuses dinner.

11. **After reviewing the last two hours of care in the intensive care unit, identify which prescription(s) the nurse did not complete correctly. Select all that apply.**

    1. Oxygen titration.
    2. Completion of labs draw.
    3. Blood glucose monitoring.
    4. Sodium nitroprusside titration.
    5. Metformin.
    6. Acetaminophen.
    7. Diet.
    8. Indwelling catheter.
    9. Baseline weight.

    Clinical Hint: To use high-level clinical judgment, begin by identifying clinical cues that establish a concern for the nurse and require additional exploration.

12. **Which priority data collected by the nurse should have been communicated to the health care provider?**

    1. Crackles, edema, jugular venous distension (JVD).
    2. Headache.
    3. Premature ventricular contractions (PVCs).
    4. Labs.

13. **The nurse gathers information and begins to prepare an SBAR telephone conversation for the health care provider. Complete each section of the communication form.**

    S – _____

    B – _____

    A – _____

    R – _____

    Clinical Hint:
    S - Situation
    B - Background
    A - Assessment
    R - Recommendation

14. **The nurse obtains additional directions from the provider to administer potassium chloride 10 mEq intravenously "now." Which action should the nurse perform first?**

    1. Input the new order into the computer.
    2. Confirm that the dosing is safe for administration.
    3. Restate the order to the provider.
    4. Review the policy on potassium administration.

15. **The pharmacy delivers KCl 10 mEq in 100 mL NS to infuse over 1 hour. Before administering the medication, what action(s) should the nurse take? Select all that apply.**

    1. Start a new IV site.
    2. Confirm the medication to the order.
    3. Confirm allergies.
    4. Check a single patient identifier.
    5. Determine the safe rate of administration.

16. **The next day, the client's blood pressure is stable and he is weaned off the nitroprusside. As the nurse reviews the intake and output record below, what assessment changes are anticipated?**

   1. Crackles will be increased.
   2. O_2 saturations will be improved.
   3. Weight will have stabilized.
   4. A fluid restriction is needed.

   Clinical Hint: The nurse must review data in trends (hours or days worth of data) to make the best clinical judgment. Anything with numbers should be explored in trends. This includes labs, weights, intake/output, vital signs, etc.

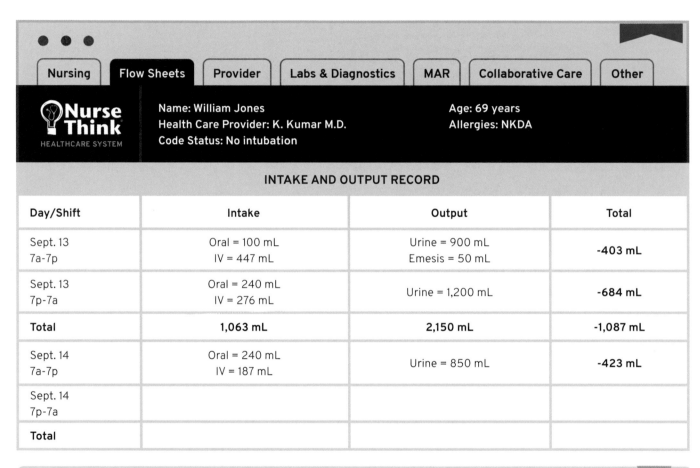

Nursing	Flow Sheets	Provider	Labs & Diagnostics	MAR	Collaborative Care	Other

Nurse Think HEALTHCARE SYSTEM

Name: William Jones
Health Care Provider: K. Kumar M.D.
Code Status: No intubation

Age: 69 years
Allergies: NKDA

INTAKE AND OUTPUT RECORD

Day/Shift	Intake	Output	Total
Sept. 13 7a-7p	Oral = 100 mL IV = 447 mL	Urine = 900 mL Emesis = 50 mL	-403 mL
Sept. 13 7p-7a	Oral = 240 mL IV = 276 mL	Urine = 1,200 mL	-684 mL
Total	1,063 mL	2,150 mL	-1,087 mL
Sept. 14 7a-7p	Oral = 240 mL IV = 187 mL	Urine = 850 mL	-423 mL
Sept. 14 7p-7a			
Total			

17. **NurseThink® Prioritization Power!**

   Mr. Jones is being discharged today. List what needs to be included in his discharge planning and teaching based on these discharge instructions:

   Discharge to home

   Furosemide 40 mg each day, orally _____

   Digoxin 0.25 mg each day, orally _____

   Continue previous medications _____

   Home care nurse to see client beginning tomorrow _____

Clinical Hint: Reviewing discharge instructions is the time for the nurse to evaluate that the instructions are comprehensive and inclusive. For example, does the client require some dietary limitations that were not specified? It is the nurse's role to seek clarification before discharge.

18. NurseThink® Time!

Complete the Medication Reconciliation form below.

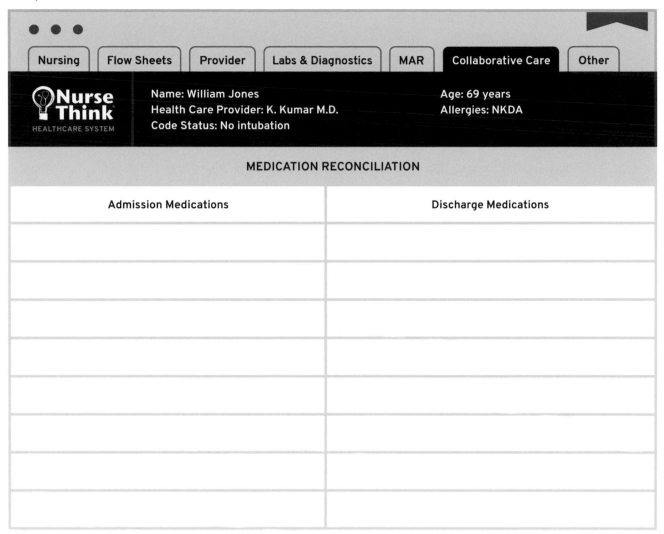

| | Nursing | Flow Sheets | Provider | Labs & Diagnostics | MAR | Collaborative Care | Other |

Nurse Think HEALTHCARE SYSTEM

Name: William Jones
Health Care Provider: K. Kumar M.D.
Code Status: No intubation

Age: 69 years
Allergies: NKDA

MEDICATION RECONCILIATION

Admission Medications	Discharge Medications

19. **During the discharge conversations, Mr. Jones shares with the nurse "I grew up in the church but lost my faith during the war. I feel my days are getting closer to the end and wonder if there's something more in the afterlife. Are you a believer?" How should the nurse begin the conversation?**

1. "It's common when someone experiences what you've been through to feel a sense of wonder."
2. "I'm a strong Christian and go to church every week."
3. "It sounds like you have questions for the hospital chaplain, let me see if she's available to see you before you go home."
4. "Do you have a church close to your home?"

20. **On the way home after the shift, the discharging nurse gets a call from a nursing colleague who happens to be Mr. Jones neighbor. The colleague is at Mr. Jones house and asks about his discharge instructions since he has some questions. How should the nurse respond?**

1. Ask the colleague to read the discharge instructions to you.
2. Provide the information being asked.
3. Ask to speak to Mr. Jones.
4. Suggest Mr. Jones call the home care nurse.

Conceptual Debriefing & Case Reflection

1. Compare the impaired perfusion that Kandice Sheridan experienced with the impaired perfusion of William Jones. How are they the same and how are they different?

   _____

   _____

2. What was your single greatest learning moment while completing the case of Kandice Sheridan? What about William Jones?

   _____

   _____

3. How did the nursing (not medical) care provided to Kandice Sheridan and William Jones change the outcome for each of them?

   _____

   _____

4. Identify safety concerns for both Kandice Sheridan and William Jones for each case.

   _____

   _____

5. Identify in each case how the nurse provided basic care and comfort to best meet the client's needs.

   _____

   _____

6. What steps in each case did the nurse take that prevented hospital-acquired injury?

   _____

   _____

7. How did the nurse provide culturally sensitive/competent care?

   _____

   _____

8. How will learning about the case of Kandice Sheridan and William Jones impact the care you provide for future clients?

   _____

   _____

Conceptual Quiz: Fundamentals and Advanced

Fundamental Quiz

1. A nurse volunteering at a first aid station during a race is caring for a participant who is feeling dizzy and light-headed. What priority action should the nurse take?
   1. Have the runner drink some water.
   2. Take the client's blood pressure.
   3. Have the client lay down.
   4. Determine how long the runner has felt poorly.

2. A client with a history of clot formation is experiencing sudden pain in the left great toe. What should the nurse do next?
   1. Determine circulation, movement, and sensation (CMS) to the feet.
   2. Offer pain medication.
   3. Assess for popliteal and dorsalis pedis pulses.
   4. Elevate the left foot.

3. The nurse is caring for a client on extended bedrest. Which action(s) should the nurse take when getting the client out of bed for the first time? Select all that apply.
   1. Medicate for pain.
   2. Request additional assistance.
   3. Obtain orthostatic blood pressure readings.
   4. Apply a gait belt.
   5. Deliver additional intravenous fluids.
   6. Raise the head of the bed.

4. The school nurse is assessing a child with a newly placed cast on the right arm. The nurse notes that the fingers are slightly cooler than those on the left hand. What should the nurse do next?
   1. Nothing, this is normal.
   2. Ask the child if the cast feels tight.
   3. Assess the fingertips on each hand for blanching.
   4. Assess the radial pulse in the right wrist.

5. The nurse is caring for a client taking clopidogrel after having an embolic event. The client shares that since starting the medication he has noticed that his stools are darker in color. What is an appropriate response by the nurse?
   1. That is typical with this medication.
   2. Tell me what you mean by "darker"?
   3. Often dietary changes can cause this.
   4. When is the last time you had a bowel movement?

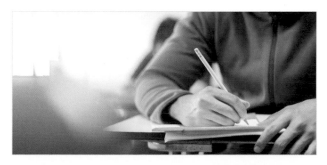

Advanced Quiz

6. The nurse is caring for a client who's mean arterial pressure has been < 60 mmHg for the last two hours. Which serum lab(s) should the nurse anticipate in response to this event?
   1. Elevation in the liver enzymes.
   2. Decrease in potassium level.
   3. Elevation in serum albumin level.
   4. Decrease in BUN and creatinine.

7. A client in the emergency department has been hydrated with normal saline over the last hour for hypovolemia. Assessment changes now include a rapid bounding pulse and shortness of breath. What action should the nurse delegate to the unlicensed assistive personnel?
   1. Raise the head of bed.
   2. Apply oxygen.
   3. Stop IV fluids.
   4. Obtain blood pressure.

8. A client has been treated with a diuretic for fluid overload and shortness of breath. After voiding 960 mL clear yellow urine over an hour, the client says she feels funny. What should the nurse do next?
   1. Reassess the oxygen saturation reading.
   2. Administer an additional dose of the diuretic.
   3. Assess the blood pressure.
   4. Obtain a serum potassium level.

9. The nurse is caring for a client who has had significant uterine bleeding after childbirth. The client is now critical. The electronic health record shows this information. What can the nurse conclude from the information? Select all that apply.

Time	BP (MAP)	HR	RR	Sats
0821	105/63	124	24	94% RA
0755	118/70	117	23	96% RA
0738	132/76	110	22	97% RA

   1. The client's condition is stabilizing.
   2. The changes indicate that an action is needed.
   3. The heart rate is increasing from the pain of delivery.
   4. The saturations are dropping because of the tachypnea.
   5. The respiratory rate and heart rate changes are a result of the loss of blood.

10. For each condition, select a potential action to take. There is only 1 priority action for each condition. Each potential action can only be used once. Not all potential actions are used.

Potential Action to Take	Condition	Priority Action
A. Hourly urine output	Hypovolemic shock	
B. Recombinant tissue plasminogen activator	Pulmonary embolism	
C. Orthostatic blood pressure	Acute coronary syndrome	
D. High flow oxygen	Raynaud's Disease	
E. Oxygen at 2 L/nasal cannula	Cardiogenic shock	
F. Norepinephrine 2 mcg/min	Embolic stroke/brain attack	
G. Blood pressure	Deep vein thrombosis	
H. Nifedipine 20 mg by mouth		
I. Enoxaparin 1 mg/kg SC		

Protection

Immunity / Inflammation / Infection

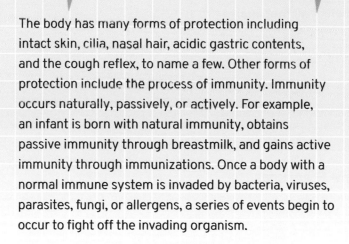

The body has many forms of protection including intact skin, cilia, nasal hair, acidic gastric contents, and the cough reflex, to name a few. Other forms of protection include the process of immunity. Immunity occurs naturally, passively, or actively. For example, an infant is born with natural immunity, obtains passive immunity through breastmilk, and gains active immunity through immunizations. Once a body with a normal immune system is invaded by bacteria, viruses, parasites, fungi, or allergens, a series of events begin to occur to fight off the invading organism.

Inflammation is a defense mechanism that occurs when the immune system recognizes damaged cells, irritants, and pathogens, and begins a biological response to remove it. Infections, wounds, and any damage to tissue would not be able to heal without an inflammatory response. Chronic inflammation, on the other hand, can cause disease and illness, including cancers and rheumatoid arthritis.

Infection is the result of the body's inability to destroy and remove an invading organism. It can be localized or systemic, acute or chronic. Keep in mind, there is usually always inflammation associated with an infection, but not always is there an infection if there is an inflammation. It is important to differentiate between the two.

Next Gen Clinical Judgment:

> What symptoms of inflammation could be observed in a client who is immune-compromised?

> How could the nurse differentiate between inflammation and infection?

> What is the difference between immunity that is acquired passively versus actively?

> Hypersensitivity reaction is a result of a malfunctioning immune system. What signs and symptoms would be observed?

> List diseases and illnesses that are related to the immune system.

Go To Clinical Case

While caring for this client, be sure to review the concept maps in chapters 3 and 4.

Case 1: Healthcare Acquired Infections: Catheter-associated urinary tract infection (CAUTI)

Related Concepts: Mobility, Perfusion, Inflammation, Immunity
Threaded Topics: Culturally Sensitive Care, Communication, Error Prevention

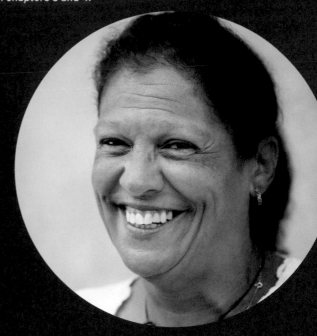

Ana Maria Martinez is a 54-year-old client with a history of rheumatoid arthritis. Her chronic illness is well controlled with daily prednisone and nonsteroidal anti-inflammatory drugs (NSAIDs). Spanish is her primary language, and she lives with her daughter, son-in-law, and two small grandchildren who assist with her activities of daily living. Two days ago, Ms. Martinez fell when going outside to get the mail. She could not get up and was found an hour later by a neighbor who called 911.

Upon arrival at the emergency department, it was determined that she had a transverse fracture of the left trochanter head and was admitted to the hospital in preparation for surgery the following day.

1. **Which factor(s) contribute to Ms. Martinez's injury? Select all that apply.**

   1. Older adult age.
   2. Chronic use of corticosteroid medication.
   3. Chronic use of NSAID medication.
   4. Limitation of movement.
   5. Lack of English proficiency.

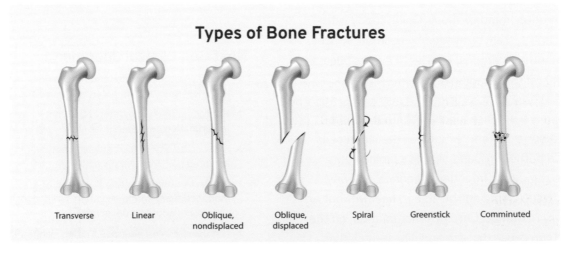

Types of Bone Fractures

Transverse   Linear   Oblique, nondisplaced   Oblique, displaced   Spiral   Greenstick   Comminuted

Admitting prescriptions include the following.

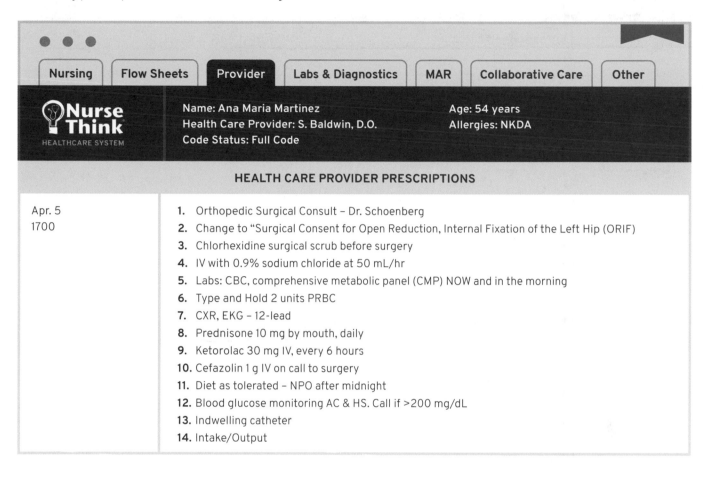

Nursing | **Flow Sheets** | **Provider** | **Labs & Diagnostics** | **MAR** | **Collaborative Care** | **Other**

Nurse Think
HEALTHCARE SYSTEM

Name: Ana Maria Martinez
Health Care Provider: S. Baldwin, D.O.
Code Status: Full Code

Age: 54 years
Allergies: NKDA

HEALTH CARE PROVIDER PRESCRIPTIONS

Apr. 5
1700

1. Orthopedic Surgical Consult – Dr. Schoenberg
2. Change to "Surgical Consent for Open Reduction, Internal Fixation of the Left Hip (ORIF)
3. Chlorhexidine surgical scrub before surgery
4. IV with 0.9% sodium chloride at 50 mL/hr
5. Labs: CBC, comprehensive metabolic panel (CMP) NOW and in the morning
6. Type and Hold 2 units PRBC
7. CXR, EKG – 12-lead
8. Prednisone 10 mg by mouth, daily
9. Ketorolac 30 mg IV, every 6 hours
10. Cefazolin 1 g IV on call to surgery
11. Diet as tolerated – NPO after midnight
12. Blood glucose monitoring AC & HS. Call if >200 mg/dL
13. Indwelling catheter
14. Intake/Output

2. **List all prescriptions that increase the risk of infection?**

_____

_____

3. **List all prescriptions that are specific for the prevention of infection?**

_____

_____

4. **The nurse is beginning preoperative teaching and realizes that Ms. Martinez lacks English language proficiency. How should the nurse best evaluate the client's level of understanding?**

   1. Ask Ms. Martinez if she understands English.
   2. Ask the family how much she understands.
   3. Have Ms. Martinez teach-back what was taught.
   4. Request an interpreter to be present.

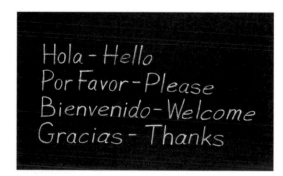

Hola – Hello
Por Favor – Please
Bienvenido – Welcome
Gracias – Thanks

5. **NurseThink® Prioritization Power!**

   The nurse is preparing the client for surgery. List the **Top 3 Priority** safety actions.

   1. _____

   2. _____

   3. _____

The nurse reviews Ms. Martinez's lab results.

● ● ●

| Nursing | Flow Sheets | Provider | Labs & Diagnostics | MAR | Collaborative Care | Other |

Name: Ana Maria Martinez
Health Care Provider: S. Baldwin, D.O.
Code Status: Full Code

Age: 54 years
Allergies: NKDA

LABORATORY REPORT

Lab	Normal	Apr. 5	Apr. 6	
WBC	4,000 - 10,000 μL	9,000	15,000 H	
Hemoglobin	12.0 - 17.0 g/dL	11.0 L	6.9 L	
Hematocrit	36.0 - 51.0%	35 L	28 L	
RBC	4.2 - 5.9 cells/L	3.8 L	2.5 L	
Platelets	150,000 - 350,000 μL	145,000 L	102,000 L	
Calcium	9 - 10.5 g/dL	8.8 L	8.7 L	
Chloride	98 - 106 mEq/L	99	98	
Magnesium	1.5 - 2.4 mEq/L	2.1	1.9	
Phosphorus	3.0 - 4.5 mg/dL	3.1	3.0	
Potassium	3.5 - 5.0 mEq/L	3.2 L	3.3 L	
Sodium	136 - 145 mEq/L	142	144	
Glucose	70 - 100 mg/dL	189 H	267 H	
BUN	8 - 20 mg/dL	39 H	25 H	
Creatinine	0.7 - 1.3 mg/dL	1.3	1.2	
Creatine Kinase (CPK)	30 - 170 U/L	422 H	304 H	
Lactic Dehydrogenase (LDH)	60 - 100 U/L	154 H	279 H	
Aminotransferase, Aspartate (AST)	0 - 35 U/L	34	33	
Aminotransferase, Alanine (ALT)	0 - 35 U/L	30	32	
GGT	9 - 48 U/L	42	36	
T. Bilirubin	1.2 mg/dL	0.9	1.0	
Cholesterol	< 200 mg/dL	259 H	246 H	
Triglycerides	< 150 mg/dL	198 H	188 H	

6. **Which lab(s) should the nurse bring to the attention of the health care provider prior to surgery? Select all that apply.**

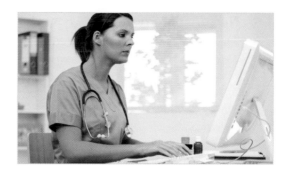

1. White blood cells.
2. Hemoglobin/Hematocrit.
3. Calcium.
4. Potassium.
5. Glucose.
6. Cholesterol/Triglycerides.

7. **Which additional lab(s) is/are concerning and should be reported to the surgeon prior to surgery?**

1. Red blood cells.
2. Platelet count.
3. Creatinine level.
4. Liver enzymes.

After alerting the surgeon of the lab reports the surgery is postponed. Intravenous antibiotics are started, potassium is replaced, and the client receives 1 unit of packed red blood cells. Because of poor venous access, a peripherally inserted central catheter (PICC) is placed in the left basilic vein. Additionally, Ms. Martinez is started on short-acting insulin to control the blood glucose levels.

The next day, on April 7, she shows improvement and is taken to surgery for an Open Reduction, Internal Fixation of the Left Hip. Ms. Martinez is now 24 hours postoperative. The nurse reviews her electronic vital sign record.

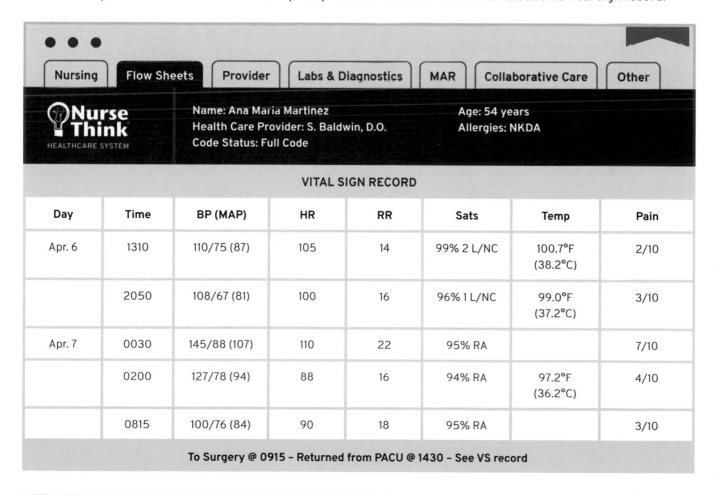

| Nursing | Flow Sheets | Provider | Labs & Diagnostics | MAR | Collaborative Care | Other |

Nurse Think — HEALTHCARE SYSTEM

Name: Ana Maria Martinez
Health Care Provider: S. Baldwin, D.O.
Code Status: Full Code

Age: 54 years
Allergies: NKDA

VITAL SIGN RECORD

Day	Time	BP (MAP)	HR	RR	Sats	Temp	Pain
Apr. 6	1310	110/75 (87)	105	14	99% 2 L/NC	100.7°F (38.2°C)	2/10
	2050	108/67 (81)	100	16	96% 1 L/NC	99.0°F (37.2°C)	3/10
Apr. 7	0030	145/88 (107)	110	22	95% RA		7/10
	0200	127/78 (94)	88	16	94% RA	97.2°F (36.2°C)	4/10
	0815	100/76 (84)	90	18	95% RA		3/10

To Surgery @ 0915 – Returned from PACU @ 1430 – See VS record

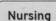

| Nursing | Flow Sheets | Provider | Labs & Diagnostics | MAR | Collaborative Care | Other |

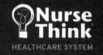

Name: Ana Maria Martinez
Health Care Provider: S. Baldwin, D.O.
Code Status: Full Code

Age: 54 years
Allergies: NKDA

VITAL SIGN RECORD (CONTINUED)

Day	Time	BP (MAP)	HR	RR	Sats	Temp	Pain
Apr. 7	1635	110/72 (85)	92	22	94% RA	98.0°F (36.6°C)	8/10
	1905	115/70 (85)	88	20	94% RA	100.0°F (37.7°C)	5/10
	2200	110/75 (87)	86	18	94% RA	97.0°F (36.2°C)	2/10
Apr. 8	0800	118/75 (89)	98	20	95% RA	98.0°F (36.6°C)	98.0°F (36.6°C)
	1620	98/56 (70)	110	22	92% RA	100.5°F (38.0°C)	6/10
	2110	89/50 (63	114	24	95% 1 L/NC	101.2°F (38.4°C)	5/10

8. **After analyzing the vital sign trends, what information is most concerning to the nurse?**
   1. Respiratory rate of 14 on April 6.
   2. Blood pressure of 145/88 (107) at 0030 on April 7.
   3. Blood pressure of 89/50 (63) at 2110 on April 8.
   4. Temperature of 101.2°F (38.4°C) at 2110 on April 8.

9. **Based on this information, what should be the nurse's priority action?**
   1. Increase oxygen for low respiratory rate at 1310 on April 6.
   2. Deliver pain meds for high blood pressure at 0300 on April 7.
   3. Increase IV fluids for low blood pressure at 2110 on April 8.
   4. Deliver acetaminophen for fever at 2110 on April 8.

10. **At 1620 on April 8, there is a change in the client's condition. What action(s) should the nurse take? Select all that apply.**

    1. Deliver pain medication with close monitoring.
    2. Stop IV fluids.
    3. Apply oxygen.
    4. Place a cool cloth on the client's forehead.
    5. Encourage coughing and deep breathing.
    6. Have the client walk in the hall.

11. **At 2110 on April 8, the nurse decides to contact the provider for additional orders. What additional assessment information should the nurse collect in preparation for the SBAR communication.**

    _____

    _____

12. **The nurse notes that there are two providers following Ms. Martinez. Which provider should the nurse contact first?**

    1. Dr. Baldwin.
    2. Dr. Schoenberg.

The nurse communicates with the provider.

S – Hi Dr. Baldwin, this is the nurse caring for Ms. Martinez at NurseThink®Healthcare System. I'm calling because her blood pressure is low at 89/50 mmHg and temperature is up to 101.2°F (38.4°C).

B– She came in on April 5th after falling and fracturing her hip. She returned from surgery 24 hours ago. She has a history of rheumatoid arthritis and takes prednisone daily. She also had an elevated WBC count prior to surgery and has been receiving cefazolin IV.

A – Her wound site is slightly reddened with clear, serous drainage, the staples are intact. Her lungs are diminished in the bases, and she has been placed on 1 L/NC to maintain her saturations at 95%. WBCs are at 13,000 without a left shift. The indwelling catheter is draining concentrated, cloudy urine. Her PICC catheter dressing is intact with an antimicrobial patch covering the insertion site.

13. **Based on the SBA(R) communication, what assessment findings indicate the most likely site(s) of infection? Select all that apply.**

    1. Wound.
    2. Lungs.
    3. Blood.
    4. Urine.
    5. PICC catheter.

14. **As the nurse, complete the "R" (Recommendation) of the SBAR report.**

    _____

    _____

The nurse receives these orders from the provider.

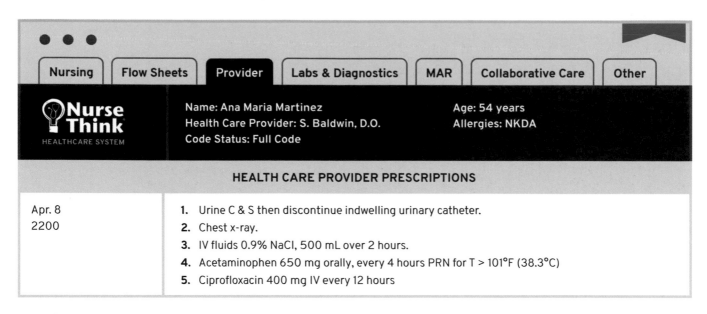

	HEALTH CARE PROVIDER PRESCRIPTIONS
Apr. 8 2200	**1.** Urine C & S then discontinue indwelling urinary catheter. **2.** Chest x-ray. **3.** IV fluids 0.9% NaCl, 500 mL over 2 hours. **4.** Acetaminophen 650 mg orally, every 4 hours PRN for T > 101°F (38.3°C) **5.** Ciprofloxacin 400 mg IV every 12 hours

Nursing | **Flow Sheets** | **Provider** | **Labs & Diagnostics** | **MAR** | **Collaborative Care** | **Other**

Name: Ana Maria Martinez
Health Care Provider: S. Baldwin, D.O.
Code Status: Full Code

Age: 54 years
Allergies: NKDA

NurseThink HEALTHCARE SYSTEM

15. **Which of these prescriptions should the nurse implement first?**

   1. Urine C&S then discontinue indwelling urinary catheter.
   2. Chest x-ray.
   3. IV fluids 0.9% NaCl, 500 mL over 2 hours.
   4. Acetaminophen 650 mg orally, every 4 hours PRN for T > 101°F (38.3°C).
   5. Ciprofloxacin 400 mg IV every 12 hours.

Next Gen Clinical Judgment:
New health care prescriptions should be prioritized and not completed sequentially. Determine the highest risk to safety, coupled with what can be completed quickly when prioritizing a long list of prescriptions.

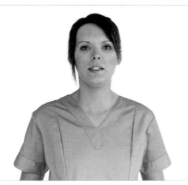

16. **THIN Thinking Time!**
   Reflect on the events that have occurred since Ana Maria Martinez came to the emergency department and apply **THIN Thinking** to what events could have prevented the current situation.

   T – _____

   H – _____

   I – _____

   N – _____

T - Top 3
H - Help Quick
I - Identify Risk to Safety
N - Nursing Process

Scan to access the 10-Minute-Mentor on THIN Thinking.

NurseThink.com/THINThinking

The diagnostic and culture reports return for Ms. Martinez. Her chest x-ray shows bilateral atelectasis and the urinalysis is positive for leukocytes, nitrite, bacteria, blood, and protein, indicating she has a bladder and kidney infection.

17. **Given this information, what priority action should the nurse take?**
    1. Implement coughing and deep breathing hourly.
    2. Ambulate in the hallway hourly.
    3. Place an indwelling catheter for accurate output measurements.
    4. Limit oral fluids.

The hospital's quality management and infection control departments notice an increase of catheter-acquired urinary tract infections (CAUTI) on the nursing unit where Ms. Martinez is a client. A chart review is conducted which leads to a mandatory training session for the nurses and other appropriate health care team members.

18. **What information should be included in the educational session about the prevention of CAUTIs? Select all that apply.**
    1. A review of the Center for Disease Control's (CDC) criteria for catheter insertion.
    2. Daily review of need for indwelling catheter.
    3. Early recognition of CAUTI symptoms.
    4. Use of aseptic technique with catheter care.
    5. Importance of securing the device and keeping bag below the level of the bladder.
    6. Frequency of indwelling catheter care.

19. **During the training session, the nurse reviews the *CDC (2009) Criteria for Indwelling Urinary Catheter (IUC) Insertion.* Using these guidelines, did Ms. Martinez meet the criteria for an indwelling catheter?**
    1. Yes.
    2. No.

CDC (2009) Criteria for Indwelling Urinary Catheter (IUC) Insertion:

> Acute urinary retention (sudden and painful inability to urinate (SUNA, 2008) or bladder outlet obstruction
> To improve comfort for end-of-life care if needed
> Critically ill and need for accurate measurements of I&O (e.g., hourly monitoring)
> Selected surgical procedures (GU surgery/colorectal surgery)
> To assist in healing open sacral or perineal wound in the incontinent patient
> Need for intraoperative monitoring of urinary output during surgery or large volumes of fluid or diuretics anticipated
> Prolonged immobilization (potentially unstable thoracic or lumbar spine, multiple traumatic injuries such as pelvic fractures)

Gould, C., Umscheid, C., et al. (2017). Guideline for prevention of catheter-associated urinary tract infections 2009. Healthcare Infection Control Practices Advisory Committee. Retrieved from https://www.cdc.gov/infectioncontrol/guidelines/cauti/index.html with permission.

20. **After the training how will the quality improvement and infection control departments identify that their training is effective?**
    1. Nurses will place fewer indwelling catheters.
    2. UAPs will follow aseptic technique when caring for catheters.
    3. The occurrence rate of CAUTIs will decrease on the nurse unit.
    4. The team will state having a deeper understanding of the process.

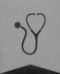
Case 2: Hypersensitivity Reaction and Abdominal Pain

Related Concepts: Cognition, Infection, Inflammation
Threaded Topic: Growth and Development

Ryan Herrill is a 6-year-old child being seen for a routine well-visit as a new patient whose family recently moved to the rural desert southwest from the eastern United States. As the nurse obtains the health history from Ryan's parents, it is apparent that Ryan's childhood has not been a healthy one.

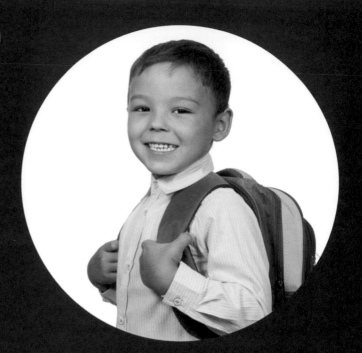

Nursing	Flow Sheets	Provider	Labs & Diagnostics	MAR	Collaborative Care	Other

Name: Ryan Herrill
Health Care Provider: J. Knight M.D.
Code Status: Full

Age: 6 years
Allergies: PCN, sulfa, latex, dairy, gluten, eggs, pet dander, nuts

HEALTH HISTORY

Medical History

> Multiple allergies

- Intolerance noted to gluten, dairy, and eggs - since age 9 months - cause severe diarrhea, nausea, and vomiting.
- Nut allergy – since age 2 years – cause difficulty breathing. Also reactive to nut "dust."
- Penicillin (PCN) and sulfa – causes severe rash.
- Latex allergy – "mild" anaphylactic reaction at age 3 years.
- Seasonal allergies to certain tree blossoms and pet dander – itching eyes, running nose, coughing.

> Asthma – since age 1.

> Reoccurring strep throat since age 2 – typically once each winter.

> Fracture of right arm and clavicle from a bicycle accident at age 5.

Surgical History

> Surgical repair of right arm fracture age 5 (outpatient).

Mental Health History

> Treated for attention-deficit/hyperactive disorder (ADHD) since age 3 – treated with cognitive-behavioral therapy and methylphenidate orally since starting school.

Hospitalizations

> Ages 9 months, 3-years, and 5-years for severe diarrhea and weight loss.

> Ages 2 and 4 for asthma.

Developmental Level

> Meets physical developmental milestones. Height 40 inches (101.6 cm) and Weighs 36 pounds (13.6 kg).

> "Slow" in school and parents are considering "special classes" or homeschooling with tutoring.

Immunization History

> Received routine immunizations at 12 months. Parents have refused all immunizations since due to severe allergy history. "We are afraid of what could happen and wonder if the immunizations could have caused all of this."

1. **Determine Ryan's percentile for height and weight.**

_____ *Height.* _____ *Weight.*

Next Gen Clinical Judgment: Go to the CDC website and compare the wide variety of Growth Charts.

Scan to link to the CDC website.
www.cdc.gov/growthcharts/cdc_charts.htm

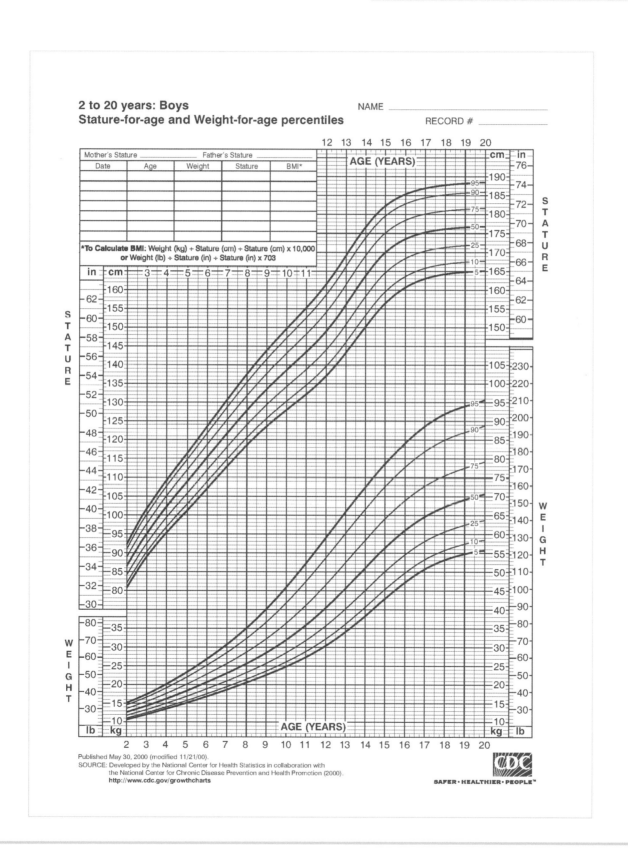

2. As the nurse reviews the health record, what condition is the priority concern?
   1. ADHD.
   2. Allergies.
   3. Asthma.
   4. Lack of immunizations.

3. The nurse reviews Ryan's list of allergies, finding many concerns. Place each allergy in order of concern from highest to lowest. ____, ____, ____, ____, ____.
   1. Gluten and dairy.
   2. Nuts.
   3. PCN and sulfa.
   4. Latex.
   5. Seasonal.

4. What is the nurse's priority teaching topic for Ryan's parents?

   _____

5. The clinic is not a latex-free zone. As the nurse prepares for Ryan's physical assessment, which item(s) require special attention? Select all that apply.
   1. Gloves.
   2. Blood pressure cuff.
   3. Oxygen saturation.
   4. Adhesive tape.
   5. Inhaler spacer.

6. As the nurse is speaking with Ryan's parents and examining him, he becomes very fidgety and won't stay on the examination table. What action should the nurse take?
   1. Tell him to sit still and he can have candy after the visit.
   2. Ask the parents to address the situation.
   3. Give Ryan a small age-appropriate toy.
   4. Ignore the behavior.

7. The nurse is concerned about Ryan's lack of immunizations. Although she wants to be respectful of the parent's personal decision, she feels it is in Ryan's best interest to pursue the topic. Relying on the recommendations of the American Academy of Pediatrics (AAP), how should the nurse begin the conversation with the parents?
   1. "Do you know that the American Academy of Pediatrics fully supports the delivery of routine immunizations for children?"
   2. "Can you tell me more about your concerns about Ryan receiving immunizations?"
   3. "Are you afraid that Ryan will get sick from the other kids at school since he's not immunized?"
   4. "It seems that you are placing Ryan in danger by not getting him immunized."

After a conversation with the nurse and health care provider, Ryan's parents provide consent for immunizations if an antihistamine is given beforehand. The nurse delivers the antihistamine, then gathers latex-free equipment for the injections and two automatic epinephrine injectors, to be safe. She then reviews the Center for Disease Control (CDC) immunization record, knowing that Ryan had all of his immunizations at 12 months.

Next Gen Clinical Judgment: Obtain the correct immunization record and determine the appropriate immunizations for Ryan.

Scan to link to the CDC website.
www.cdc.gov/vaccines/schedules/index.html

8. **Which immunization(s) should Ryan receive? Select all that apply.**

    1. Hepatitis B.
    2. DTaP.
    3. PCV13.
    4. IPV.
    5. MMR.
    6. Tdap.

Clinical Hint: There are several charts for immunizations based on age. Always be certain that you are looking at the correct one for your client.

9. **After the immunizations, the clinic continues to monitor Ryan for 1 hour for signs of an immediate hypersensitivity reaction. Which symptoms should the nurse anticipate should this occur? Select all that apply.**

    1. Rash.
    2. Difficulty breathing.
    3. Sleepiness.
    4. Runny nose.
    5. Eye swelling.

10. **NurseThink® Prioritization Power!**
    As the nurse prepares to discharge Ryan from the clinic, what are the **Top 3 Priority** discharge instructions for his parents?

    1. _____

    2. _____

    3. _____

Two weeks after the immunizations, Ryan gets home from school, telling his mother that he feels "yucky. He has a low-grade fever and says his tummy hurts. His mom feeds him a snack, thinking he may be hungry and gives him some ibuprofen for the fever. She lays him down for a nap while watching cartoons.

Ryan wakes up crying with pain. He says "my tummy hurts, my tummy hurts" but cannot identify where the pain is. His mother takes him to urgent care. They complete an assessment and find his pain is worse in the right lower quadrant. They decide to send Ryan to the emergency room for diagnostic tests.

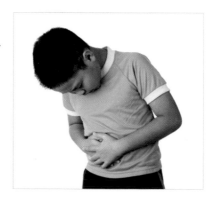

Review the emergency room record.

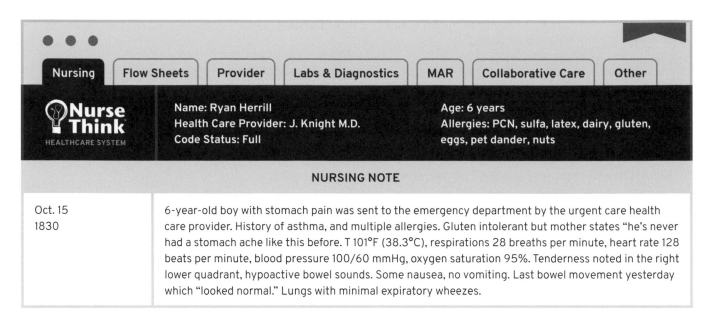

| Nursing | Flow Sheets | Provider | Labs & Diagnostics | MAR | Collaborative Care | Other |

NurseThink HEALTHCARE SYSTEM

Name: Ryan Herrill
Health Care Provider: J. Knight M.D.
Code Status: Full

Age: 6 years
Allergies: PCN, sulfa, latex, dairy, gluten, eggs, pet dander, nuts

NURSING NOTE

| Oct. 15 1830 | 6-year-old boy with stomach pain was sent to the emergency department by the urgent care health care provider. History of asthma, and multiple allergies. Gluten intolerant but mother states "he's never had a stomach ache like this before. T 101°F (38.3°C), respirations 28 breaths per minute, heart rate 128 beats per minute, blood pressure 100/60 mmHg, oxygen saturation 95%. Tenderness noted in the right lower quadrant, hypoactive bowel sounds. Some nausea, no vomiting. Last bowel movement yesterday which "looked normal." Lungs with minimal expiratory wheezes. |

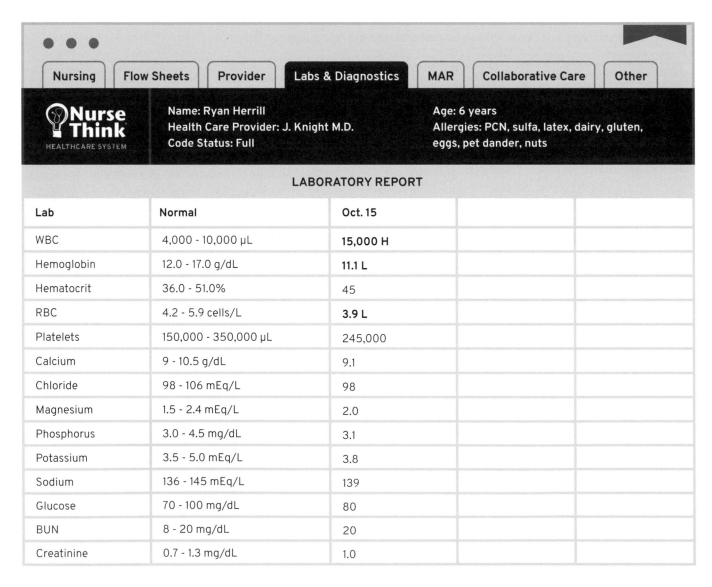

| Nursing | Flow Sheets | Provider | Labs & Diagnostics | MAR | Collaborative Care | Other |

NurseThink HEALTHCARE SYSTEM

Name: Ryan Herrill
Health Care Provider: J. Knight M.D.
Code Status: Full

Age: 6 years
Allergies: PCN, sulfa, latex, dairy, gluten, eggs, pet dander, nuts

LABORATORY REPORT

Lab	Normal	Oct. 15		
WBC	4,000 - 10,000 µL	**15,000 H**		
Hemoglobin	12.0 - 17.0 g/dL	**11.1 L**		
Hematocrit	36.0 - 51.0%	45		
RBC	4.2 - 5.9 cells/L	**3.9 L**		
Platelets	150,000 - 350,000 µL	245,000		
Calcium	9 - 10.5 g/dL	9.1		
Chloride	98 - 106 mEq/L	98		
Magnesium	1.5 - 2.4 mEq/L	2.0		
Phosphorus	3.0 - 4.5 mg/dL	3.1		
Potassium	3.5 - 5.0 mEq/L	3.8		
Sodium	136 - 145 mEq/L	139		
Glucose	70 - 100 mg/dL	80		
BUN	8 - 20 mg/dL	20		
Creatinine	0.7 - 1.3 mg/dL	1.0		

11. **What hypothesis can the nurse make, given this information?**
    1. Ryan has a delayed reaction to his immunizations.
    2. Ryan ate a food to which he is allergic.
    3. He is having a difficult time at school and wants to stay home.
    4. It is possible that Ryan has developed appendicitis.

12. **The nurse enters Ryan's room. What observation is most concerning?**

    _____

    _____

    _____

    _____

    _____

    _____

13. **Ryan has a ruptured appendix and surgery is scheduled within the hour. Complete the chart below pertaining to the preoperative care.**

	Indicated	Non-essential	Contraindicated
Delivery of IV antibiotic.			
Preoperative teaching with family.			
Parenteral signature on consent.			
Confirmation of correct ID band.			
Verbal hand-off to operating room nurses and anesthesiologist about allergies.			
Confirmation that IV is patent			
Instruction of postoperative pain management options.			
Oral medication for prevention of allergic reaction.			
Prophylactic placement of an indwelling catheter.			

14. **After surgery, the post-anesthesia care unit calls the nurse to give report. Ryan's surgery went well and he is stable. They'd like to know which room he will be going to after surgery. The charge nurse evaluates the room choices on the unit. Which is the best bed placement for Ryan? Check the best option.**

Room 245 ☐	Room 246 ☐	Room 247 ☐
Bed 1: Open **Bed 2:** 15-month-old girl with asthma	**Bed 1:** 14-year-old boy with a fracture, in traction. **Bed 2:** 16-year-old boy with a football head injury.	**Bed 1:** 7-year-old boy on neutropenic precautions. **Bed 2:** Open
Room 248 ☐	Room 249 ☐	**Room 250 – 4 Bed Ward** ☐
Bed 1: 3-year-old girl with pneumonia – lots of visitors **Bed 2:** Open	**Bed 1:** 6-year-old girl post-appendectomy. **Bed 2:** Open	**Bed 1:** 9-year-old boy with newly diagnosed diabetes. **Bed 2:** 8-year-old boy to be discharged this afternoon. **Bed 3:** Open **Bed 4:** 10-year-old boy with a MRSA infection.
Room 251 ☐	Room 252 ☐	
Bed 1: Open **Bed 2:** Open	**Bed 1:** Open **Bed 2:** 7-year-old boy newly diagnosed with Crohn's disease.	

15. **The nurse reflects on the assessment over the last 6 hours since surgery. What information requires additional action?**

    1. Bowel sounds are absent.
    2. Pain was worse before surgery.
    3. Lung sounds with wheezes throughout.
    4. Abdominal incision with a dime-sized drop of dried blood.

16. **NurseThink®Prioritization Power!**

    Evaluate the assessment change above and pick the **Top 3 Priority** assessments required at this time.

    1. _____

    2. _____

    3. _____

With further assessment, the nurse discovers that Ryan's oxygen saturation is 92%, his breathing is mildly labored, and his eyes are "puffy." The nurse places Ryan on 2 L of oxygen per nasal cannula and decides to contact the health care provider.

17. The nurse gathers a full set of vital signs and begins to prepare SBAR for the health care provider. Complete each section of the communication form.

S – _____

B – _____

A – _____

R – _____

> **Clinical Hint:**
> **S** - Situation
> **B** - Background
> **A** - Assessment
> **R** - Recommendation

18. The nurse receives an order for epinephrine 0.01 mg/kg (1:1,000 solution) subcutaneous x 1 dose. Available in 1 mg/mL (1:1,000 solution). What sized syringe will the nurse use to pull up the medication?

_____ mL   _____ sized syringe

Ryan's condition improves after the dose of epinephrine. Once he is stabilized, the nurse reviews the medication administration record to determine what may have caused the allergic reaction.

Next Gen Clinical Judgment:
> How does the nurse know that the epinephrine is effective?
> What action would the nurse take, should the initial dose of epinephrine not be effective?
> What is the worst-case scenario should the epinephrine not work?

Nursing	Flow Sheets	Provider	Labs & Diagnostics	MAR	Collaborative Care	Other

Nurse Think HEALTHCARE SYSTEM

Name: Ryan Herrill
Health Care Provider: J. Knight M.D.
Code Status: Full

Age: 6 years
Allergies: PCN, sulfa, latex, dairy, gluten, eggs, pet dander, nuts

MEDICATION ADMINISTRATION RECORD

Oct. 16 0400	1. Piperacillin 100 mg/tazobactam 12.5 mg per kg IV every 8 hours. 2. Vancomycin 10 mg/kg IV every 6 hours. 3. Morphine sulfate 0.15–0.3 mg/kg IV every 4 hours PRN for severe pain. 4. Acetaminophen 15 mg/kg/dose IV every 6 hours PRN for mild pain or temperature > 100.5°F (38°C).

19. Which medication from the MAR is most concerning?
   1. Piperacillin/tazobactam.
   2. Vancomycin.
   3. Morphine sulfate.
   4. Acetaminophen.

20. As Ryan is discharged, his mother says "None of this would have happened if Ryan wouldn't have had those immunizations." How should the nurse respond?

_____

_____

Conceptual Debriefing & Case Reflection

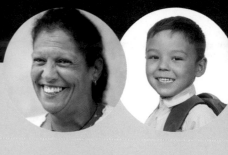

1. Compare the impaired protection that Ana Maria Martinez experienced with the impaired protection of Ryan Herrill. How are they the same and how are they different?

   _____

   _____

2. What was your single greatest learning moment while completing the case of Ana Maria Martinez? What about Ryan Herrill?

   _____

   _____

3. How did the nursing care provided to Ana Maria Martinez and Ryan Herrill change the outcome for each of them?

   _____

   _____

4. Identify safety concerns for both Ana Maria Martinez and Ryan Herrill for each case.

   _____

   _____

5. In what areas of each case study was basic care and comfort utilized?

   _____

   _____

6. What steps in each case did the nurse take that prevented hospital-acquired injury?

   _____

   _____

7. How did the nurse provide culturally sensitive/competent care?

   _____

   _____

8. How will learning about the case of Ana Maria Martinez and Ryan Herrill impact the care you provide for future clients?

   _____

   _____

Fundamental Quiz

1. **A postoperative client's temperature is 95.9°F (35.5°C). What additional assessment findings should the nurse anticipate? Select all that apply.**
   1. Cool fingers and toes.
   2. Capillary refill < 3 seconds.
   3. Diaphoresis.
   4. Perioral cyanosis.
   5. Goosebumps.

2. **A client is receiving the first dose of chemotherapy. What priority teaching point should the nurse include before discharge?**
   1. "You will be more tired than usual and need to rest frequently."
   2. "You may have some vomiting from the medication and should maintain hydration."
   3. "You are at a higher risk for infection and should not be around anyone that is ill."
   4. "You'll want to eat small frequent meals to maintain your nutrition."

3. **A client experiencing chronic inflammation of the joints is asking about some natural home remedies. What could the nurse suggest? Select all that apply.**
   1. Increased intake of Omega-3 fatty acids.
   2. Cardiovascular exercise like running or distance bike riding.
   3. Mind-body activities like yoga and tai-chi.
   4. Reduce exposure to toxins within the environment.
   5. Get at least 7 hours of sleep each night.

4. **A nurse is teaching about the use and over-use of antibiotics. Which statement is correct?**
   1. Antibiotic use is contraindicated in bacterial infections.
   2. Overuse of antibiotics can lead to antibiotic resistance.
   3. Antibiotics should be taken until symptoms subside.
   4. Antibiotics have a low incidence of allergic reactions.

5. **The nurse is determining immunizations for a 5-year-old preparing for school. Use the immunization record on the CDC website to determine which immunization the child requires. Select all that apply.**
   1. DTap.
   2. IPV.
   3. MMR.
   4. VAR.
   5. Hep A.
   6. IIV.

Advanced Quiz

6. **The nurse is caring for a client who "doesn't feel very well." Assessment includes temperature 100.9°F (38.3°C); heart rate 110; respirations 24 breaths per minute. The nurse reviews the labs below. What actions should the nurse take next?**

Lab	Normal	August 5	August 6
WBC	4,000-10,000 cells/mL	9,000	15,100 H
Hemoglobin	12-17 g/dL	11.0 L	10.9 L
Hematocrit	36-51%	38 L	34 L
RBC	4.2-5.9 cells/L	3.80 L	3.6 L

   1. Evaluate which antibiotics the client is receiving.
   2. Assess the blood pressure.
   3. Request a serum lactate level.
   4. Ask the client to describe 'not feeling well.'

7. **A client with a pale-yellow productive cough tells the nurse that the sputum is becoming thicker and a darker yellow. The client does not have a fever or elevations of the white blood cells. The lung sounds are course crackles that clear with coughing. What actions should the nurse take next?**
   1. Collect a sputum specimen and obtain an order for a culture and sensitivity.
   2. Obtain suction for the bedside.
   3. Obtain an order for an incentive spirometer.
   4. Encourage the client to drink more water.

8. **The nurse is evaluating the head and neck of a client and discovers a grape-sized lump where the lymph nodes are located. What question(s) should the nurse ask next? Select all that apply.**
   1. "Do you have a family history of cancer?"
   2. "Have you had a recent infection?"
   3. "Is this painful?"
   4. "Have you noticed this lump before?"
   5. "Do you have other lumps like this?"

9. **The nurse is taking care of a critical client whose body temperature is 103.9°F (39.9°C). Which interventions should the nurse consider? Select all that apply.**
   1. Remove covers.
   2. Place on cooling blanket or place ice packs in the armpits and groin.
   3. Deliver acetaminophen 1,000 mg IV.
   4. Cool the room.
   5. Place a fan on the client.

10. **An immune-compromised client is being treated for a leg wound infection which has minimal redness and is unchanged since admission. The client's temperature has increased to 99.9°F (37.7°C). What should be the nurse's next action?**
    1. Document the findings.
    2. Assess the white blood cell count.
    3. Deliver acetaminophen 650 mg orally.
    4. Elevate the leg on 2 pillows.

CHAPTER

8

Homeostasis

Fluid and Electrolyte Balance / Acid-Base Balance

Think of homeostasis as a process of balance. For proper function, the cells, tissues, and organs in the body are maintained and regulated to a point of stability. Homeostasis is a normal state of functioning and is supported by the constant fluctuations of biochemical and physiological processes. Five body functions work to maintain homeostasis: temperature, glucose, blood pressure, toxins, and pH. In this chapter's case studies, the focus is on fluid and electrolyte balance and acid-base balance.

Next Gen Clinical Judgment:

Answer these questions:

> What assessment changes are found in fluid volume excess? What about fluid volume deficit?

> Consider each system of the body, one-by-one and how it is impacted by fluid volume excess or deficit.

> Which electrolytes are most affected by fluid volume excess or deficit?

> What assessment changes will be seen with each of the 4 acid-base abnormalities?

> List 3 nursing interventions for each of the following:
  - fluid volume excess
  - fluid volume deficit
  - electrolytes imbalance
  - respiratory acidosis
  - respiratory alkalosis
  - metabolic acidosis
  - metabolic alkalosis

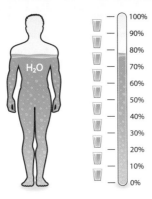

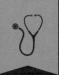

Go To Clinical Case

While caring for this client, be sure to review the concept maps in chapters 3 and 4.

Case 1: Acid-Base Imbalance from Aspirin Overdose

Related Concepts: Circulation; Respiration, Comfort, Cognition
Threaded Topics: Older Adult, Risk for Injury, Environmental Assessment, Communication, Sensory Perception

Millie Marten is an 83-year-old female that lives with her cat, Sam, in a senior apartment. She suffers from rheumatoid and osteoarthritis, cataracts, and adrenal insufficiency (Addison's disease). She no longer drives but takes the bus to the market three times a week for groceries. Her church is at the end of the block, and she never misses a Sunday service. The home care nurse comes to see Millie once a week since she came home from the skilled care rehabilitation facility three weeks ago after fracturing her hip. Her physical therapist also comes to her home twice a week. Her rehabilitation is going well, and she's independent with the use of a walker when she is outside of the house. Millie's daughter and son live out of the state but stayed with her the first week after she returned home.

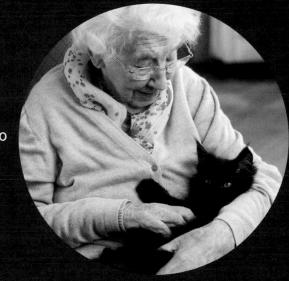

During the visit, the nurse reviews Millie's medication bottles.

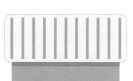

Rx
Prednisone
5 mg tablets

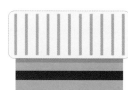

Rx
Furosemide
20 mg tablets

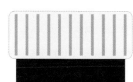

Rx
ASA/Oxycodone
Hydrochloride tabs

Rx
Aspirin
Extra Strength

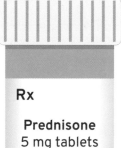

1. Determine the specifics of each of Millie's medications. For each shaded box in the table select the correct answer.

Medication	Dose, Route, Frequency	Drug Class	Patient Teaching
Prednisone	5 mg p.o. daily	1. Mineralocorticoid 2. Glucocorticoid 3. Loop diuretic 4. Osmotic diuretic	Increase dose during times of stress
Furosemide	20 mg p.o. daily	Diuretic	**Select all that apply** 1. Report signs of infection. 2. Monitor potassium levels. 3. Weigh self, daily. 4. Increase oral fluid intake.
ASA and oxycodone hydrochloride	1 to 2 tablets every 4-6 hours for pain as needed	**Select all that apply** 1. Nonsteroidal anti-inflammatory 2. Narcotic 3. Analgesic 4. Antiplatelet	Surgical site pain
Aspirin Extra-Strength	1. 325 mg p.o. 2 tabs every 4 hours PRN 2. 500 mg p.o. 2 tabs every 6 hours PRN 3. 650 mg p.o. 2 tabs every 4 hours PRN 4. 1000 mg 2 tabs every 6 hours PRN	Analgesic, antipyretic, antiinflammatory, and platelet aggregation inhibitors	Arthritis pain

2. As the nurse reviews the medications, what is concerning?

_____

_____

_____

3. THIN Thinking Time!
   Reflect on the information the nurse has collected and apply **THIN Thinking**.

   T – _____

   H – _____

   I – _____

   N – _____

T - Top 3
H - Help Quick
I - Identify Risk to Safety
N - Nursing Process

Scan to access the 10-Minute-Mentor on THIN Thinking.

NurseThink.com/THINThinking

4. **As the nurse evaluates Millie's home environment for safety, what should the nurse include?**
    1. Frequency in which her children visit.
    2. Types of foods she eats.
    3. Presence of stairs.
    4. Sleeping quality.

The nurse asks about Millie's pain since surgery. She says the pain is worse in the mornings and at bedtime, so she's been taking extra pain medication. The nurse completes a physical examination and finds that Millie is not aware of the day or time, but can identify self and the president. She says she's been sick to her stomach lately. Millie's skin is bronze in appearance from adrenal insufficiency. Her temperature is 99.4°F (37.4°C), heart rate 98, respirations 26, blood pressure 99/47 (64) lying and 78/40 (53) standing with reported dizziness. Millie tells the nurse she has this strange ringing in her ears. The incision on her hip is almost healed.

---

5. **NurseThink® Prioritization Power!**
    Evaluate the information within the nurse's assessment and pick the **Top 3 Priority** assessment findings.

    1. _____

    2. _____

    3. _____

---

6. **What would the nurse determine is/are the reason(s) for Millie's orthostatic hypotension? Select all that apply.**
    1. Furosemide.
    2. Prednisone.
    3. ASA and oxycodone hydrochloride.
    4. Adrenal insufficiency.
    5. Osteoarthritis.
    6. Older adult age.

    Clinical Hint: Orthostatic hypotension is a drop in blood pressure of at least 20 mmHg systolic or 10 mmHg diastolic when someone stands from a lying position. Common causes include dehydration and autonomic dysfunction.

7. **The nurse is concerned about Millie's confusion, hyperventilation, vomiting, and tinnitus. What could cause these findings?**
    1. Reaction to the pain medication.
    2. Dehydration.
    3. Acetylsalicylic acid overdose.
    4. Poor dietary intake.

8. **The nurse hypothesizes that Millie's hyperventilation is a result of metabolic acidosis from the acetylsalicylic acid ingestion. What action would be appropriate?**
    1. Encourage her to take slow, deep breaths.
    2. Have her breathe into a paper bag.
    3. Moisten her lips and continue to allow the hyperventilation.
    4. Offer her some pain medication.

9. The home care nurse gathers information and begins to prepare an SBAR telephone conversation for the HCP. Complete each section of the SBAR communication.

S - _____

B - _____

A - _____

R - _____

Clinical Hint:
S - Situation
B - Background
A - Assessment
R - Recommendation

10. The nurse arranges for Millie to be transported to the emergency department. She's very concerned about Sam, her cat and does not want to leave him. What should the nurse do?

1. Find a neighbor to feed the cat.
2. Take the cat home.
3. Leave the cat.
4. Send the cat with Millie.

Upon arrival to the emergency department, the health care provider writes these prescriptions.

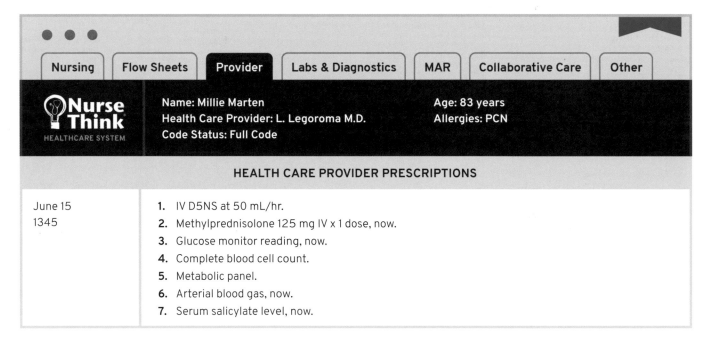

| Nursing | Flow Sheets | Provider | Labs & Diagnostics | MAR | Collaborative Care | Other |

NurseThink HEALTHCARE SYSTEM

Name: Millie Marten
Health Care Provider: L. Legoroma M.D.
Code Status: Full Code

Age: 83 years
Allergies: PCN

HEALTH CARE PROVIDER PRESCRIPTIONS

June 15
1345

1. IV D5NS at 50 mL/hr.
2. Methylprednisolone 125 mg IV x 1 dose, now.
3. Glucose monitor reading, now.
4. Complete blood cell count.
5. Metabolic panel.
6. Arterial blood gas, now.
7. Serum salicylate level, now.

11. Explain each of the prescriptions and its purpose, specific to Millie's care. In other words, why is it being ordered?

1. IV D5NS at 50 mL/hr. _____

2. Methylprednisolone 125 mg IV x 1 dose, now. _____

3. Glucose monitor reading, now. _____

4. Complete blood cell count. _____

5. Metabolic panel. _____

6. Arterial blood gas, now. _____

7. Serum salicylate level, now. _____

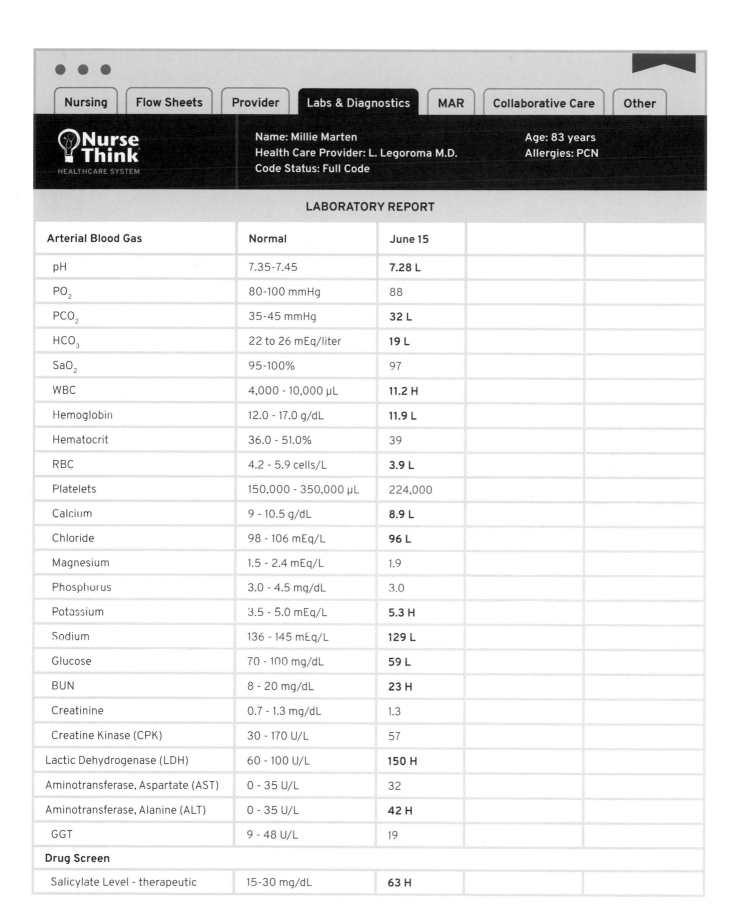

LABORATORY REPORT

Name: Millie Marten
Health Care Provider: L. Legoroma M.D.
Code Status: Full Code
Age: 83 years
Allergies: PCN

Arterial Blood Gas	Normal	June 15		
pH	7.35-7.45	**7.28 L**		
PO$_2$	80-100 mmHg	88		
PCO$_2$	35-45 mmHg	**32 L**		
HCO$_3$	22 to 26 mEq/liter	**19 L**		
SaO$_2$	95-100%	97		
WBC	4,000 - 10,000 µL	**11.2 H**		
Hemoglobin	12.0 - 17.0 g/dL	**11.9 L**		
Hematocrit	36.0 - 51.0%	39		
RBC	4.2 - 5.9 cells/L	**3.9 L**		
Platelets	150,000 - 350,000 µL	224,000		
Calcium	9 - 10.5 g/dL	**8.9 L**		
Chloride	98 - 106 mEq/L	**96 L**		
Magnesium	1.5 - 2.4 mEq/L	1.9		
Phosphorus	3.0 - 4.5 mg/dL	3.0		
Potassium	3.5 - 5.0 mEq/L	**5.3 H**		
Sodium	136 - 145 mEq/L	**129 L**		
Glucose	70 - 100 mg/dL	**59 L**		
BUN	8 - 20 mg/dL	**23 H**		
Creatinine	0.7 - 1.3 mg/dL	1.3		
Creatine Kinase (CPK)	30 - 170 U/L	57		
Lactic Dehydrogenase (LDH)	60 - 100 U/L	**150 H**		
Aminotransferase, Aspartate (AST)	0 - 35 U/L	32		
Aminotransferase, Alanine (ALT)	0 - 35 U/L	**42 H**		
GGT	9 - 48 U/L	19		
Drug Screen				
Salicylate Level - therapeutic	15-30 mg/dL	**63 H**		

Clinical Hint: When caring for a client with an Acid-Base concern, remember ROME. Respiratory Opposite - Metabolic Equal. Find an online video that explains ROME.

From the lab report, Millie has salicylate toxicity. The health care provider orders activated charcoal orally, every 4 hours until the charcoal is eliminated through the stool. Although the HCP considers alkaline diuresis, it is held because of the hypotension.

12. **Which laboratory finding(s) is/are consistent with salicylate toxicity? Select all that apply.**

   1. Hyperkalemia.
   2. Metabolic acidosis.
   3. Leukocytosis.
   4. Hypoglycemia.
   5. Salicylate level.

Refresh your ABG Interpretation skills.
www.rnceus.com/abgs/abgmethod.html →

13. **What is the purpose of the activated charcoal and how does it work?**

   _____

   _____

   _____

14. **Arterial Blood Gas Review. Match the ABG on the left to its name on the right. May use the names more than once; not all names are used.**

ABG	Name
_____ pH 7.21; CO$_2$ 33; HCO$_3$ 22	1. Respiratory Acidosis
_____ pH 7.47; CO$_2$ 34; HCO$_3$ 26	2. Respiratory Alkalosis
_____ pH 7.46; CO$_2$ 40; HCO$_3$ 28	3. Metabolic Acidosis
_____ pH 7.32; CO$_2$ 36; HCO$_3$ 18	4. Metabolic Alkalosis
_____ pH 7.38; CO$_2$ 43; HCO$_3$ 22	5. Respiratory Acidosis - Compensated
_____ pH 7.49; CO$_2$ 30; HCO$_3$ 21	6. Respiratory Alkalosis - Compensated
_____ pH 7.48; CO$_2$ 44; HCO$_3$ 30	7. Metabolic Acidosis - Compensated
_____ pH 7.42; CO$_2$ 49; HCO$_3$ 29	8. Metabolic Alkalosis – Compensated
	9. Normal ABG

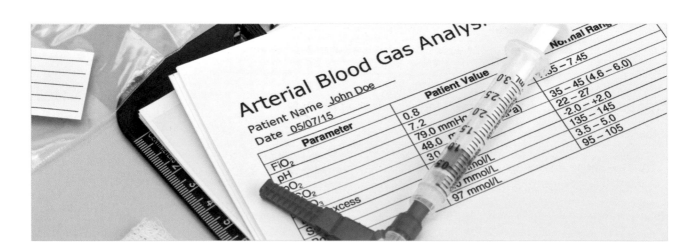

Millie is admitted to the medical unit for monitoring. Over the next 24 hours with the use of activated charcoal every 4 hours, her labs show these trends.

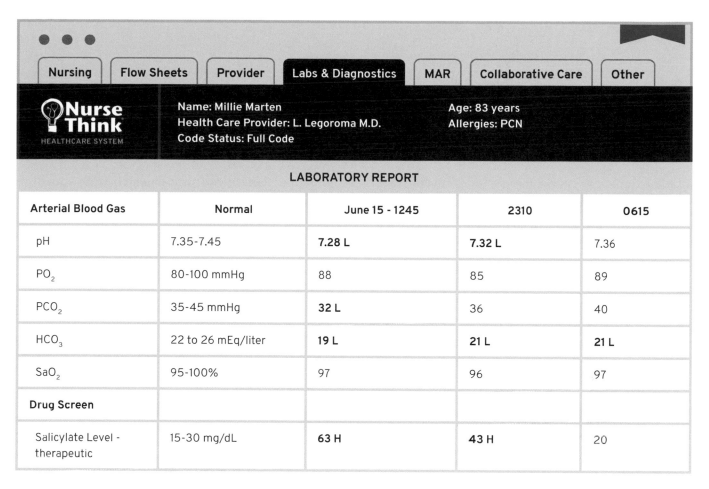

Nursing | Flow Sheets | Provider | **Labs & Diagnostics** | MAR | Collaborative Care | Other

Nurse Think HEALTHCARE SYSTEM

Name: Millie Marten
Health Care Provider: L. Legoroma M.D.
Code Status: Full Code

Age: 83 years
Allergies: PCN

LABORATORY REPORT

Arterial Blood Gas	Normal	June 15 - 1245	2310	0615
pH	7.35-7.45	**7.28 L**	**7.32 L**	7.36
PO_2	80-100 mmHg	88	85	89
PCO_2	35-45 mmHg	**32 L**	36	40
HCO_3	22 to 26 mEq/liter	**19 L**	**21 L**	**21 L**
SaO_2	95-100%	97	96	97
Drug Screen				
Salicylate Level - therapeutic	15-30 mg/dL	**63 H**	**43 H**	20

15. **What assumption can the nurse make about the laboratory trends?**
   1. The acidosis is worsening.
   2. The alkalosis is improving.
   3. There has been no change.
   4. The acid-base imbalance has resolved.

Millie is preparing for discharge. She is no longer confused and will be discharged to home. The home care nurse will see her daily to confirm she is following the discharge instructions.

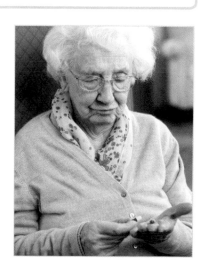

16. **In preparation for discharge teaching, what is the priority?**
   1. Complete a medication reconciliation.
   2. Check with the neighbor that her cat is all right.
   3. Have physical therapy evaluate her ability to go home.
   4. Arrange for her children to come and care for her at home.

17. As the acute care nurse, complete an SBAR hand-off report to the home care nurse. Complete each section of the communication form.

S – _____

B – _____

A – _____

R – _____

18. The home care nurse makes her first visit since Millie got home from the hospital. In which order should the nurse perform these actions after entering the home? _____, _____, _____, _____, _____.

1. Review Millie's hospital discharge orders.
2. Perform hand hygiene.
3. Complete a focused assessment.
4. Document the visit.
5. Remove medications from Millie's pillbox that are no longer prescribed.

19. The nurse asks Millie a series of questions to determine her ability to live safely by herself. For each item determine its appropriateness for this assessment.

	Appropriate	Non-Appropriate
"Do you enjoy living alone?"		
"Do you ever feel unsafe living alone?"		
"Do you have enough money to live in a group home?"		
"Can your children move in with you?"		
"Have you ever thought about getting rid of Sam, so you don't trip on him?"		
"Tell me what types of meals you fix for yourself."		
"Are there any specific resources you may need?"		

20. In review of the acid-base disorders, list common causes for each imbalance.

Respiratory Acidosis	Respiratory Alkalosis	Metabolic Acidosis	Metabolic Alkalosis

Case 2: Electrolyte imbalance and fluid overload from acute renal insufficiency

Related Concepts: Elimination, Hormonal, Perfusion, Oxygenation
Threaded Topics: Culture, Language Barrier, Dialysis, Diet Education, Diabetes, Community Resources

Alfredo Hernandez is a 38-year-old male who lives in southern Texas. He and his family migrated to the United States from Guatemala a few years ago and live together in a small house. His primary language is Spanish, but he has acquired the ability to understand and speak some English in his three years here. Like his mother, father, sisters, and cousins, he has Type II diabetes. His diabetes is poorly controlled, and he is now insulin dependent. He has hypertension, decreased vision and his feet are often "cold and numb." His family brings him to the community hospital today because he's having a hard time breathing.

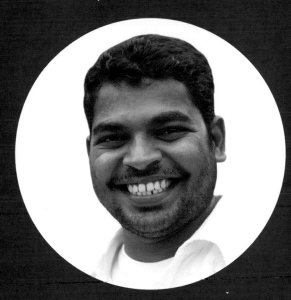

1. **What should be the nurse's first action after placing Alfredo in a hospital gown?**

   1. Obtain a glucose monitor reading.
   2. Assess the blood pressure.
   3. Take an oxygen saturation reading.
   4. Place Alfredo on an EKG monitor.

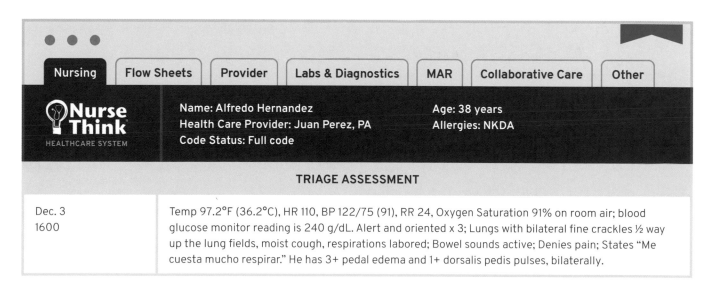

Nursing	Flow Sheets	Provider	Labs & Diagnostics	MAR	Collaborative Care	Other

Nurse Think HEALTHCARE SYSTEM

Name: Alfredo Hernandez
Health Care Provider: Juan Perez, PA
Code Status: Full code

Age: 38 years
Allergies: NKDA

TRIAGE ASSESSMENT

Dec. 3 1600	Temp 97.2°F (36.2°C), HR 110, BP 122/75 (91), RR 24, Oxygen Saturation 91% on room air; blood glucose monitor reading is 240 g/dL. Alert and oriented x 3; Lungs with bilateral fine crackles ½ way up the lung fields, moist cough, respirations labored; Bowel sounds active; Denies pain; States "Me cuesta mucho respirar." He has 3+ pedal edema and 1+ dorsalis pedis pulses, bilaterally.

2. **NurseThink® Prioritization Power!**

   Reflect on Alfredo's assessment findings and identify the **Top 3 Priority** assessment concerns that indicate fluid volume excess.

   1. _____

   2. _____

   3. _____

3. **What should be the nurse's priority nursing action?**
   1. Obtain an order for insulin.
   2. Raise the head of the bed.
   3. Place oxygen at 2 L/nasal cannula.
   4. Obtain a translator.

Clinical Hint: Healthcare organizations that receive Medicare, Medicaid, or other sources of federal funds have a legal obligation to provide oral interpreters and written translated documents. Failing to provide language access services to limited English proficiency patients is a form of national origin discrimination. There was case law in the United States Supreme Court (Lau v. Nichols. 1974) that established this basic principle.

The nurse obtains prescriptions from the HCP.

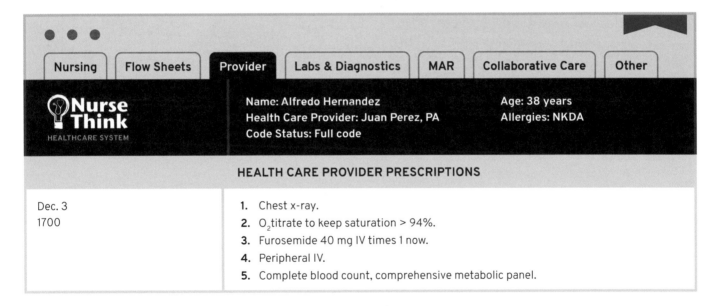

| Nursing | Flow Sheets | Provider | Labs & Diagnostics | MAR | Collaborative Care | Other |

Name: Alfredo Hernandez
Health Care Provider: Juan Perez, PA
Code Status: Full code
Age: 38 years
Allergies: NKDA

HEALTH CARE PROVIDER PRESCRIPTIONS

Dec. 3
1700

1. Chest x-ray.
2. O_2 titrate to keep saturation > 94%.
3. Furosemide 40 mg IV times 1 now.
4. Peripheral IV.
5. Complete blood count, comprehensive metabolic panel.

4. **Place the prescriptions in order of the priority in which the nurse should complete them.** ___, ___, ___, ___.
   1. Request chest x-ray and lab draw.
   2. Place O_2 at 2 L/nasal cannula.
   3. Deliver furosemide 40 mg IV dose.
   4. Place IV line.

5. **The nurse reassesses the oxygen saturation reading after 15 minutes, and it is 94%. What should the nurse do next?**
   1. Nothing, this is acceptable.
   2. Notify the HCP.
   3. Increase the O_2 to 3 L/nasal cannula.
   4. Place Alfredo on a simple mask.

6. The chest x-ray is completed. The radiologist calls the nurse to say "the lungs have fluffy consolidation bilaterally." How should the nurse interpret this report?

   1. There is pneumonia in both lungs.
   2. Atelectasis is present.
   3. There is fluid accumulation in both lungs.
   4. A pneumothorax is present.

7. The nurse is evaluating the client's response to the furosemide. Which finding determines the dose was effective?

   1. Urine output of 200 mL over 4 hours.
   2. Crackles bilaterally in the lower bases.
   3. Jugular venous distension evident.
   4. Potassium level decreases.

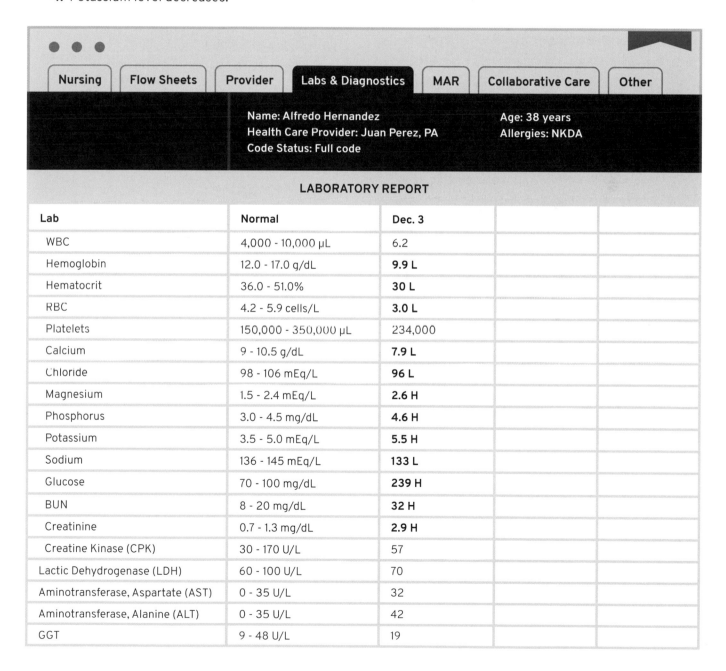

| Nursing | Flow Sheets | Provider | Labs & Diagnostics | MAR | Collaborative Care | Other |

Name: Alfredo Hernandez
Health Care Provider: Juan Perez, PA
Code Status: Full code

Age: 38 years
Allergies: NKDA

LABORATORY REPORT

Lab	Normal	Dec. 3		
WBC	4,000 - 10,000 µL	6.2		
Hemoglobin	12.0 - 17.0 g/dL	9.9 L		
Hematocrit	36.0 - 51.0%	30 L		
RBC	4.2 - 5.9 cells/L	3.0 L		
Platelets	150,000 - 350,000 µL	234,000		
Calcium	9 - 10.5 g/dL	7.9 L		
Chloride	98 - 106 mEq/L	96 L		
Magnesium	1.5 - 2.4 mEq/L	2.6 H		
Phosphorus	3.0 - 4.5 mg/dL	4.6 H		
Potassium	3.5 - 5.0 mEq/L	5.5 H		
Sodium	136 - 145 mEq/L	133 L		
Glucose	70 - 100 mg/dL	239 H		
BUN	8 - 20 mg/dL	32 H		
Creatinine	0.7 - 1.3 mg/dL	2.9 H		
Creatine Kinase (CPK)	30 - 170 U/L	57		
Lactic Dehydrogenase (LDH)	60 - 100 U/L	70		
Aminotransferase, Aspartate (AST)	0 - 35 U/L	32		
Aminotransferase, Alanine (ALT)	0 - 35 U/L	42		
GGT	9 - 48 U/L	19		

8. **What hypothesis can the nurse make from the lab and chest x-ray reports?**
    1. Alfredo has renal insufficiency causing fluid overload.
    2. Alfredo has signs of liver failure causing fluid shifting.
    3. Alfredo has an infection that is likely pneumonia.
    4. Alfredo has poor myocardial contractility causing fluid excess.

9. **What should the nurse include in Alfredo's plan of care? Select all that apply.**
    1. Daily weights.
    2. Strict intake and output.
    3. Encourage oral fluids.
    4. Monitor pulse for irregularity.
    5. Restrict dietary sodium and potassium.

Alfredo is admitted to the medical unit with dyspnea and renal insufficiency. A nephrologist is consulted and prescribes a 24-hour urine collection for creatinine clearance.

10. **The nurse requests a translator to instruct Alfredo about the process of collection. What should the nurse include in the teaching? Select all that apply.**
    1. All urine must go into the container over the next 24 hours.
    2. The container with urine must be kept at room temperature.
    3. Only this dark container can be used to collect the urine.
    4. Empty your bladder now, before we begin the test.
    5. There will be signs in the bathroom alerting the staff of this test.

11. **Alfredo is placed on a fluid restriction of 1 liter per 24 hours. He is asking for something to drink at 2245. Based on the intake and output record, what is the nurse's best response?**
    1. "No, I'm sorry, but you've had your allotment of fluid for the day. I can bring you some oral swabs."
    2. "You have met your allotment of fluid for the day. Let me listen to your lungs to see if I can give you something more."
    3. "You have almost met your fluid restriction for the day; I'll bring you some ice chips."
    4. "You can have a glass of juice, water or milk. Which would you prefer?"

Time	Intake	Output
2300-0700	> 100 mL juice	> 50 mL
0700-1500	> 240 mL soup > 120 mL gelatin > 6 oz. milk	> 250 mL > 100 mL
1500-2300	> 150 mL juice > 110 mL flavored ice > 2 oz. water	> 50 mL
Totals		

12. **The nurse is mentoring a second-semester nursing student who is studying fluid assessment findings. Help the student match each finding with its appropriate fluid status.**

_____ Hepatomegaly	_____ Weight gain	**A. Fluid Overload**
_____ Cerebral edema	_____ Puffy eyes	**B. Fluid Deficit**
_____ Orthostatic hypotension	_____ Cool skin	**C. Either Overload or Deficit**
_____ Tachycardia	_____ Edema	
_____ Thready pulse	_____ Distended jugular veins	
_____ Thirst		

Two days after admission, the nurse caring for Alfredo learns through an interpreter that his family is frustrated that he is getting weaker. Not familiar with Alfredo, the nurse reviews the medical record to better understand what is happening in order to address the family's concerns.

Nursing | **Flow Sheets** | **Provider** | **Labs & Diagnostics** | **MAR** | **Collaborative Care** | **Other**

NurseThink
HEALTHCARE SYSTEM

Name: Alfredo Hernandez
Health Care Provider: Juan Perez, PA
Code Status: Full code

Age: 38 years
Allergies: NKDA

LABORATORY REPORT

Lab	Normal	Dec. 3	Dec. 4	Dec. 5
WBC	4,000 - 10,000 μL	6.2	10.2	12.3 H
Hemoglobin	12.0 - 17.0 g/dL	9.9 L	9.4 L	9.0 L
Hematocrit	36.0 - 51.0%	30 L	29 L	30 L
RBC	4.2 - 5.9 cells/L	3.0 L	2.9 L	2.8 L
Platelets	150,000 - 350,000 μL	234,000	249,000	300,000
Calcium	9 - 10.5 g/dL	7.9 L	7.9 L	7.8 L
Chloride	98 - 106 mEq/L	96 L	95 L	96 L
Magnesium	1.5 - 2.4 mEq/L	2.6 H	1.4 L	1.3 L
Phosphorus	3.0 - 4.5 mg/dL	4.6 H	4.6 H	4.8 H
Potassium	3.5 - 5.0 mEq/L	5.5 H	5.7 H	5.8 H
Sodium	136 - 145 mEq/L	133 L	132 L	131 L
Glucose	70 - 100 mg/dL	239 H	201 H	168 H
BUN	8 - 20 mg/dL	32 H	29 H	34 H
Creatinine	0.7 - 1.3 mg/dL	2.9 H	3.0 H	3.3 H
Glomerular Filtration Rate (GFR)	> 60 mL/min/1.73m2			16 L
Daily Weight		65.9 kg	66.8 kg	68.2 kg
Oxygen Saturation		94%	95%	94%
Oxygen		2 L/NC	3 L/NC	4 L/NC
Blood Pressure (MAP)		122/75 (91)	139/88 (105)	145/92 (110)
Heart Rate		110	115	117

13. **NurseThink® Prioritization Power!**

    Reflect on Alfredo's trends in data and identify the **Top 3 Priority** concerns.

    1. _____

    2. _____

    3. _____

14. Knowing that Alfredo's condition is worsening, what potential complication(s) should the nurse be monitoring for? Select all that apply.

    1. Cardiac dysrhythmias.
    2. Pulmonary edema.
    3. Sepsis.
    4. Liver failure.
    5. Deep vein thrombosis.

15. It is determined that Alfredo will be started on hemodialysis. A temporary dialysis catheter is placed into his right internal jugular. What should the nurse assess with this type of dialysis catheter?

    1. Bruit and thrill.
    2. Circulation to the extremity.
    3. Dressing intactness.
    4. Radial pulse.

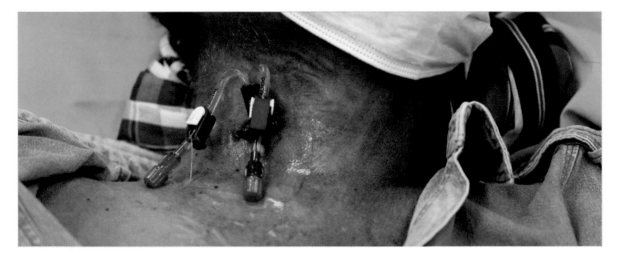

16. The nurse learns that Alfredo is going to dialysis in 3 hours. He has several medications due, which ones should the nurse hold before dialysis? Select all that apply.

    1. Regular insulin, 5 units subcutaneously.
    2. Metoprolol 25 mg orally.
    3. Furosemide 80 mg orally.
    4. Calcium acetate 667 mg orally.
    5. Amoxicillin 250 mg orally.

Alfredo completed his first hemodialysis treatment and returns to the medical unit. Upon return, the nurse assesses that he is sleepy but arousable and cooperative; warm to touch but afebrile; heart rate is 115 beats per minute, respirations are 18 with an oxygen saturation of 96% on room air, and blood pressure is 89/45 (60). His glucose monitor reading is 65 g/dL. The dressing to his temporary dialysis catheter is intact, and the red and blue clamps are closed.

17. **THIN Thinking Time!**
    Reflect on the post-dialysis information and apply **THIN Thinking**.

    T – _____

    H – _____

    I – _____

    N – _____

    T - Top 3
    H - Help Quick
    I - Identify Risk to Safety
    N - Nursing Process

    Scan to access the 10-Minute-Mentor → *on THIN Thinking.*

    NurseThink.com/THINThinking

18. **What action should the nurse take in response to the post-dialysis assessment? Select all that apply.**
    1. Lower the head of the bed.
    2. Deliver fluids – wide open.
    3. Have Alfredo drink juice.
    4. Apply a cooling blanket.
    5. Apply oxygen.

19. **Over a few days, Alfredo's condition improves. The nurse is preparing him for discharge. What is important to include? Complete the discharge instructions on the following page.**

20. **Using the interpreter for the discharge instructions, the nurse identifies that Alfredo is concerned about complying with the renal and diabetic diet with his preference of traditional Hispanic foods. Which action should the nurse take?**
    1. Plan to have the hospital prepare his meals.
    2. Identify a Spanish-speaking dietitian in the community that Alfredo can consult.
    3. Teach his family about the dietary restrictions, encouraging him to stay compliant.
    4. Arrange for meals-on-wheels to deliver his meals.

	Types	Frequency	Access Site	Complications
Hemodialysis At home or in a center	Short daily	2-3 hours, 6 days/ week	> Arteriovenous (AV) fistula > AV graft > A catheter	> Infection > Blood clots > Water and/or electrolytes imbalance
	Traditional	3-4 hours, 3 times/ week		
	Nocturnal	6-8 hours 3+ days/ week		
Peritoneal dialysis	Continuous ambulatory peritoneal dialysis (CAPD)	4-5 times/day	> Peritoneal catheter	> Peritonitis
	Automated peritoneal dialysis	6-8 hours every night		

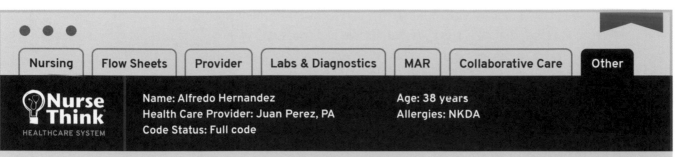

Name: Alfredo Hernandez
Health Care Provider: Juan Perez, PA
Code Status: Full code

Age: 38 years
Allergies: NKDA

DISCHARGE INSTRUCTIONS

Discharge

Diet

_____
_____

Oral fluid intake

_____
_____

Activity

_____
_____

Dialysis catheter care

_____
_____

Follow-up with dialysis

_____
_____

Diabetes management

_____
_____

Daily self-monitoring

_____
_____

Problems to report to HCP

_____
_____

Medication instructions
> Regular insulin
> NPH insulin
> Metoprolol
> Renal vitamins
> Aluminum hydroxide
> Famotidine

Conceptual Debriefing & Case Reflection

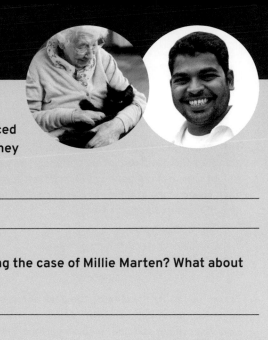

1. Compare the impaired homeostasis that Millie Marten experienced with the impaired homeostasis of Alfredo Hernandez. How are they the same and how are they different?

    _____

    _____

2. What was your single greatest learning moment while completing the case of Millie Marten? What about Alfredo Hernandez?

    _____

    _____

3. How did the nursing care provided to Millie Marten and Alfredo Hernandez change the outcome for each of them?

    _____

    _____

4. Identify safety concerns for both Millie Marten and Alfredo Hernandez for each case.

    _____

    _____

5. In what areas of each case study was basic care and comfort utilized?

    _____

    _____

6. What steps in each case did the nurse take that prevented hospital-acquired injury?

    _____

    _____

7. How did the nurse provide culturally sensitive/competent care?

    _____

    _____

8. How will learning about the case of Millie Marten and Alfredo Hernandez impact the care you provide for future clients?

    _____

    _____

Fundamental Quiz

1. The nurse is reviewing admission orders for a newly admitted client with bounding peripheral pulses, stated weight gain of three pounds overnight, pitting ankle edema, and moist crackles bilaterally. Which action should the nurse perform first?

   1. Obtain an oxygen saturation reading.
   2. Administer furosemide 40 mg IV push.
   3. Determine the respiratory rate.
   4. Obtain a serum potassium level.

2. The nurse realizes that twice the dose of furosemide was delivered to an older adult with dementia. Which vital sign assessment should the nurse perform first?

   1. Oxygen saturation.
   2. Respiratory rate.
   3. Heart rate.
   4. Blood pressure.

3. The nurse is caring for a client with metabolic acidosis. Which finding needs immediate attention?

   1. Respiratory rate of 28 breath per minute.
   2. Client reports palpitations.
   3. Client reports feeling of nausea.
   4. Hypoactive bowel sounds.

4. Which client should the nurse see first?

   1. 42-year-old with a K+ of 3.2 mEq/L.
   2. 85-year-old with a pH of 7.31.
   3. 16-year-old with a Na+ of 125 mEq/L.
   4. 67-year-old with 3+ pedal edema.

5. The nurse is about to deliver spironolactone 100 mg to a client whose potassium is 3.3 mEq/L. What should be the nurse's next action?

   1. Hold the medication.
   2. Notify the health care provider.
   3. Deliver the spironolactone.
   4. Assess for dysrhythmias.

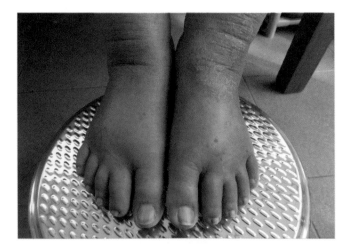

Advanced Quiz

6. The nurse is caring for a client receiving intravenous albumin for low serum protein levels and fluid shift. Which change indicates an anticipated response? Select all that apply.

   1. A change in blood pressure from 97/52 (67) mmHg to 115/69 (78) mmHg.
   2. A decrease in urinary output.
   3. A change in peripheral edema from 3+ to 4+.
   4. An increase in abdominal ascites fluid.
   5. A decrease in the hematocrit.

7. The nurse is admitting a patient with a temperature of 102.9°F (39.4°C), heart rate of 125, blood pressure of 90/44 (59) mmHg, respiratory rate of 24 and oxygen saturation of 95% on room air. Which nursing action is the highest priority?

   1. Apply oxygen at 2 L/NC.
   2. Deliver 0.9% normal saline at 250 mL/hr.
   3. Elevate the head of the bed.
   4. Administer acetaminophen.

8. The nurse is caring for an older adult client. Vitals include T 99.8°F (37.6°C), HR 96, RR 28, BP 170/90 (117) mmHg. The client is restless, has dyspnea and is anxious. His oxygen saturation drops to 87% when he pulls his oxygen cannula off. Which action should the nurse take after reapplying the oxygen?

   1. Administer an anti-anxiety medication.
   2. Auscultate the lung sounds.
   3. Check recent labs.
   4. Administer an anti-hypertensive medication.

9. A client is on the 5th day of nasogastric suctioning. Which assessment finding raises the greatest concern?

   1. Tenting skin.
   2. Irregular pulse.
   3. Extreme tiredness.
   4. Decreasing urine output.

10. The nurse is performing the 0800 assessment on a stable client with fluid and electrolytes imbalance. The blood pressure reading from the non-invasive blood pressure cuff is 189/99 (129) mmHg. The nurse reviews the chart and finds this information.

Today at 0400	Yesterday at 2300	Yesterday at 1900	Yesterday at 1600	Yesterday at 1300
128/56 (80)	132/59 (83)	125/60 (82)	135/70 (92)	134/68 (90)

What should be the nurse's next action?

   1. Deliver the PRN blood pressure medication.
   2. Complete a neurological assessment.
   3. Reevaluate the blood pressure.
   4. Ask the client if they have been hypertensive before.

Respiration

Oxygenation / Gas Exchange

The process of respiration includes both oxygenation and gas exchange. Oxygenation is the process of providing cells with oxygen through pulmonary ventilation (breathing) and perfusion (the movement of blood to the tissues). Gas exchange is the process by which oxygen moves passively by diffusion across the capillaries to the cells while carbon dioxide is removed from the body through the respiratory system. Nurses encounter alterations in oxygenation and gas exchange in all ages of clients and must identify problems and intervene quickly to prevent life-threatening complications.

Next Gen Clinical Judgment:

> What are the different assessment findings for a client with oxygenation problems versus perfusion problems?

> Can a client have adequate respirations but inadequate oxygenation? Explain.

> Why is "airway" first when talking about airway-breathing-circulation?

> What is the role of respirations in the acid-base balance of the body?

> List diseases and illnesses that are related to the respiratory system.

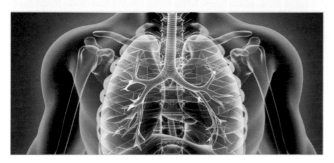

_____

_____

_____

_____

_____

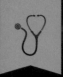

Go To Clinical Case

While caring for this client, be sure to review the concept maps in chapters 3 and 4.

Case 1: Impaired Oxygenation with Secondary Infection

Related Concepts: Acid-Base Balance, Infection
Threaded Topics: Medication Calculations, Delegation, Health Promotion

Luanne Yazzie is a 56-year-old who has lived her life around second-hand smokers. Her parents smoked in the home she grew up in, her first husband smoked before dying from complications of diabetes, and she works as a card dealer in a Nevada casino which allows smoking. Although she has never smoked, Luanne learned a year ago that she had developed early symptoms of emphysema.

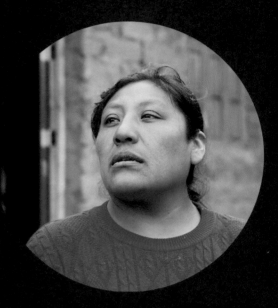

1. **Which symptoms does Luanne demonstrate that indicate early signs of emphysema? Select all that apply.**

   1. Increasing shortness of breath when climbing stairs.

   2. Production of dark yellow-green sputum.

   3. Wheezing with exhalation.

   4. Increased morning mucus production.

   5. Barrel chest.

2. **Luanne comes to the clinic for increasing shortness of breath and worsening symptoms. The health care provider considers several pulmonary lab and diagnostic tests. Match the diagnostic test on the left with the appropriate client teaching on the right.**

_____ Arterial Blood Gases (ABGs)	A. Be sure your sample is sputum from the lungs and not saliva.
_____ Oxygen Saturation	B. You will breathe forcefully into a machine to determine the volume of air in your lungs.
_____ Pulmonary Function Tests (PFTs)	C. A tube will pass into your lungs while you are asleep to visualize the structures and take samples of the tissue if needed.
_____ Serum Hemoglobin Level (Hgb)	D. A clip will be placed on your finger to determine the oxygen level in your blood.
_____ Chest X-Ray (CXR)	E. You will lay still on your back and be placed in a large machine for scanning.
_____ Computerized Tomography (CT)	F. A blood sample is taken from your wrist, and it can be painful.
_____ Sputum Culture & Sensitivity (C&S)	G. A blood test that helps your ability to carry oxygen in your blood.
_____ Bronchoscopy	H. A test that can determine the shape of your expanded lungs.

3. Luanne's provider prescribes a chest x-ray (CXR) and pulmonary function tests (PFT). These confirm that she is at a moderate (Stage 2) disease with a forced expiratory volume in one second (FEV1) of 65% of normal. Luanne has many questions for the nurse about what this means. How should the nurse respond?

   1. The chest x-ray shows damage to the air sacs of your lungs.
   2. Your lungs are not functioning at full capacity any longer, explaining your shortness of breath.
   3. Your disease has improved from when the symptoms started a year ago.
   4. This information needs to be explained by your provider.

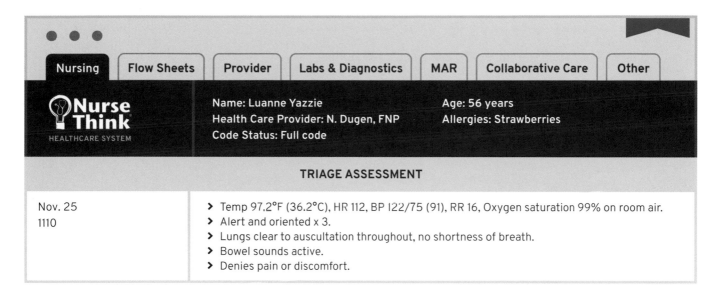

| Nursing | Flow Sheets | Provider | Labs & Diagnostics | MAR | Collaborative Care | Other |

Nurse Think
HEALTHCARE SYSTEM

Name: Luanne Yazzie
Health Care Provider: N. Dugen, FNP
Code Status: Full code

Age: 56 years
Allergies: Strawberries

TRIAGE ASSESSMENT

| Nov. 25 1110 | > Temp 97.2°F (36.2°C), HR 112, BP 122/75 (91), RR 16, Oxygen saturation 99% on room air.
> Alert and oriented x 3.
> Lungs clear to auscultation throughout, no shortness of breath.
> Bowel sounds active.
> Denies pain or discomfort. |

4. The registered nurse reviews the assessment documented by the LPN/LVN and diagnostic findings. Which assessment inconsistencies require re-evaluation by the RN? Select all that apply.

   1. Temperature, heart rate, blood pressure.
   2. Respiratory rate and oxygen saturation.
   3. Orientation.
   4. Lung sounds.
   5. Bowel sounds.
   6. Pain level.

   Clinical Hint: The RN is responsible for confirming the client is safe. If the data or assessment information provided by the LPN or UAP is questionable, the RN should reassess.

5. For each assessment selected, determine why it would be important for the RN to reevaluate.

   _____
   _____
   _____
   _____
   _____

6. **NurseThink® Prioritization Power!**

   Reflect on Luanne's diagnosis and identify the **Top 3 Priority** teaching needs.

   1. _____

   2. _____

   3. _____

Luanne is discharged from the clinic with these new prescriptions.

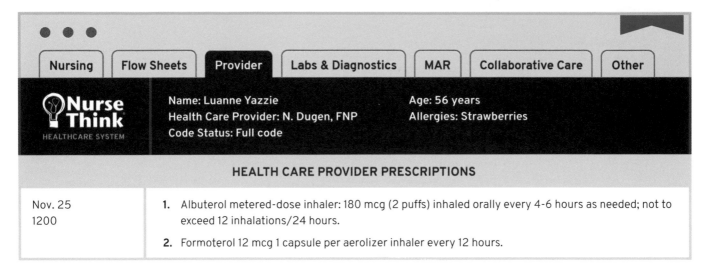

| Nursing | Flow Sheets | Provider | Labs & Diagnostics | MAR | Collaborative Care | Other |

Name: Luanne Yazzie
Health Care Provider: N. Dugen, FNP
Code Status: Full code

Age: 56 years
Allergies: Strawberries

HEALTH CARE PROVIDER PRESCRIPTIONS

| Nov. 25 1200 | 1. Albuterol metered-dose inhaler: 180 mcg (2 puffs) inhaled orally every 4-6 hours as needed; not to exceed 12 inhalations/24 hours. |
| | 2. Formoterol 12 mcg 1 capsule per aerolizer inhaler every 12 hours. |

7. **Luanne does not understand the need for two inhalers. How should the nurse explain the differences?**

   1. They both work to expand your lungs and improve your ability to breathe.
   2. One will help your breathing; the other will repair the damage to your lungs.
   3. One is a short-term for immediate relief, and the other is for long-term control.
   4. One opens your airways, and the other decreases the inflammation.

> **Clinical Hint:** Inhaler considerations:
> › Incorrect use of inhalers reduces their benefit.
> › Teaching should take place when the inhaler is prescribed.
> › The technique of self-administration should be assessed routinely.
> › With children or older adults who may not have the dexterity or capacity to properly use an inhaler the caregiver should demonstrate their correct use.

Luanne is managed well on the two inhalers for over a year. One morning she awakens feeling more short of breath than usual. She goes to work but has to leave early since her breathing is more difficult and the cough is getting worse despite the use of her albuterol inhaler every 1-2 hours. She goes to the urgent care on the way home.

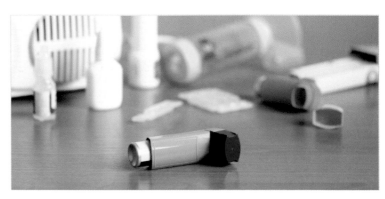

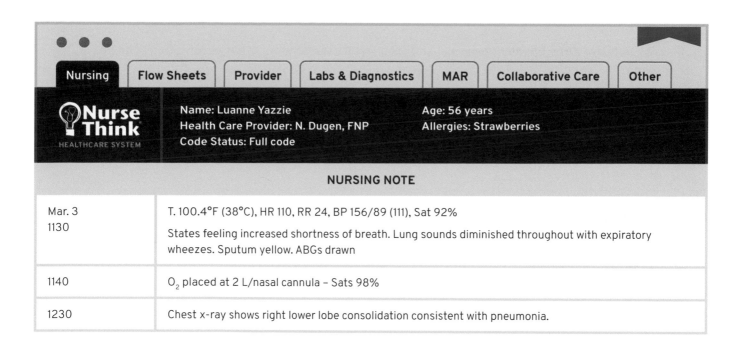

NURSING NOTE

Mar. 3 1130	T. 100.4°F (38°C), HR 110, RR 24, BP 156/89 (111), Sat 92%
	States feeling increased shortness of breath. Lung sounds diminished throughout with expiratory wheezes. Sputum yellow. ABGs drawn
1140	O₂ placed at 2 L/nasal cannula – Sats 98%
1230	Chest x-ray shows right lower lobe consolidation consistent with pneumonia.

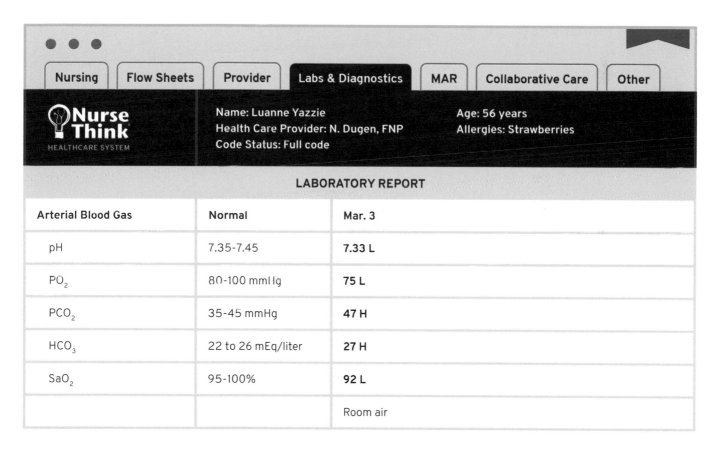

LABORATORY REPORT

Arterial Blood Gas	Normal	Mar. 3
pH	7.35-7.45	7.33 L
PO_2	80-100 mmHg	75 L
PCO_2	35-45 mmHg	47 H
HCO_3	22 to 26 mEq/liter	27 H
SaO_2	95-100%	92 L
		Room air

Next Gen Clinical Judgement: Find an app on your phone that shows you how to understand arterial blood gases.

8. The nurse reviews Luanne's physical and diagnostic assessments. What assumptions can be made?

    1. Luanne's current medications are ineffective for her worsening COPD.

    2. Luanne has a secondary infection that's impairing her ability to breathe.

    3. Luanne requires intubation with mechanical ventilation.

    4. Luanne is unable to compensate for her acid-base imbalance.

9. The health care provider prescribes albuterol per small volume nebulizer (SVN). Luanne asks the nurse how it's different from the metered dose inhaler (MDI) she takes at home. How should the nurse respond?

    1. The MDI is less portable to use.

    2. The SVN uses compressed air to distribute the medication into your lungs.

    3. The SVN provides oxygen during delivery of the medication.

    4. The MDI has a lower dosage and is less potent.

10. The nurse is instructing Luanne on how to use the nebulizer. What should be included in the instructions? Select all that apply.

    1. Fully exhale before taking the medication.

    2. Rinse your mouth after use.

    3. Firmly place your lips around the mouthpiece.

    4. Take normal breaths during administration.

    5. You may feel your heartbeat increase with administration.

    6. Let me know if you feel lightheaded or dizzy.

    Clinical Hint: Spacers can be especially helpful to adults and children who find a regular metered dose inhaler hard to use. People who use corticosteroid inhalers should use a spacer to prevent getting the medicine in their mouth, where oral yeast infections can occur.

Luanne is discharged after her oxygen saturation increased to 94% on room air. She was started on an oral antibiotic and told to get rest and not to return to work for 7 days. She returned to work after 2 days since she was feeling better, and could not afford to take 7 days off of work.

11. What else could the nurse suggest that would be helpful for Luanne's recovery? Select all that apply.

    1. Increase fluid intake.

    2. Ambulate around the block twice each day.

    3. Complete the full dose of antibiotics.

    4. Consume at least 2000 calories each day.

    5. Avoid smoky environments.

After a week the shortness of breath has returned. Her son notices that she seems mildly confused. He takes her to the emergency department. The triage nurse takes her vital signs and performs a focused assessment.

Clinical Hint: When a client is experiencing a new onset of confusion, first, rule out hypoxia as the cause.

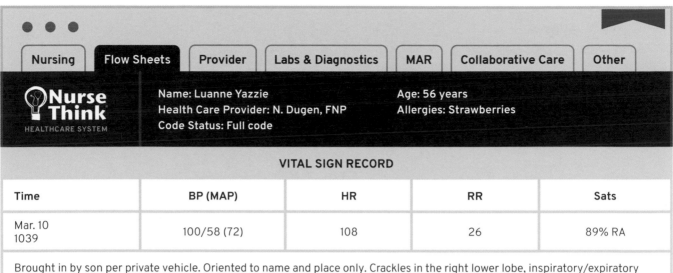

VITAL SIGN RECORD

Name: Luanne Yazzie
Health Care Provider: N. Dugen, FNP
Code Status: Full code
Age: 56 years
Allergies: Strawberries

Time	BP (MAP)	HR	RR	Sats
Mar. 10 1039	100/58 (72)	108	26	89% RA

Brought in by son per private vehicle. Oriented to name and place only. Crackles in the right lower lobe, inspiratory/expiratory wheezes. Moist cough. Some use of accessory muscles. States having a hard time breathing.

12. **THIN Thinking Time!**

Reflect on the events that have occurred since Luanne Yazzie came to the emergency department and apply **THIN Thinking.**

T – _____

H – _____

I – _____

N – _____

T - Top 3
H - Help Quick
I - Identify Risk to Safety
N - Nursing Process

Scan to access the 10-Minute-Mentor on THIN Thinking.

NurseThink.com/THINThinking

13. **What should be the nurse's next action? Place in order of priority.** _____, _____, _____, _____ .
    1. Raise the head of the bed.
    2. Apply oxygen at 2 L/nasal cannula.
    3. Complete a more comprehensive assessment.
    4. Notify the health care provider.
    5. Encourage pursed-lip breathing.

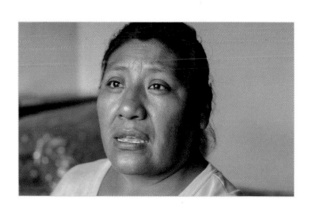

14. **Luanne's son asks why she is so confused. How should the nurse respond?**
    1. The medications that your mom is taking can sometimes cause confusion.
    2. She may have had a stroke, and we'll run some tests.
    3. She's probably just tired of being sick.
    4. Her oxygen levels are low which can cause confusion.

Clinical Hint: Confusion from hypoxia will occur after the oxygen saturation drops. If your client is adequately oxygenating and they are confused, explore other reasons for the confusion (medications, acid/base imbalance, metabolic issue).

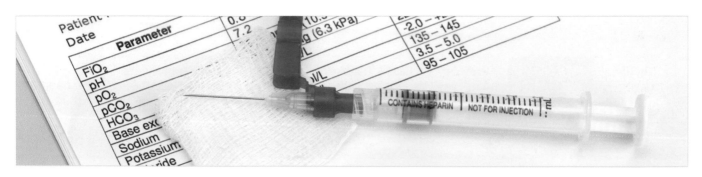

Nursing	Flow Sheets	Provider	**Labs & Diagnostics**	MAR	Collaborative Care	Other

NurseThink
HEALTHCARE SYSTEM

Name: Luanne Yazzie
Health Care Provider: N. Dugen, FNP
Code Status: Full code

Age: 56 years
Allergies: Strawberries

LABORATORY REPORT

Arterial Blood Gas	Normal	Mar. 3	Mar. 10 – 1100	
pH	7.35-7.45	7.33 L	7.25 L	
PO$_2$	80-100 mmHg	75 L	71 L	
PCO$_2$	35-45 mmHg	47 H	51 H	
HCO$_3$	22 to 26 mEq/liter	27 H	28H	
SaO$_2$	95-100%	92 L	90 L	
		Room air	2 L/NC	

15. **Provide rationale for each of these abnormal findings.**

Tachypnea: _____

Respiratory Acidosis: _____

Adventitious Breath Sounds:_____

16. **The nurse gathers information and begins to prepare an SBAR telephone conversation for the health care provider. Complete each section of the communication form.**

S – _____

B – _____

A – _____

R – _____

Clinical Hint:
S - Situation
B - Background
A - Assessment
R - Recommendation

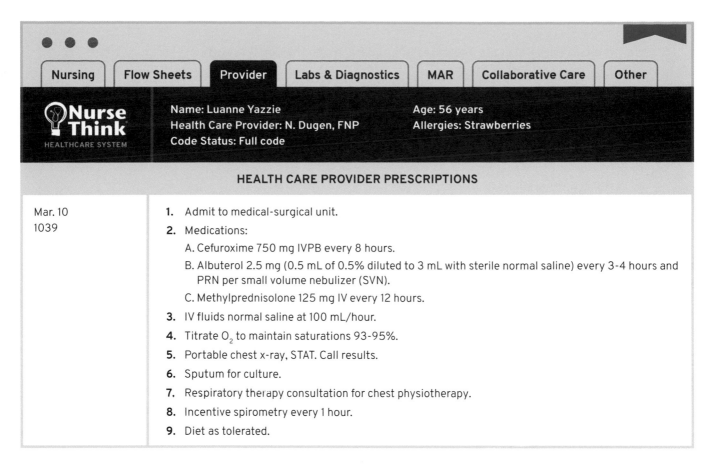

HEALTH CARE PROVIDER PRESCRIPTIONS

Mar. 10 1039	

1. Admit to medical-surgical unit.

2. Medications:

A. Cefuroxime 750 mg IVPB every 8 hours.

B. Albuterol 2.5 mg (0.5 mL of 0.5% diluted to 3 mL with sterile normal saline) every 3-4 hours and PRN per small volume nebulizer (SVN).

C. Methylprednisolone 125 mg IV every 12 hours.

3. IV fluids normal saline at 100 mL/hour.

4. Titrate O_2 to maintain saturations 93-95%.

5. Portable chest x-ray, STAT. Call results.

6. Sputum for culture.

7. Respiratory therapy consultation for chest physiotherapy.

8. Incentive spirometry every 1 hour.

9. Diet as tolerated.

Before initiating the orders, the nurse performs another focused assessment on Luanne.

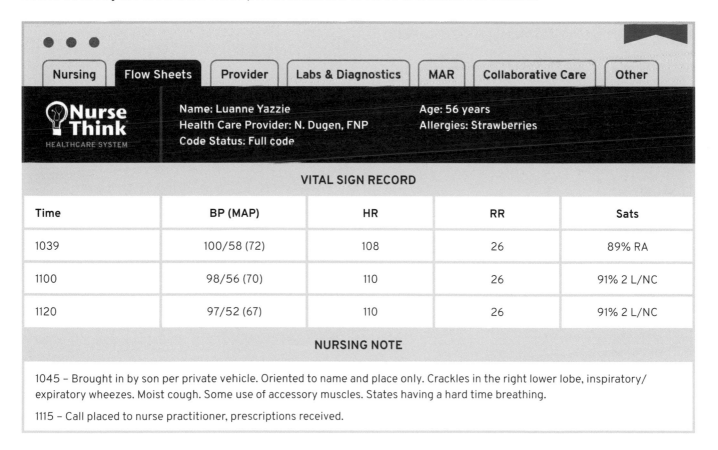

VITAL SIGN RECORD

Time	BP (MAP)	HR	RR	Sats
1039	100/58 (72)	108	26	89% RA
1100	98/56 (70)	110	26	91% 2 L/NC
1120	97/52 (67)	110	26	91% 2 L/NC

NURSING NOTE

1045 – Brought in by son per private vehicle. Oriented to name and place only. Crackles in the right lower lobe, inspiratory/expiratory wheezes. Moist cough. Some use of accessory muscles. States having a hard time breathing.

1115 – Call placed to nurse practitioner, prescriptions received.

17. With the current vital signs and assessment data, place the Top 3 Priority prescriptions in the order the nurse should initiate them. _____, _____, _____.

1. Cefuroxime 750 mg IVPB every 8 hours.

2. Albuterol 2.5 mg (0.5 mL of 0.5% diluted to 3 mL with sterile normal saline) every 3-4 hours and PRN per small volume nebulizer (SVN).

3. Methylprednisolone 125 mg IV every 12 hours.

4. IV fluids normal saline at 100 mL/hour.

5. Titrate O_2 to maintain saturations 93-95%.

6. Portable chest x-ray, STAT. Call results.

7. Sputum for culture.

8. Respiratory therapy consultation for chest physiotherapy (CPT).

9. Incentive spirometry every 1 hour.

18. Luanne's O_2 is increased to 3 L/NC. She's received a treatment of albuterol per small volume nebulizer (SVN) and chest physiotherapy (CPT) from the respiratory therapist. Her IV fluids have been initiated at 100 mL/hr. How will the nurse know if the treatments have been effective? Select all that apply.

1. O_2 saturation is 92%.

2. Respiratory rate is 24 breaths per minute.

3. She is coughing up yellow-green phlegm.

4. Heart rate is 112 beats per minute.

5. Blood pressure is 102/60 (74) mmHg.

Over the next 24 hours, Luanne's condition improves. Read the nurse's notes and answer the questions below.

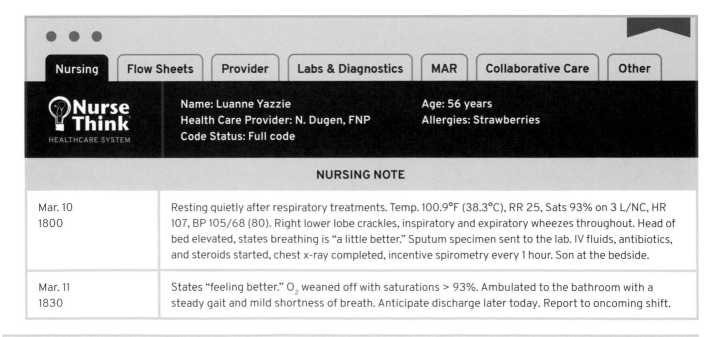

| | Nursing | Flow Sheets | Provider | Labs & Diagnostics | MAR | Collaborative Care | Other |

Nurse Think HEALTHCARE SYSTEM

Name: Luanne Yazzie
Health Care Provider: N. Dugen, FNP
Code Status: Full code

Age: 56 years
Allergies: Strawberries

NURSING NOTE

Mar. 10 1800	Resting quietly after respiratory treatments. Temp. 100.9°F (38.3°C), RR 25, Sats 93% on 3 L/NC, HR 107, BP 105/68 (80). Right lower lobe crackles, inspiratory and expiratory wheezes throughout. Head of bed elevated, states breathing is "a little better." Sputum specimen sent to the lab. IV fluids, antibiotics, and steroids started, chest x-ray completed, incentive spirometry every 1 hour. Son at the bedside.
Mar. 11 1830	States "feeling better." O_2 weaned off with saturations > 93%. Ambulated to the bathroom with a steady gait and mild shortness of breath. Anticipate discharge later today. Report to oncoming shift.

19. On the day of admission, what additional information would be most important for the nurse to document?

1. Urinary output.
2. Results of the sputum culture.
3. Orientation.
4. Last bowel movement.

The nurse reviews the oxygen titration record.

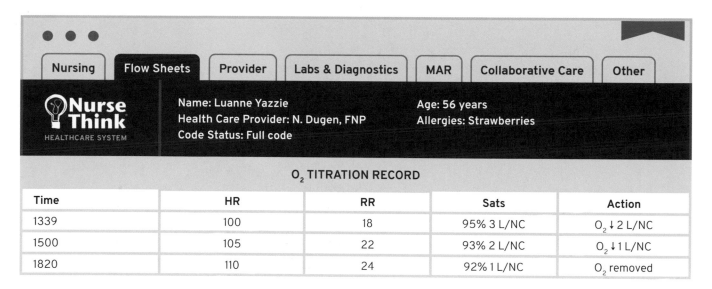

Nursing	Flow Sheets	Provider	Labs & Diagnostics	MAR	Collaborative Care	Other

Name: Luanne Yazzie
Health Care Provider: N. Dugen, FNP
Code Status: Full code

Age: 56 years
Allergies: Strawberries

O_2 TITRATION RECORD

Time	HR	RR	Sats	Action
1339	100	18	95% 3 L/NC	O_2 ↓ 2 L/NC
1500	105	22	93% 2 L/NC	O_2 ↓ 1 L/NC
1820	110	24	92% 1 L/NC	O_2 removed

20. The night nurse reviews the oxygen titration record. What evaluation can be made?

1. The nurse made the appropriate decisions about titration.
2. The client has become oxygen dependent.
3. The health care provider needs to be urgently notified.
4. The client is not ready to be without oxygen.

Clinical Hint: Identifying errors and evaluation of the effectiveness of a treatment is an important part of clinical judgment.

OXYGEN DELIVERY DEVICES

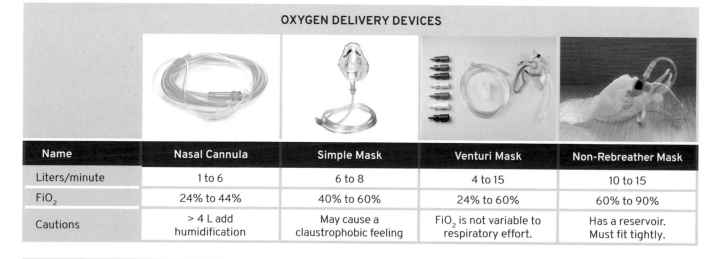

Name	Nasal Cannula	Simple Mask	Venturi Mask	Non-Rebreather Mask
Liters/minute	1 to 6	6 to 8	4 to 15	10 to 15
FiO_2	24% to 44%	40% to 60%	24% to 60%	60% to 90%
Cautions	> 4 L add humidification	May cause a claustrophobic feeling	FiO_2 is not variable to respiratory effort.	Has a reservoir. Must fit tightly.

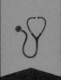

Go To Clinical Case

While caring for this client, be sure to review the concept maps in chapters 3 and 4.

Case 2: Impaired Oxygenation and Gas Exchange from Fluid Accumulation

Related Concepts: Comfort, Cellular Regulation, Nutrition, Protection
Threaded Concepts: Legal Issues, Communication, Delegation,
Medication Calculation, Use of Social Media

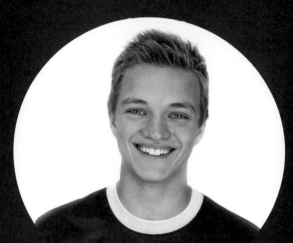

Eric Van Sickle is a 16-year-old with a history of Non-Hodgkin's Lymphoma. He was treated aggressively with chemotherapy and radiation and has been in remission for three years. He considers lymphoma a problem of the past and is working hard to live a healthy lifestyle. He sleeps 6-7 hours a night and eats a diet of lean proteins, fruits, and vegetables. He also commits to running 1-2 miles each morning. He is active at school, an honor student, and class president. He tells his mom that he is having trouble taking a deep breath, just over the last week. She makes a clinic appointment.

1. The admitting nurse assesses his oxygenation/gas exchange status. What should the nurse include? **Select all that apply.**

   1. Lung sounds.
   2. Oxygen saturation.
   3. Lymph node palpation.
   4. Capillary refill.
   5. Depth and symmetry of respiration.

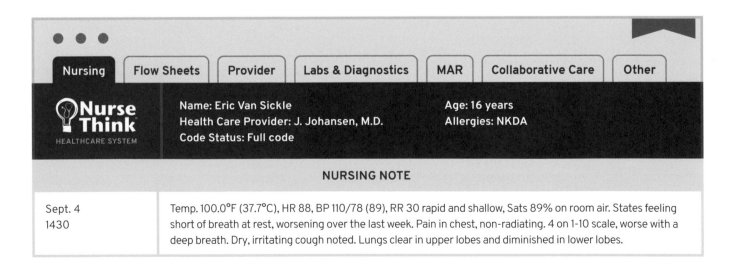

| Nursing | Flow Sheets | Provider | Labs & Diagnostics | MAR | Collaborative Care | Other |

NurseThink HEALTHCARE SYSTEM

Name: Eric Van Sickle
Health Care Provider: J. Johansen, M.D.
Code Status: Full code

Age: 16 years
Allergies: NKDA

NURSING NOTE

| Sept. 4 1430 | Temp. 100.0°F (37.7°C), HR 88, BP 110/78 (89), RR 30 rapid and shallow, Sats 89% on room air. States feeling short of breath at rest, worsening over the last week. Pain in chest, non-radiating. 4 on 1-10 scale, worse with a deep breath. Dry, irritating cough noted. Lungs clear in upper lobes and diminished in lower lobes. |

2. **The registered nurse reviews the assessment information. Which finding is most concerning?**
   1. Temperature, heart rate, blood pressure.
   2. Respiratory rate and oxygen saturation.
   3. Chest pain.
   4. Lung sounds.

3. **NurseThink® Prioritization Power!**
   Reflect on Eric's assessment data and identify the **Top 3 Priority** Interventions.

   1. _____

   2. _____

   3. _____

Eric's health care provider orders a chest x-ray. Review the report below.

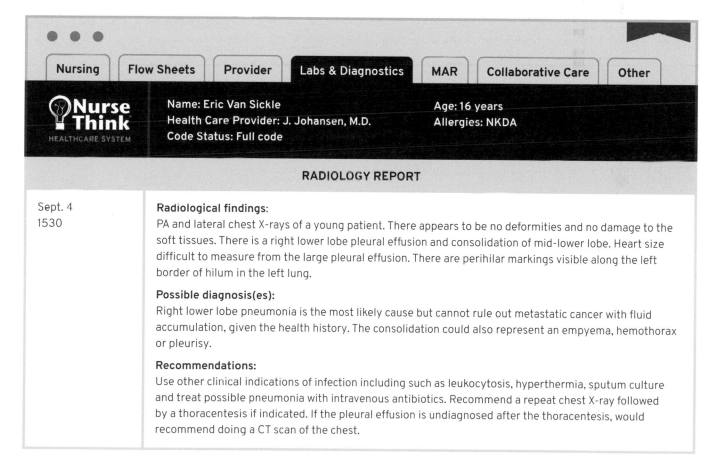

| Nursing | Flow Sheets | Provider | **Labs & Diagnostics** | MAR | Collaborative Care | Other |

Nurse Think HEALTHCARE SYSTEM

Name: Eric Van Sickle
Health Care Provider: J. Johansen, M.D.
Code Status: Full code

Age: 16 years
Allergies: NKDA

RADIOLOGY REPORT

Sept. 4
1530

Radiological findings:
PA and lateral chest X-rays of a young patient. There appears to be no deformities and no damage to the soft tissues. There is a right lower lobe pleural effusion and consolidation of mid-lower lobe. Heart size difficult to measure from the large pleural effusion. There are perihilar markings visible along the left border of hilum in the left lung.

Possible diagnosis(es):
Right lower lobe pneumonia is the most likely cause but cannot rule out metastatic cancer with fluid accumulation, given the health history. The consolidation could also represent an empyema, hemothorax or pleurisy.

Recommendations:
Use other clinical indications of infection including such as leukocytosis, hyperthermia, sputum culture and treat possible pneumonia with intravenous antibiotics. Recommend a repeat chest X-ray followed by a thoracentesis if indicated. If the pleural effusion is undiagnosed after the thoracentesis, would recommend doing a CT scan of the chest.

4. **What assumptions can the nurse make from the x-ray report?**
    1. Eric's lungs have an infection and should resolve with antibiotics.
    2. Additional tests are needed to determine the problem.
    3. Eric's x-ray is inadequate and needs to be repeated.
    4. Eric's x-ray report is normal.

5. **Given the information that the nurse knows about Eric's condition, which nursing intervention would be contraindicated?**
    1. Cough and deep breathing to increase expectoration.
    2. Increase oral fluids to liquefy secretions.
    3. Heating pad for chest wall pain.
    4. Ambulation to mobilize secretions.

After consulting a pulmonologist, Eric is admitted to the children's hospital for further workup. A thoracentesis is performed using IV conscious sedation in interventional radiology. He returns to the medical floor after the procedure.

Handoff Report

Eric Van Sickle received a thoracentesis under fluoroscopy where 800 mL cloudy pink fluid was removed from his right lower lobe and sent to the lab for cytology, and culture & sensitivity. He received midazolam 2 mg IV. His vital signs have been stable throughout the procedure. He's now on room air. He's arousable to touch. His parents are at the bedside.

6. **The nurse enters the room and notes that Eric's respirations are 10 per minute, even, and unlabored, the oxygen saturation reading is 99% and the head of the bed is flat. What should be the nurses next action?**
    1. Continue to allow him to sleep.
    2. Gently arouse him by touching his arm.
    3. Place him on oxygen.
    4. Raise the head of the bed.

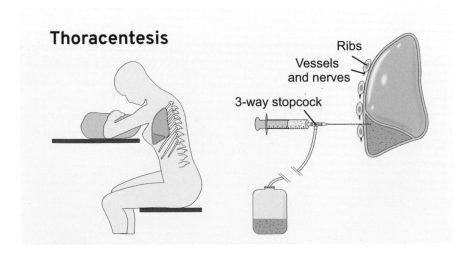

Over the next hour, the nurse records post-procedural care.

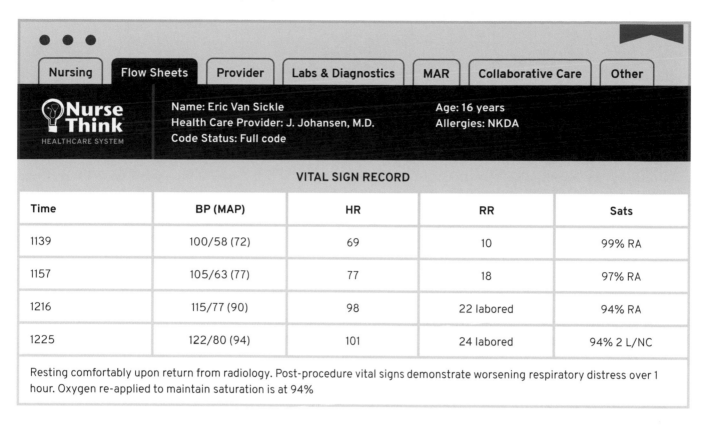

Time	BP (MAP)	HR	RR	Sats
1139	100/58 (72)	69	10	99% RA
1157	105/63 (77)	77	18	97% RA
1216	115/77 (90)	98	22 labored	94% RA
1225	122/80 (94)	101	24 labored	94% 2 L/NC

Resting comfortably upon return from radiology. Post-procedure vital signs demonstrate worsening respiratory distress over 1 hour. Oxygen re-applied to maintain saturation is at 94%

7. **Before the nurse contacts the health care provider, what additional assessments are priority? Select all that apply.**
   1. Auscultation of lung sounds.
   2. Assessment of thoracentesis dressing.
   3. Assessment for a tracheal shift.
   4. Measurement of urine output.
   5. Orientation to person, place, and time.

8. **After further assessment, the nurse discovers a tracheal shift to the left and absent breath sounds on the right side. A call is placed to the health care provider. Complete the communication form.**

S – _____

_____

B – _____

_____

A – _____

_____

R – _____

_____

Clinical Hint:
S - Situation
B - Background
A - Assessment
R - Recommendation

Next Gen Clinical Judgement: Practice giving this report to another person. Talk into a cell phone to make it more 'real'.

These verbal orders are received, and the provider says he will arrange with interventional radiology for a chest tube placement.

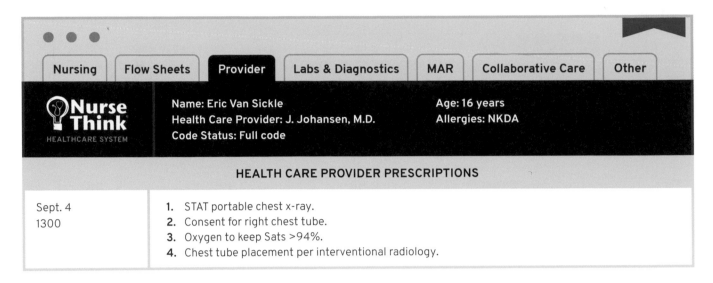

9. **The nurse returns to the room and finds Eric is anxious and afraid. His parents went to the cafeteria for a cup of coffee. The nurse needs to explain what is going on and obtain consent for the chest tube placement. How should the nurse proceed?**
   1. See if Eric has a sedative ordered.
   2. Tell him you will get his parents from the cafeteria.
   3. Explain the situation to Eric and obtain consent.
   4. Stay with Eric and send someone else to get his parents.

Once Eric's parents return to the room, the nurse pulls up a chair to the bedside, sits down, and explains the situation to the family. "Eric is having more difficulty breathing as you can see. We think he may have experienced a pneumothorax from the thoracentesis. I've spoken with the health care provider, and we are getting another x-ray. If it confirms a pneumothorax, Eric will need to have a chest tube with a closed chest drainage system. Here is the consent that you need to sign for the procedure. What questions do you have?"

10. **Critique how the nurse communicated with the family and determine what should/could have been done differently.**

   _____

   _____

   _____

11. **The x-ray showed a 70% pneumothorax, and a chest tube is placed. Eric returns to the floor with a right-sided 20 french chest tube connected to a chest tube drainage system at -20 cm H_2O of suction. Prioritize the sequence of assessments. _____, _____, _____, _____.**
   1. Drainage System: setting for suction, fluid in the collection chamber, bubbles in the water seal chamber.
   2. Respiratory Status: rate and depth, saturation level, lung sounds.
   3. Dressing: chest tube dressing intactness.
   4. Pain: discomfort in chest from tube.

The next day, the nurse is reviewing the chest tube assessment flow sheet for the previous 24 hours.

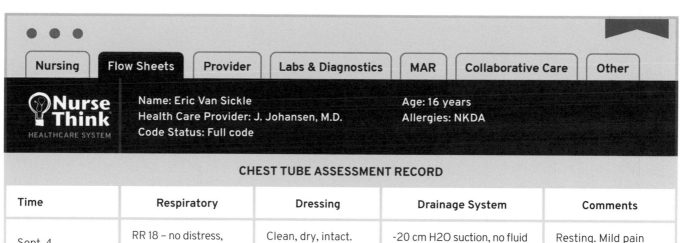

| Nursing | Flow Sheets | Provider | Labs & Diagnostics | MAR | Collaborative Care | Other |

NurseThink HEALTHCARE SYSTEM

Name: Eric Van Sickle
Health Care Provider: J. Johansen, M.D.
Code Status: Full code

Age: 16 years
Allergies: NKDA

CHEST TUBE ASSESSMENT RECORD

Time	Respiratory	Dressing	Drainage System	Comments
Sept. 4 1500	RR 18 – no distress, Sats 98% on RA, Lungs with RLL crackles	Clean, dry, intact. Pressure dressing secure	-20 cm H2O suction, no fluid in collection chamber, rare bubble in water seal chamber	Resting. Mild pain with movement 2/10
Sept. 4 2330	RR 16 – no distress, Sats 98% on RA, Lungs with RLL crackles	Clean, dry, intact. Pressure dressing secure	-20 cm H2O suction, 25 mL serous fluid in collection chamber, rare bubble in water seal chamber	Pain 4/10, medicated with PO pain med.
Sept. 5 0730	RR 18 – no distress, Sats 96% on RA, Lungs with RLL and LLL crackles	Clean, dry, intact. Pressure dressing rolling up around edges	-20 cm H2O suction, 75 mL serous fluid in collection chamber, occasional bubble in water seal chamber	Pain 5/10 with movement. Medicated with PO pain med. Ambulated in hall with 1 assist
Sept. 5 1450	RR 22. shallow, Sats 94% on RA, Lungs with crackles bilaterally	Clean, dry, intact. Pressure dressing loose around edges	-20 cm H2O suction, 175 mL serous fluid in collection chamber, occasional bubble in water seal chamber	Pain 7/10 with movement. States PO pain med is not helpful.

12. **THIN Thinking Time!**

    Reflect on the care of the chest tube over the last 24 hours and apply **THIN Thinking.**

    T – _____

    H – _____

    I – _____

    N – _____

T - Top 3
H - Help Quick
I - Identify Risk to Safety
N - Nursing Process

Scan to access the
10-Minute-Mentor →
on THIN Thinking.

NurseThink.com/THINThinking

13. **The nurse is evaluating the fluid within the collection chamber and the intermittent bubbling in the water seal chamber. What conclusion can be made?**

   1. The color of the fluid is concerning.
   2. The amount of the fluid is concerning.
   3. The bubbling is concerning.
   4. The findings are to be expected.

14. **The nurse identifies the need for several interventions. Which can be delegated to the UAP? Select all that apply.**

   1. Changing the chest tube dressing.
   2. Obtaining an incentive spirometer.
   3. Positioning the client for the dressing change.
   4. Obtaining pain medication.
   5. Instructing about the importance of taking deep breaths.

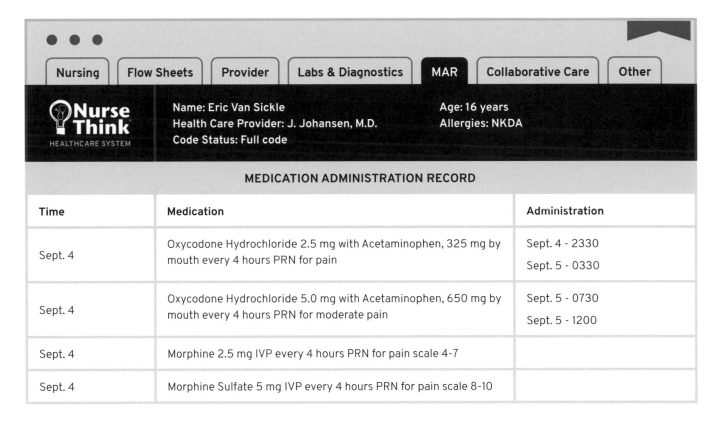

| Nursing | Flow Sheets | Provider | Labs & Diagnostics | MAR | Collaborative Care | Other |

Nurse Think HEALTHCARE SYSTEM

Name: Eric Van Sickle
Health Care Provider: J. Johansen, M.D.
Code Status: Full code

Age: 16 years
Allergies: NKDA

MEDICATION ADMINISTRATION RECORD

Time	Medication	Administration
Sept. 4	Oxycodone Hydrochloride 2.5 mg with Acetaminophen, 325 mg by mouth every 4 hours PRN for pain	Sept. 4 - 2330 Sept. 5 - 0330
Sept. 4	Oxycodone Hydrochloride 5.0 mg with Acetaminophen, 650 mg by mouth every 4 hours PRN for moderate pain	Sept. 5 - 0730 Sept. 5 - 1200
Sept. 4	Morphine 2.5 mg IVP every 4 hours PRN for pain scale 4-7	
Sept. 4	Morphine Sulfate 5 mg IVP every 4 hours PRN for pain scale 8-10	

15. **The nurse reviews the medication administration record to identify the best options for pain control. What consideration(s) are priority in making a safe decision? Select all that apply.**

   1. Risk of narcotic dependence.
   2. Adequate pain control.
   3. Compromised respiratory status.
   4. Last bowel movement.
   5. Acetaminophen dosing.

The nurse decides to deliver morphine sulfate (MS) 2.5 mg IVP for pain rated at a 6 on a 1-10 scale and re-evaluate the response after 15 minutes (peak time 20 minutes).

16. **The morphine pre-filled syringe includes morphine sulfate 5 mg in 2 mL of solution. The nurse draws up 2.5 mg, then further dilutes the MS to a total of 10 mL of solution. It is recommended that the dose of 2.5 mg be administered over 5 minutes. At what rate should the nurse deliver the IV push pain medicine?**

    _____ mL/minute

17. **After 15 minutes, the nurse performs an evaluation. Which finding will determine the medication was effective?**
    1. Pain is tolerable.
    2. Respiratory rate of 16 breaths per minute.
    3. Client is sleeping.
    4. Blood pressure is 110/67 (81) mmHg.

18. **The UAP tells the nurse that Eric has a temporal temperature of 100.4°F (38°C). What should be the nurse's next action?**
    1. Deliver a dose of acetaminophen.
    2. Ask the UAP to retake the temperature orally.
    3. Auscultate the lung sounds.
    4. Observe the chest tube collection chamber drainage.

19. **NurseThink® Prioritization Power!**
    Reflect on Eric's pulmonary status and identify the **Top 3 Priority** Respiratory Interventions.

    1. _____

    2. _____

    3. _____

20. **A couple of days later, Eric's chest tube was pulled, and he was ready for discharge. His cytology report came back positive for malignancy, and he was scheduled to see the oncologist the next day for treatment options. Eric asks the nurse if he can "friend" her on social media so they can stay in touch. How should the nurse respond?**
    1. "Sure, why not. I'd like to hear how you do with your cancer."
    2. "I'm not on social media."
    3. "It's not considered professional for me to "friend" my patients on social media."
    4. "Let me check with my manager; I'm not sure."

    Next Gen Clinical Judgment: The National Council State Boards of Nursing (NCSBN) has established guidelines about social media for nurses, as inappropriate posts by nurses have resulted in licensure and legal repercussions.

    Scan this QR code to watch a video about the policies of social media. www.ncsbn.org

Conceptual Debriefing & Case Reflection

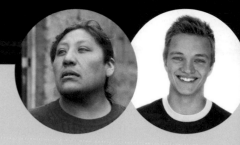

1. Compare the impaired respiration that Luanne Yazzie experienced with the impaired respiration of Eric Van Sickle. How are they the same and how are they different?

   _____

   _____

2. What was your single greatest learning moment while completing the case of Luanne Yazzie? What about Eric Van Sickle?

   _____

   _____

3. How did the nursing care provided to Luanne Yazzie and Eric Van Sickle change the outcome for each of them?

   _____

   _____

4. Identify safety concerns for both Luanne Yazzie and Eric Van Sickle for each case.

   _____

   _____

5. In what areas of each case study was basic care and comfort utilized?

   _____

   _____

6. What steps in each case did the nurse take that prevented hospital-acquired injury?

   _____

   _____

7. How did the nurse provide culturally sensitive/competent care?

   _____

   _____

8. How will learning about the case of Luanne Yazzie and Eric Van Sickle impact the care you provide for future clients?

   _____

Fundamental Quiz

1. The nurse is making rounds on a client after lunch. The client states, "It's strange, I feel like I cannot catch my breath." What should the nurse do next?
   1. Observe if the client shows signs of respiratory distress.
   2. Obtain an oxygen saturation reading.
   3. Auscultate the breath sounds.
   4. Reassure the client that they are all right.

2. While assessing a sleeping client with a closed head injury, the nurse notices that the breathing pattern is shallow and irregular. What should the nurse do next?
   1. Obtain an oxygen saturation reading to measure oxygenation.
   2. Call the health care provider to report the finding.
   3. Arouse the client to see if the pattern continues.
   4. Obtain a heart rate and blood pressure reading.

3. While assessing the client who feels short of breath the nurse finds this Information: respirations 22 breaths per minute and labored; oxygen saturation 93% on room air; bilateral crackles in the bases of the lungs. Which action should the nurse perform first?
   1. Apply oxygen at 2 L by cannula.
   2. Elevate the head of the bed.
   3. Deliver furosemide as ordered.
   4. Encourage the client to cough and deep breathe.

4. An older adult is admitted with a cough of thick yellow sputum, a fever and new onset of confusion. The nurse attempts to obtain an oxygen saturation reading and respiratory rate, but the combative client is uncooperative. How should the nurse proceed?
   1. Apply oxygen as ordered.
   2. Obtain orders to restrain the client.
   3. Leave the client alone until she is more cooperative.
   4. Obtain an order to sedate the client.

5. The nurse has finished delivering a bronchodilator via small volume nebulizer. Which documented assessment(s) indicates the treatment was effective? Select all that apply.

Time	BP (MAP)	HR	RR	Sat	Lung Sounds
Before Treatment	105/63 (77)	99	24	94% 2 L/NC	Expiratory Wheezes
After Treatment	118/70 (86)	112	20	94% 2 L/NC	Clear to Auscultation

   1. Blood pressure.
   2. Heart rate.
   3. Respiratory rate.
   4. Oxygen saturation.
   5. Lung sounds.

Advanced Quiz

6. The nurse is caring for a ventilated client. The ventilator settings are assist control (AC), 12; tidal volume (TV), 600; positive end-expiratory pressure (PEEP), 5; and FiO_2, 40%. The ventilator alarm begins to sound "low pressure." What should be the nurse's next action?
   1. Increase the FiO_2 to 50%.
   2. Decrease the PEEP to 3.
   3. Suction the client.
   4. Confirm that all connections are tight.

7. The family member of a client runs out of the room yelling, "Help! My dad is choking!" The nurse arrives in the room and finds the client unconscious and blue. Abdominal thrusts are quickly performed, and a piece of meat is removed from the client's mouth. The client's airway is opened, and the client begins to breathe on his own and responds slowly. What should the nurse do next?
   1. Apply 100% oxygen per non-rebreather mask.
   2. Place O_2 at 2 L/NC.
   3. No oxygen is needed.
   4. Obtain an oxygen saturation reading.

8. The nurse is caring for an older adult with neurological impairment who is receiving mechanical ventilation. Based on the information within the collaborative note, determine the category for each listed intervention.

COLLABORATIVE CARE NOTE	
Time	**Note**
0915	Albuterol 2.5 mg in 0.5 mL NS delivered via inline nebulizer. HR 110 after treatment, lungs with coarse crackles, oxygen saturation is 94%
0945	High-pressure alarms sounding, client coughing forcefully. Appears agitated. Oxygen saturation 89%.

Determine the priority for each option listed in the next table based on the following key:

> **Indicated:** an action that should be taken by the nurse.

> **Non-essential:** an action that the nurse could take that would not be harmful, but is not the priority at this time.

> **Contraindicated:** an action could harm the client.

	Indicated	Nonessential	Contraindicated
Suction the client			
Disconnect the ventilator and manually ventilate the client			
Determine if the client is biting on the endotracheal tube			
Request a chest x-ray			
Administer sedation			
Check the endotracheal cuff pressure			
Disconnect the tubing connection to the oxygen supply			

9. For each finding, select a potential action to take. There is only 1 priority action for each condition. Each potential action can only be used once. Not all potential actions are used.

Potential Action to Take	Finding	Priority Action
A. Chest tube	Oxygen saturation 88%	
B. Cough and deep breathing	Loose productive cough	
C. Intubation	Atelectasis	
D. Oxygen	Fine crackles in bilateral lung fields	
E. Diuretics	Tracheal shift	
F. Incentive spirometry	Apnea	
G. Percussion and postural drainage		

10. A client is admitted to the emergency department with severe flank pain. Vital signs include Temp. 101°F (38.3°C), HR 120, RR 28, and BP 81/50 (60) mmHg, oxygen saturation of 91%, pain of 9/10. What should the nurse do first?

   1. Begin IV fluid administration.
   2. Deliver oxygen.
   3. Pain control.
   4. Raise the head of the bed.

Regulation

Cellular / Intracranial / Thermo

Like homeostasis, regulation is a normal and automatic function within the body. The cells of the body work continually to maintain a stable internal environment of temperature, heart rate, respiratory rate, blood glucose levels, and blood pressure. Cellular regulation is maintained by the regulation of hormones and neurotransmitters. The growth and function of cells is an important part of this process. Intracranial regulation, for example, is the balance of mechanisms that protect the brain from toxins that cause injury, pressures, and chemicals.

Thermoregulation, on the other hand, includes the processes of sweating and shivering to maintain a normal body temperature. In this chapter, we will address patient cases of abnormal cell growth and intracranial pressure.

Next Gen Clinical Judgment:

> What observations can the nurse make with a client experiencing abnormal cellular, intracranial, and thermoregulation?

> How could abnormal cellular regulation impact thermoregulation?

> How could abnormal intracranial regulation impact thermoregulation?

> List nursing interventions for a client experiencing abnormal intracranial regulation.

_____

> List nursing interventions for a client experiencing abnormal thermoregulation.

_____

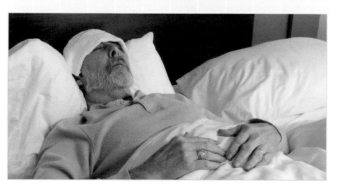

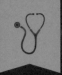
Case 1: Abnormal Cell Growth

Related Concepts: Adaptation: Coping, Emotion: Mood, Anxiety, Grief
Threaded Topics: Family Dynamics, Central Lines, Medications, Alternative and Complementary Therapies, Advanced Directives, End-of-life

Britta Nilsson is a 32-year-old female of Scandinavian descent. She has fair skin with freckles, blue eyes, and blonde hair. She has a slender build. Many of her summer vacations as a teen were spent at the ocean shore, enjoying the salty water and sandy beaches. This is where she met her husband. Jim and Britta have been married for 12 years and have 3 children, Erik, Caryn, and Andrea. They live in a large metropolitan city where Britta works in a chemical plant as a chemist.

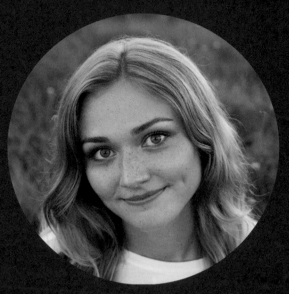

She smokes two cigarettes a day, but only as a stress release at work. Britta is diligent about getting an annual physical examination by her health care provider, mostly because her mother died of cancer at an early age. Twice in the past five years, she's had a mole removed, both being benign. She sees this as a nuisance but she's not concerned.

1. **Which non-controllable risk factor(s) does Britta have for abnormal cell growth? Select all that apply.**
   1. Her Scandinavian heritage.
   2. Fair skin with freckles.
   3. Family history of cancer.
   4. Blue eyes.
   5. Blonde hair.

2. **Which lifestyle decision(s) increase(s) her risk for abnormal cell growth? Select all that apply.**
   1. Vacations on the beach.
   2. Metropolitan living.
   3. Chemical exposure.
   4. Cigarette smoke.
   5. Mole removal.

Britta noticed a strange freckle on her back that seemed to look different than it used to. Anticipating that is was nothing important, she chose to continue to watch it. Seven months later during her annual physical, her health care provider asked about it.

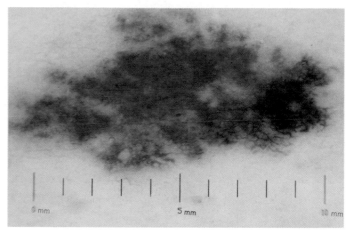

Image: Measured in milliliters (mm).

3. Match the assessment descriptions of a skin lesion on the left, to the correct definition on the right.

Description:	Definition:
_____Asymmetry	1. Size.
_____Border	2. Outline of the lesion.
_____Color	3. Changes over time.
_____Diameter	4. Shape and/or pattern of the lesion.
_____Evolving	5. Shade of darkness.

4. How should the nurse document Britta's lesion?

_____

_____

_____

5. Which observations of Britta's mole would alert the nurse that it could be cancerous? Select all that apply.
   1. Regular symmetry.
   2. Irregular border.
   3. Varying shades of light and dark brown.
   4. 3 mm in diameter.
   5. Itchy.

Clinical Hint: Often, clients are not able to see skin changes in 'hidden' areas of the body. Nurses should observe for abnormal lesions with each assessment. Do not assume that the client is aware of the abnormality.

Next Gen Clinical Judgment: Perform an Internet search for abnormal skin lesion and describe 5 images you observe. Describe them using the 5 descriptions discussed.

The mole is removed, and the tissue is sent for pathology.

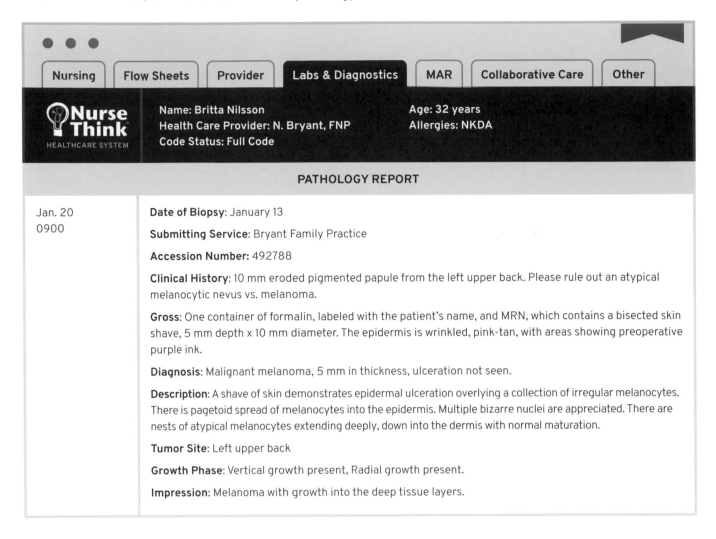

Nursing | Flow Sheets | Provider | **Labs & Diagnostics** | MAR | Collaborative Care | Other

NurseThink
HEALTHCARE SYSTEM

Name: Britta Nilsson
Health Care Provider: N. Bryant, FNP
Code Status: Full Code

Age: 32 years
Allergies: NKDA

PATHOLOGY REPORT

Jan. 20
0900

Date of Biopsy: January 13

Submitting Service: Bryant Family Practice

Accession Number: 492788

Clinical History: 10 mm eroded pigmented papule from the left upper back. Please rule out an atypical melanocytic nevus vs. melanoma.

Gross: One container of formalin, labeled with the patient's name, and MRN, which contains a bisected skin shave, 5 mm depth x 10 mm diameter. The epidermis is wrinkled, pink-tan, with areas showing preoperative purple ink.

Diagnosis: Malignant melanoma, 5 mm in thickness, ulceration not seen.

Description: A shave of skin demonstrates epidermal ulceration overlying a collection of irregular melanocytes. There is pagetoid spread of melanocytes into the epidermis. Multiple bizarre nuclei are appreciated. There are nests of atypical melanocytes extending deeply, down into the dermis with normal maturation.

Tumor Site: Left upper back

Growth Phase: Vertical growth present, Radial growth present.

Impression: Melanoma with growth into the deep tissue layers.

---

6. **From the pathology report, what assumptions can be made?**
    1. Britta should not be concerned; the mole is benign.
    2. The tissue is cancerous and requires further diagnostic testing for metastasis.
    3. The cancerous tissue is contained and not a threat.
    4. The report is not conclusive.

Britta is asked to return to the provider's office with her husband. The news is delivered that the mole is malignant melanoma, the deadliest form of skin cancer and it has invaded the underlying tissue. Additional tests are needed to determine if the cancer has spread to other areas of the body and if it has, they will be referred to an oncologist for further treatment. Jim and Britta are devastated and terrified.

Weeks later, Britta and Jim learn that Britta's cancer is in Stage IV, in the lymph nodes with metastasis to both the lungs and the brain. Immunotherapy will be started, followed by aggressive chemotherapy if there is no response. Britta asks what her prognosis is but the oncologist avoids the question, saying every case is different. This makes Britta even more afraid.

7. On the way out of the office, Britta asks the nurse why the doctor did not give her a specific prognosis. How should the nurse respond?

   1. "I'm sure you will be fine, I wouldn't worry about it."
   2. "He's that way with everyone; you are not unique."
   3. "I can see this is bothering you; let's go back and ask him again."
   4. "Do an internet search when you get home; you can find the answer."

8. Britta is immediately placed on immunotherapy. The provider suggests a combination therapy of anti-PD-1 and anti-CTLA4 antibodies. During instructions about the new medications, Britta is confused and asks if immunotherapy is the same as chemotherapy. Which statement by the nurse is correct?

   1. "Immunotherapy is safer than chemotherapy in killing the unhealthy cells."
   2. "Immunotherapy is given before chemotherapy to decrease the side effects."
   3. "Immunotherapy strengthens the body to heal itself."
   4. "Immunotherapy suppresses the body to create better outcomes from chemotherapy."

9. After three months of immunotherapy, Britta's tumors in her lungs and brain continue to grow. The oncologists decide to implant a long-term central catheter and begin chemotherapy. Britta shares with the nurse that her husband has immersed himself into work and won't share his feelings with her, the kids are acting out and, she feels depressed all of the time. Which resource(s) should the nurse provide? Select all that apply.

   1. Hospice services.
   2. Dietary counseling.
   3. Palliative care services.
   4. Family counseling.
   5. Cancer support group.

10. Britta has a tunneled, implanted port placed in her left upper chest. Explain what actions the nurse needs to take and why.

   _____   _____
   _____
   _____
   _____
   _____

11. NurseThink® Prioritization Power!
    Evaluate the information in the image above and pick the **Top 3 Priority** actions.

    1. _____
    2. _____
    3. _____

12. **Britta begins chemotherapy that includes dacarbazine and temozolomide. The nurse reviews the medications given to minimize the side effects of the chemotherapy. Complete the colored boxes in the chart below.**

Medication	Dose, Route, Frequency	Purpose	Drug Class	Patient Teaching
Ondansetron	8 mg orally twice a day	Nausea	5-ht3 antagonist	
Filgrastim	5 mcg/kg/day subcutaneously, in a single-dose, daily	Increase the number of white blood cells		Report any signs of allergic reaction or shortness of breath. Must come to the clinic daily for injection. Report pain in the left upper stomach or left shoulder. Report signs of infection.
Epoetin Alfa	50 units/kg subcutaneously 3 times weekly		Erythropoiesis-stimulating agents	Report any signs of allergic reaction. Monitor for signs of clot formation. Report a high blood pressure.
Lorazepam	0.5 mg orally twice a day as needed		Benzodiazepines	May make you sleepy and lethargic. Do not drive after taking. Can slow respirations. Follow instructions and do not exceed dose.

13. **Britta asks the nurse about complementary and alternative therapies. Connect the therapy to its description.**

Therapy	Description
_____Meditation	1. State of human consciousness involving focused attention and reduced peripheral awareness and an enhanced capacity to respond to suggestion.
_____Aromatherapy	2. Herb that is believed to improve mental functioning.
_____Acupuncture	3. Therapies are based on complex herbal compounds, minerals, and metal substances, originating in India.
_____Ginkgo	4. Mind-body intervention by which a trained practitioner helps a patient to generate mental images that simulate positive sensory perception.
_____Ayurveda	5. Holistic system of coordinated body posture and movement, breathing, and meditation used for the purposes of health, spirituality, and martial arts training.
_____Tai chi	6. Martial art that uses the forces of the yin and yang for its health benefits.
_____Qigong	7. Thin needles are inserted into the body to alter neuropathways.
_____Guided imagery	8. Uses plant materials and aromatic plant oils, including essential oils, and other aroma compounds to improve well-being.
_____Hypnosis	9. Believed to be a medicinal herb with antidepressant activity.
_____St. John's Wort	10. The use of hands-on healing through which a "universal energy" is transferred through the palms of the practitioner to the patient for healing.
_____Reiki	11. Focusing the mind on a particular object, thought or activity, to achieve a mentally clear and emotionally calm state.

Three weeks after the start of the chemotherapy, Britta feels so tired and weak she has a hard time getting out of bed each day. The provider orders blood work.

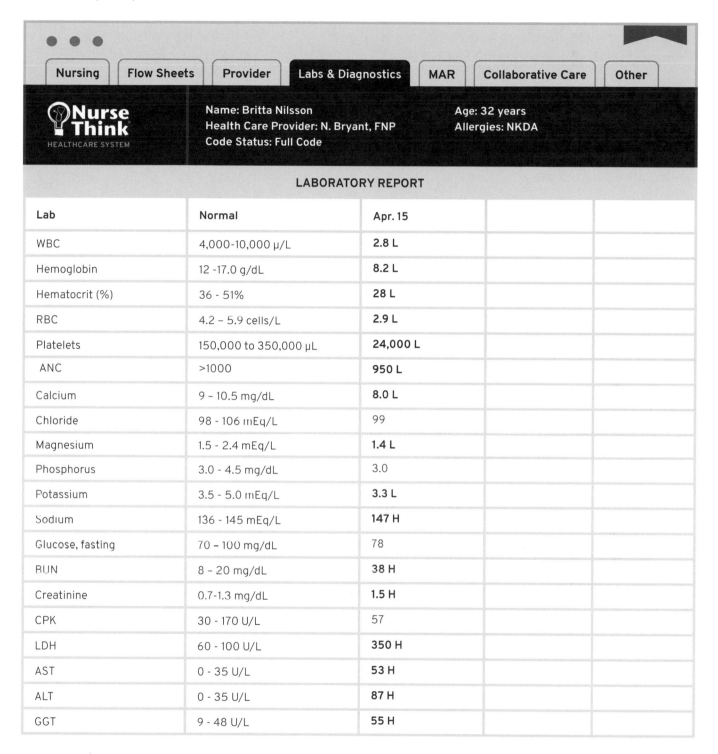

| Nursing | Flow Sheets | Provider | Labs & Diagnostics | MAR | Collaborative Care | Other |

NurseThink HEALTHCARE SYSTEM

Name: Britta Nilsson
Health Care Provider: N. Bryant, FNP
Code Status: Full Code

Age: 32 years
Allergies: NKDA

LABORATORY REPORT

Lab	Normal	Apr. 15		
WBC	4,000-10,000 µ/L	2.8 L		
Hemoglobin	12 -17.0 g/dL	8.2 L		
Hematocrit (%)	36 - 51%	28 L		
RBC	4.2 – 5.9 cells/L	2.9 L		
Platelets	150,000 to 350,000 µL	24,000 L		
ANC	>1000	950 L		
Calcium	9 – 10.5 mg/dL	8.0 L		
Chloride	98 - 106 mEq/L	99		
Magnesium	1.5 - 2.4 mEq/L	1.4 L		
Phosphorus	3.0 - 4.5 mg/dL	3.0		
Potassium	3.5 - 5.0 mEq/L	3.3 L		
Sodium	136 - 145 mEq/L	147 H		
Glucose, fasting	70 – 100 mg/dL	78		
BUN	8 – 20 mg/dL	38 H		
Creatinine	0.7-1.3 mg/dL	1.5 H		
CPK	30 - 170 U/L	57		
LDH	60 - 100 U/L	350 H		
AST	0 - 35 U/L	53 H		
ALT	0 - 35 U/L	87 H		
GGT	9 - 48 U/L	55 H		

14. **Which body system(s) is/are identified as being impacted by the illness and treatment? Select all that apply.**
    1. Kidneys.
    2. Liver.
    3. Heart.
    4. Bone marrow.
    5. Pancreas.

> **Clinical Hint:** You can make learning labs easier by grouping them by body system.

15. **Which assessment finding by the nurse is most concerning?**

    1. Bleeding gums when brushing teeth.
    2. Temperature of 100.1°F (37.8°C).
    3. Decreased urine output to 50 mL per hour.
    4. Sleepy but arousable.

16. **Based on the lab report, Britta is admitted to the hospital's oncology unit. Which precautions should the nurse implement upon admission? Select all that apply.**

    1. Neutropenic precautions.
    2. Bleeding precautions.
    3. Contact precautions.
    4. Fall precautions.
    5. Seizure precautions.

17. **As Britta is sleeping, Jim pulls the nurse aside and says, "I just don't know what I will do if she doesn't make it. I don't think I can raise three kids without her, what will I do?" How should the nurse reply?**

    1. "Lots of dads are single parents; I'm sure you will be great at it!"
    2. "Do you have other family that could raise the kids for you?"
    3. "What support systems do you have?"
    4. "How old are your children?"

18. **Britta continues to get weaker as she develops a pulmonary infection. The family considers placing her under the care of hospice. Jim says that Britta is asking to see Erik, Caryn, and Andrea in the hospital. He says "she looks so bad, I don't want the kids to be frightened." What suggestion should the nurse give?**

    1. Place an infection control mask on Britta so the children won't be afraid.
    2. Talk to the children ahead of time about what to expect.
    3. Wait until she gets to hospice to visit.
    4. Encourage Jim to take pictures rather than bringing them to the hospital.

19. **The nurse approaches Jim to ask if he or Britta have ever discussed advanced directives. Jim asks what that is. How should the nurse describe this?**

    1. It gives verbal directions for her care at the end-of-life.
    2. It is a legal document that directs her end-of-life wishes if she is not able.
    3. It makes her a do-not-resuscitate (DNR) should her heart stop.
    4. It will automatically place her under the care of hospice.

20. **Britta takes her final breath under the care of hospice with her husband, children, parents, and siblings by her side. Her family asks if they can donate her organs, so "something good" can come from this horrific tragedy. How should the nurse respond?**

    1. "She's not a candidate since she has cancer. They won't be able to use anything."
    2. "Her organs cannot be donated after death; that needs to be determined ahead of her death."
    3. "I'll contact the tissue and organ bank to see if there are any organs they are able to take."
    4. "You cannot have an open casket after organ donation; are you sure you want to do that?"

Go To Clinical Case

While caring for this client, be sure to review the concept maps in chapters 3 and 4.

Case 2: Intracranial Regulation with Brain Injury

Adaptation: Emotion: Grief, Cognition: Cognitive Functioning, Emotion: Anxiety, Grief, Adaptation: Coping, Movement: Nerve Conduction
Threaded Topics: Family Dynamics, Advanced Directives, Seizures

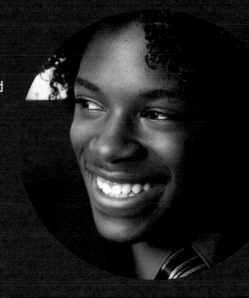

Lakisha Johnson will never forget the day her son's life changed forever. Just three days ago, her only son, Jordan was involved in a head-on collision by a drunk driver while coming home from work after a 12-hour night shift. "Jordan is such a great kid. He graduated from high school last June and got hired into the automobile factory right away. He was so excited to get his own apartment and recently started dating a sweet girl. No one deserves this, especially not him." Jordan lays still in the bed next to her with the sound of the ventilator breathing for him.

Jordan, a 19-year-old, was captain of his high school football team. Over the years he took multiple helmet-to-helmet hits, experiencing three concussions. One experience during his senior year caused him to be unconscious for 15 minutes. Lakisha felt helpless on the sidelines as the ambulance took him away.

1. As the nurse assessing Jordan in the emergency room, which finding(s) is/are consistent with a concussion from a football injury? Select all that apply.

    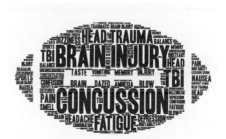

    1. Loss of consciousness.
    2. Blurred vision.
    3. Headache.
    4. Nausea and vomiting.
    5. Hypertension.

2. How should the nurse describe a concussion to Lakisha?

    1. A decrease in blood flow to the brain causing cell death.
    2. Rapid movement of the brain which can stretch and damage brain cells.
    3. Small areas of arterial bleeding upon the brain's surface.
    4. Deep hemorrhages within the brainstem.

3. Lakisha tells the nurse that Jordan experienced post-concussion syndrome after his concussion. Which symptoms typically support this diagnosis?

    1. Lethargy, depression, and a flat affect.
    2. Anxiety, insomnia, and migraines.
    3. Confusion, difficulty speaking, and tinnitus.
    4. Mental alertness, hyperactivity, and restlessness.

As Lakisha reminisces about his years playing football, she says, "At the time I thought that it was so painful and unfair that Jordan had to experience that. I now realize that this head injury from the automobile accident is much worse! I wish that Jordan would wake up and come off the breathing machine."

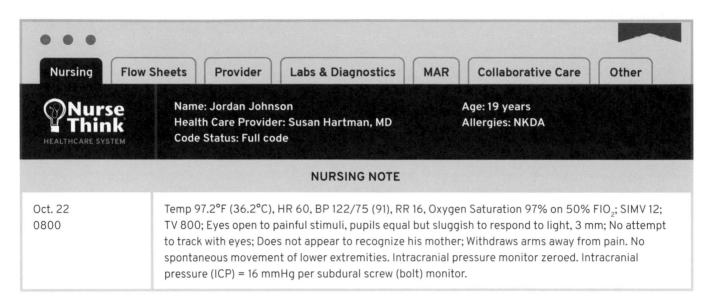

| | Nursing | Flow Sheets | Provider | Labs & Diagnostics | MAR | Collaborative Care | Other |

NurseThink HEALTHCARE SYSTEM

Name: Jordan Johnson
Health Care Provider: Susan Hartman, MD
Code Status: Full code

Age: 19 years
Allergies: NKDA

NURSING NOTE

| Oct. 22 0800 | Temp 97.2°F (36.2°C), HR 60, BP 122/75 (91), RR 16, Oxygen Saturation 97% on 50% FIO_2; SIMV 12; TV 800; Eyes open to painful stimuli, pupils equal but sluggish to respond to light, 3 mm; No attempt to track with eyes; Does not appear to recognize his mother; Withdraws arms away from pain. No spontaneous movement of lower extremities. Intracranial pressure monitor zeroed. Intracranial pressure (ICP) = 16 mmHg per subdural screw (bolt) monitor. |

4. The nurse completes the neurological assessment on Jordan. How should the nurse rate his condition using the Glasgow Coma Scale (GCS)?

   1. 3
   2. 5
   3. 7
   4. 9

Behavior	Response	
Eye-Opening	4. Spontaneously 3. To speech 2. To pain 1. No response	
Verbal	5. Oriented to time, person and place 4. Confused 3. Inappropriate words 2. Incomprehensible sounds 1. No response	**Total Score** Best Score: 15 Comatose: 8 or less Unresponsive: 3
Motor	6. Obeys command 5. Moves to localized pain 4. Flex to withdraw from pain 3. Abnormal flexion 2. Abnormal extension 1. No response	

5. **What assumptions can the nurse make, based on the GCS?**
    1. The number fluctuates hourly and is inaccurate.
    2. The number shows a minimal amount of brain damage.
    3. Jordan's number correlates with severe brain injury.
    4. Jordan will likely make a full recovery.

Next Gen Clinical Judgment: Contrast assessment findings of increased intracranial pressure in the infant, toddler, school-aged, teenaged, adult, and older adult client.

6. **The nurse recognizes the signs of increased intracranial pressure from the baseline assessment. Which assessment finding(s) support(s) this assumption? Select all that apply.**
    1. Heart rate 58 beats per minute.
    2. Widened pulse pressure.
    3. Decreased mental abilities.
    4. Intracranial pressure of 16 mmHg.
    5. Temperature.

7. **NurseThink® Prioritization Power!**

    Reflect on Jordan's assessment findings and identify the **Top 3 Priority** actions the nurse should take.

    1. _____

    2. _____

    3. _____

8. **The nurse has each of these medications prescribed. Which medication should the nurse hold and why?**
    1. Mannitol 5% 1.5 g/kg IV infused over 30-60 minutes.
    2. Phenobarbital 2 mg/kg/day IV.
    3. Acetaminophen 650 mg PR.
    4. Labetalol 20 mg IV.

    Why should the medication be held? _____

9. **The nurse is reflecting on possible complications of the bolt intracranial pressure monitor. What should be the nurses highest concern?**
    1. Fever of 101.6°F (38.6°C).
    2. Mean arterial pressure of 67 mmHg.
    3. Clear drainage at the insertion site.
    4. Urine output changes from 35 mL/ hour to 40 mL/hour.

Over the next few hours, the nurse continues to monitor Jordan closely.

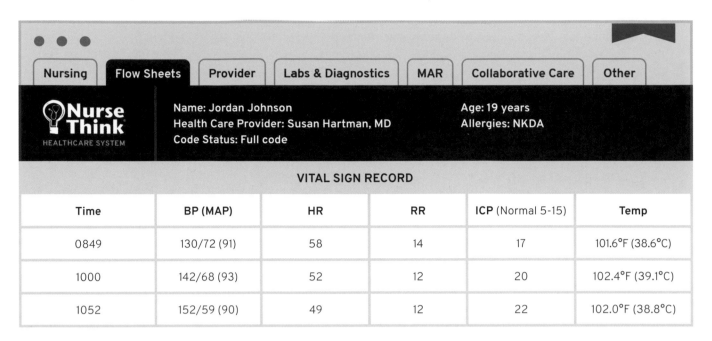

Time	BP (MAP)	HR	RR	ICP (Normal 5-15)	Temp
0849	130/72 (91)	58	14	17	101.6°F (38.6°C)
1000	142/68 (93)	52	12	20	102.4°F (39.1°C)
1052	152/59 (90)	49	12	22	102.0°F (38.8°C)

VITAL SIGN RECORD

Name: Jordan Johnson
Health Care Provider: Susan Hartman, MD
Code Status: Full code
Age: 19 years
Allergies: NKDA

10. **Calculate Jordan's Cerebral Perfusion Pressure (MAP – ICP = CPP).**

0849 = _____

1000 = _____

1052 = _____

11. **The health care provider would like Jordan's CPP to be > 70 mmHg to maintain adequate perfusion to his traumatized brain tissue. Was this sustained during this time?**

   1. Yes.

   2. No.

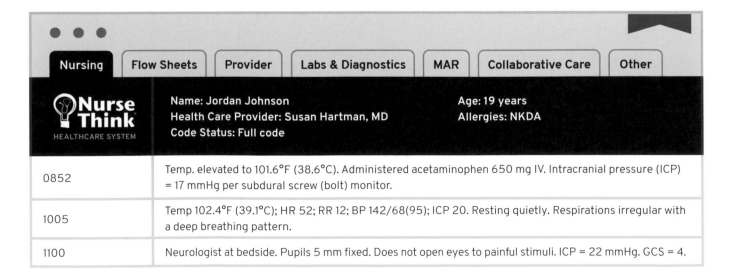

Name: Jordan Johnson
Health Care Provider: Susan Hartman, MD
Code Status: Full code
Age: 19 years
Allergies: NKDA

0852	Temp. elevated to 101.6°F (38.6°C). Administered acetaminophen 650 mg IV. Intracranial pressure (ICP) = 17 mmHg per subdural screw (bolt) monitor.
1005	Temp 102.4°F (39.1°C); HR 52; RR 12; BP 142/68(95); ICP 20. Resting quietly. Respirations irregular with a deep breathing pattern.
1100	Neurologist at bedside. Pupils 5 mm fixed. Does not open eyes to painful stimuli. ICP = 22 mmHg. GCS = 4.

12. THIN Thinking Time!

Reflect on the information the nurse has collected and apply **THIN Thinking.**

T – _____

H – _____

I – _____

N – _____

T - Top 3
H - Help Quick
I - Identify Risk to Safety
N - Nursing Process

Scan to access the
10-Minute-Mentor →
on THIN Thinking.

NurseThink.com/THINThinking

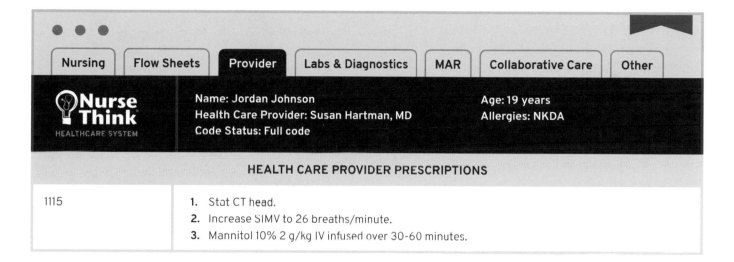

Nursing	Flow Sheets	Provider	Labs & Diagnostics	MAR	Collaborative Care	Other

Nurse Think
HEALTHCARE SYSTEM

Name: Jordan Johnson
Health Care Provider: Susan Hartman, MD
Code Status: Full code

Age: 19 years
Allergies: NKDA

HEALTH CARE PROVIDER PRESCRIPTIONS

1115	1. Stat CT head.
	2. Increase SIMV to 26 breaths/minute.
	3. Mannitol 10% 2 g/kg IV infused over 30-60 minutes.

13. In what order should the nurse perform the provider's prescriptions? _____, _____, _____.

    1. Stat CT head.
    2. Increase SIMV to 26 breaths/minute.
    3. Mannitol 10% 2 g/kg IV infused over 30-60 minutes.

14. The nurse returns to the unit with Jordan after the CT scan. The radiologist told the nurse that the scan shows a herniation of the brainstem. The prognosis is very poor. Lakisha is waiting in his room and asks the nurse what the CT scan shows. How should the nurse answer her question?

    1. "The report is very bad; you'll have to talk to the neurologist."
    2. "I'm not sure."
    3. "The radiologist will need to read the scan before we know anything."
    4. "I asked the neurologist to come and speak with you so you can get some answers."

15. The neurologist comes to the unit to talk to Jordan's mother. He begins to speak to Lakisha at the bedside. What action should the nurse take?

    1. Offer for them to go to a private family waiting area.
    2. Stay at the beside and listen to what the neurologist has to say.
    3. Give them some privacy by pulling the curtain.
    4. Ask if they'd like a hospital chaplain to be present.

16. After speaking with the neurologist, Lakisha shares that she feels empty and alone and doesn't feel she can live without Jordan. She is terrified of losing her only son. How should the nurse respond?

    1. "Do you have other children besides Jordan?"
    2. "Do you feel you may hurt yourself?"
    3. "I can see how much you love your son."
    4. "Tell me more about what Jordan means to you."

17. Later that shift, Lakisha yells out to the nurse, "Something is wrong, come quick." As the nurse enters the room, she sees that Jordan is having a clonic-tonic seizure. What observations led the nurse to think this? Select all that apply.

    1. Stiff, jerky movements.
    2. Fluttering eye-opening.
    3. Biting on the endotracheal tube.
    4. Loss of bowel control.
    5. Irregular heart rhythm.

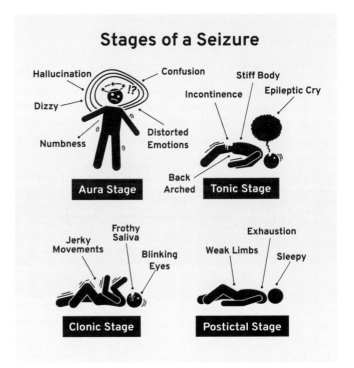

Stages of a Seizure

18. What should the nurse prioritize upon entering the room?

    1. Getting Lakisha out of the room.
    2. Calling for more help.
    3. Protecting Jordan from injury.
    4. Silencing the ventilator alarms.

19. NurseThink® Prioritization Power!

    What are the **Top 3 Priority** actions the nurse should take after protecting Jordan from injury?

    1. _____

    2. _____

    3. _____

20. After the seizure is over, the nurse cleans Jordan up and changes his bedding. What should the nurse document? Select all that apply.

    1. Type of body movement observed.
    2. Length of the seizure.
    3. Medications given to shorten the seizure.
    4. Any injuries that occurred during the seizure.
    5. Who was in the room during the seizure.

Conceptual Debriefing & Case Reflection

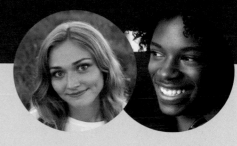

1. Compare the impaired regulation that Britta Nilsson experienced with the impaired regulation of Jordan Johnson. How are they the same and how are they different?

   _____

   _____

2. What was your single greatest learning moment while completing the case of Britta Nilsson? What about Jordan Johnson?

   _____

   _____

3. How did the nursing care provided to Britta Nilsson and Jordan Johnson change the outcome for each of them?

   _____

   _____

4. Identify safety concerns for both Britta Nilsson and Jordan Johnson for each case.

   _____

   _____

5. In what areas of each case study was basic care and comfort utilized?

   _____

   _____

6. What steps in each case did the nurse take that prevented hospital-acquired injury?

   _____

   _____

7. How did the nurse provide culturally sensitive/competent care?

   _____

   _____

8. How will learning about the case of Britta Nilsson and Jordan Johnson impact the care you provide for future clients?

   _____

   _____

Fundamental Quiz

1. The nurse checks a client's temperature using an oral, electronic thermometer. The morning temperature is 96.0°F (35.5°C), and the other vital signs are within the normal range. What should the nurse do next?
   1. Check the client's temperature history.
   2. Document the results; the temperature is normal.
   3. Check the temperature again.
   4. Get another thermometer, since the temperature is an error.

2. The nurse is caring for a client with a blood cancer. The client states, "I have twice the number of bruises today than I had yesterday." What action should the nurse take next?
   1. Evaluate the morning lab report.
   2. Document the number of bruises that the client has.
   3. Outline the bruises with a marker.
   4. Implement bleeding precautions.

3. The nurse is caring for a client with a high hemoglobin and hematocrit level from lung disease. Which statement by the client is most concerning?
   1. "I have a tender spot behind my left knee."
   2. "I get short of breath when climbing the stairs."
   3. "I need to drink more water each day."
   4. "I've cut my smoking down to 1 cigarette each day."

4. The nurse sees a UAP enter a client's room who is neutropenic without a mask. What should the nurse do?
   1. Assume the client is no longer on precautions.
   2. Report the incident to the charge nurse.
   3. Speak directly to the UAP about the observation.
   4. Continue to watch the UAP to see if the behavior is repeated.

5. A school nurse is told that the parent of a student said, "I feel like I'm going to have another seizure." What should the school nurse do next?
   1. Call 9-1-1.
   2. Determine if the parent is in a safe environment.
   3. Ask the parent to go to the hospital.
   4. Perform a physical assessment on the parent.

Advanced Quiz

6. The nurse is caring for an unidentified client who was found unresponsive in the back seat of a car in the summer. The client's core temperature is 106.9°F (41.1°C). What is the nurse's priority?
   1. Determine the client's identity.
   2. Find the client's next of kin to obtain a code status.
   3. Cool the body temperature to an acceptable number.
   4. Secure the airway.

7. The nurse is speaking with her neighbor who shares that her mother died at a young age from cancer of the "female parts." What additional question is most important for the nurse ask?
   1. "Which "female parts" were those?"
   2. "Did you know that female organ cancers are sometimes genetic?"
   3. "Do you have routine exams for cancer?"
   4. "How old was your mother when she died?"

8. A teenager with an absolute neutrophil count (ANC) of zero is exhausted and nauseated. Which nursing action(s) is/are priority? Select all that apply.
   1. Administer antiemetics.
   2. Complete a nutrition and hydration assessment.
   3. Limit visitors to two at a time.
   4. Place in a positive pressure room.
   5. Assess for sources of bleeding.
   6. Begin energy-conserving techniques.

9. The nurse receives hand-off report on each of these clients. Which client should the nurse assess first?
   1. 6-month-old with neutropenia and a temperature of 101.7°F (38.7°C).
   2. 17-year-old who is receiving the second dose of chemotherapy for bone cancer.
   3. 42-year-old with petechiae all over the abdomen and back.
   4. 80-year-old with a hemoglobin of 6.5 g/dL.

10. Place the actions on the left next to the correct condition on the right. Not all actions will be used. Each condition only has one best answer.

Action	Condition
1. Deliver nonsteroidal anti-inflammatory medications.	_____ Anemia
2. Administer intravenous fluids.	_____ Hypothermia
3. Deliver packed red blood cells.	_____ Polycythemia
4. Apply warmed blankets.	_____ Hyperthermia
5. Seizure precautions.	_____ Thrombocytopenia
6. Initiate bleeding precautions.	_____ Leukopenia
7. Initiate neutropenic precautions.	_____ Increased intracranial pressure
8. Administer pain medication.	
9. Initiate strict intake and output.	

Nutrition

Digestion / Elimination

The digestive system includes the digestive tract and its accessory organs. This consists of the structures of the mouth, pharynx, esophagus, stomach, small, and large intestines. Additionally, the salivary glands, liver, gallbladder, and pancreas play a significant role in the process of digestion through their contribution of fluids and enzymes.

The process of digestion breaks down food molecules so that they can be absorbed and utilized by the cells of the body. After food is broken down into molecules, they are small enough to be absorbed or become bodily waste that is eliminated.

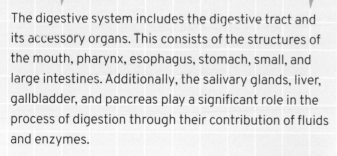

Next Gen Clinical Judgment:

> Compare the function of the structures of the GI tract in the process of digestion and elimination. Include the mouth, pharynx, esophagus, stomach, small, and large intestine.

> Consider the impact on the client if one of these structures is not working at an optimal level.

> Consider what impacts a person's hunger.

> Consider the impact on the body when nutritional needs are not met.

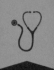

Go To Clinical Case

While caring for this client, be sure to review the concept maps in chapters 3 and 4.

Case 1: Weight Loss and Constipation

Related Concepts: Fluid and Electrolytes, Mobility, Nutrition, Elimination
Threaded Topics: Dietary Assessment, Fall Assessment, NG Tube,
Older Adult Care

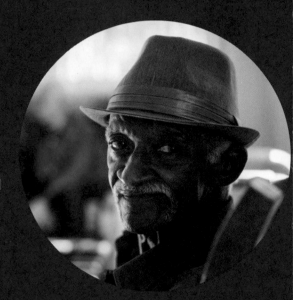

Lincoln Stark is an 82-year-old client with a 30-year history of type 2 diabetes mellitus. His blood pressure is controlled by taking both an ACE inhibitor and a beta blocker. During his last colonoscopy 10 years ago, he learned he has diverticulosis. He walks 1 mile each day to the coffee shop but sometimes feels unsteady on his feet due to the neuropathy and lack of feeling in his feet. He's married to June, his wife for over 50 years. They have 6 children, 27 grandchildren, and 5 great-grandchildren. Lincoln and June live on a meager retirement income since he retired from his ministry position at the First Baptist Church ten years ago. He tells the nurse that he misses being able to read his Bible each day because of his poor vision but is still able to play cards with friends.

Lincoln comes to the health care provider today for a routine appointment. The provider notes that his weight is down 15 pounds since his visit eleven months ago. Lincoln admits that his pants feel looser and he has to wear a belt to keep them up. He also shares that his appetite is not what it used to be and he's more constipated lately. He's more tired than usual and feels cold much of the time.

1. **NurseThink® Prioritization Power!**
   Evaluate the information in the case above and pick the **Top 3 Priority** concerns or cues.

   1. _____

   2. _____

   3. _____

2. **Based on the priority concerns, what action(s) should the nurse perform? Select all that apply.**
   1. Complete a 24-hour food recall.
   2. Obtain a finger sample blood glucose level.
   3. Gather an oxygen saturation reading.
   4. Take a blood pressure.
   5. Complete a fall risk assessment.

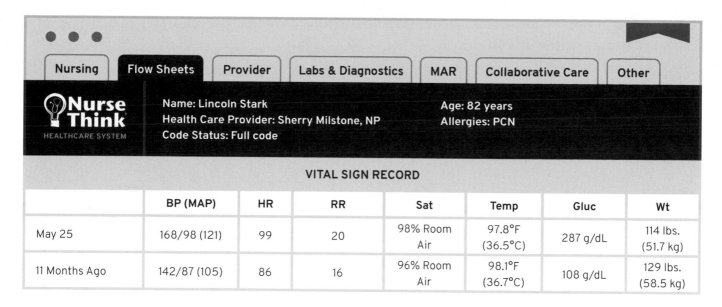

VITAL SIGN RECORD							
	BP (MAP)	HR	RR	Sat	Temp	Gluc	Wt
May 25	168/98 (121)	99	20	98% Room Air	97.8°F (36.5°C)	287 g/dL	114 lbs. (51.7 kg)
11 Months Ago	142/87 (105)	86	16	96% Room Air	98.1°F (36.7°C)	108 g/dL	129 lbs. (58.5 kg)

The nurse is concerned about Lincoln's stated neuropathy and inquires further about his mobility. He admits that he fell once a few months ago when getting out of the bathtub. He bumped his forehead but felt "lucky."

3. **Complete the Fall Risk Assessment. Record Lincoln's risk to fall score:**

_____

Name: Lincoln Stark
Health Care Provider: Sherry Milstone, NP
Code Status: Full code
Age: 82 years
Allergies: PCN

FALL RISK ASSESSMENT

Category		Points
Age	> 60-69 years (1 point) > 70-79 years (2 points) > Greater than or equal to 80 years (3 points)	
Fall History	> One fall within 6 months before admission (5 points)	
Elimination	> Incontinence (2 points) > Urgency/Frequency (2 points)	
Medications	> 1 High Fall Risk Medication (3 points) > 2 or More High-Risk Medications (5 points)	
Mobility	> Requires assistance for mobility, transfer, or ambulation (2 points) > Unsteady gain (2 points) > Visual or auditory impairment (2 points)	
Cognition	> Alerted awareness (1 point) > Impulsive (2 points) > Lack of understanding of limitations (4 points)	

4. **The nurse decides to assess Lincoln's abdominal and nutritional status. For each assessment finding, list the rationale as to why it is concerning.**

1. Hyperactive bowel sounds in upper abdomen, hypoactive bowel sounds in lower abdomen.

   _____

2. 2+ pedal edema. _____

3. Lack of abdominal fat. _____

4. Body mass index = 16. _____

5. Loss of appetite. _____

6. Pale gums and tissues. _____

5. **The nurse obtains additional information, documented in the chart, on the left. Determine if the findings are related or not related to his current situation.**

Medical History:
a 30-year history of type 2 diabetes mellitus, hypertension, diverticulosis, neuropathy, decreased vision.

Vital Signs:
97.8°F (36.5°C); pulse; 99; respiratory rate 20; 168/98 (121)

Labs:
Hemoglobin 10.2 g/dL; K+ 3.4 mEq/L; Na+ 146 mEq/L; Albumin 3.2 g/dL; A1C 7.0%

Weight:
Loss of 15 pounds in 11 months; BMI 16.

Finding	Related	Not Related
Weight change		
Irregular pulse		
No bowel movement x 3 days		
Right shoulder pain		
Pain in left posterior leg		
Intermittent diarrhea		
Red flat rash on back and abdomen		

6. **THIN Thinking Time!**

   Reflect on the nurse's collection of information for Mr. Stark and apply **THIN Thinking.**

   T – _____

   H – _____

   I – _____

   N – _____

   T - Top 3
   H - Help Quick
   I - Identify Risk to Safety
   N - Nursing Process

   Scan to access the 10-Minute-Mentor on THIN Thinking.

   NurseThink.com/THINThinking

7. **Based on the 24-hour diet recall, what hypothesis can the nurse make?**

   1. It is balanced and adequate.
   2. It is excessive in fat and sugar.
   3. It lacks a range of vitamins.
   4. It is rich in fiber.

Lincoln's 24-hour Dietary Recall
Breakfast: Oatmeal, black coffee, dry rye toast.
Lunch: Ham sandwich with mustard, black coffee.
Dinner: Pork roast, canned corn, black coffee.

Lincoln is discharged with new prescriptions for metoclopramide, docusate sodium, iron tablets, a high protein drink twice a day and a physical therapy consultation to evaluate the need for a walker.

8. **Explain the presenting symptom(s) that support(s) the need for each of the discharge prescriptions.**

   1. Metoclopramide: _____

   2. Docusate sodium: _____

   3. Iron tablets: _____

   4. High protein drink: _____

   5. Physical therapy consultation: _____

9. **For teaching, the nurse reviews material about each medication. Mark the reason(s) why the nurse should question the appropriateness of one or both of these medications for Lincoln.**

Metoclopramide	Docusate Sodium
Classification: Dopamine antagonist	**Classification:** Sulfonic acid
Administration: Take 30 minutes before meals and at bedtime.	**Administration:** Take this medication by mouth, usually at bedtime with a full glass (8 ounces or 240 milliliters) of water or juice.
Side effects: Drowsiness, dizziness, trouble sleeping, agitation, headache, and diarrhea.	**Side effects:** Stomach pain, diarrhea, or cramping.
Precautions: Consult your practitioner before using if you have: movement/muscle disorders caused by a medication, bleeding or blockage in the intestines/stomach, breast cancer, high blood pressure, kidney problems, heart failure, depression, Parkinson's disease, liver problems, or seizures.	**Precautions:** Consult your practitioner before using this medication if you have: severe abdominal pain, nausea, vomiting, a sudden change in bowel habits over the previous 2 weeks.
Dosage: 10 mg orally 4 times a day.	**Dosage:** 100 mg oral, daily.
Assessment: Monitor bowel sounds, appetite, and for side effects.	**Assessment:** Monitor stool frequency and consistency. Assess bowel sounds and for signs of abdominal pain, cramping, and nausea.

Lincoln returns home with June and begins his prescriptions. The consultation with the physical therapist leads to the use of a walker. June is concerned about Lincoln falling and arranges for one of their friends to drive Lincoln to the coffee shop each day.

A few weeks later, Lincoln begins feeling nauseous and vomiting. He and June assume it is something he ate. Twenty-four hours later, he develops stomach pain and gets lightheaded while getting out of bed. They call one of their children to take them to the emergency department where an admission assessment, labs, and diagnostic tests are completed.

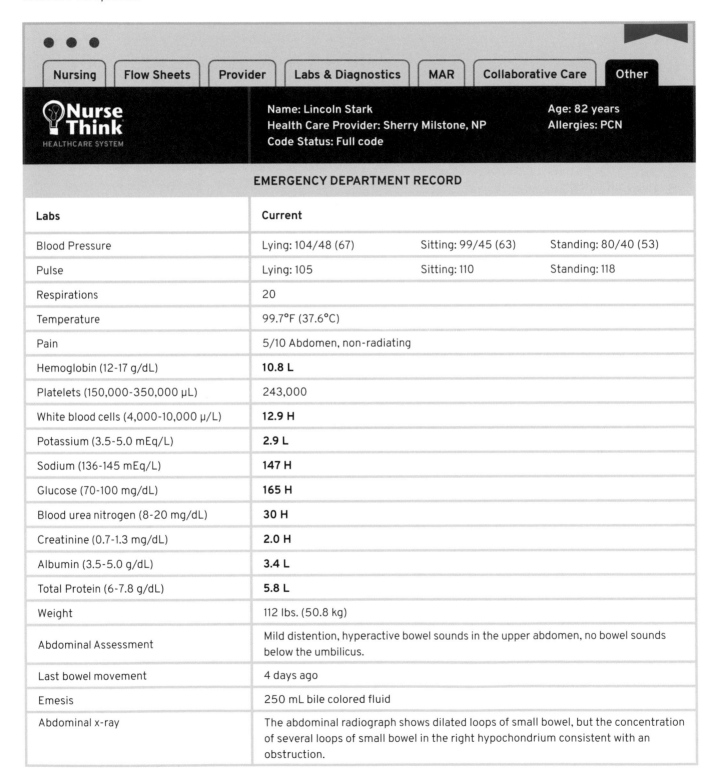

| Nursing | Flow Sheets | Provider | Labs & Diagnostics | MAR | Collaborative Care | Other |

NurseThink
HEALTHCARE SYSTEM

Name: Lincoln Stark
Health Care Provider: Sherry Milstone, NP
Code Status: Full code

Age: 82 years
Allergies: PCN

EMERGENCY DEPARTMENT RECORD

Labs	Current		
Blood Pressure	Lying: 104/48 (67)	Sitting: 99/45 (63)	Standing: 80/40 (53)
Pulse	Lying: 105	Sitting: 110	Standing: 118
Respirations	20		
Temperature	99.7°F (37.6°C)		
Pain	5/10 Abdomen, non-radiating		
Hemoglobin (12-17 g/dL)	**10.8 L**		
Platelets (150,000-350,000 µL)	243,000		
White blood cells (4,000-10,000 µ/L)	**12.9 H**		
Potassium (3.5-5.0 mEq/L)	**2.9 L**		
Sodium (136-145 mEq/L)	**147 H**		
Glucose (70-100 mg/dL)	**165 H**		
Blood urea nitrogen (8-20 mg/dL)	**30 H**		
Creatinine (0.7-1.3 mg/dL)	**2.0 H**		
Albumin (3.5-5.0 g/dL)	**3.4 L**		
Total Protein (6-7.8 g/dL)	**5.8 L**		
Weight	112 lbs. (50.8 kg)		
Abdominal Assessment	Mild distention, hyperactive bowel sounds in the upper abdomen, no bowel sounds below the umbilicus.		
Last bowel movement	4 days ago		
Emesis	250 mL bile colored fluid		
Abdominal x-ray	The abdominal radiograph shows dilated loops of small bowel, but the concentration of several loops of small bowel in the right hypochondrium consistent with an obstruction.		

10. **NurseThink® Prioritization Power!**

    Evaluate the information in the previous documentation and pick the **Top 3 Priority** concerns or cues.

    1. _____

    2. _____

    3. _____

11. **The emergency department nurse identifies the need for safety. Which action(s) would be most appropriate? Select all that apply.**

    1. Prepare suction at the bedside.
    2. Place on contact precautions.
    3. Raise the head of the bed.
    4. Do not allow ambulation.
    5. Place on an EKG monitor.

Lincoln is admitted to the medical unit for a small bowel obstruction.

12. **The nurse receives an order to place a nasogastric tube (NG). June asks why Lincoln needs this placed. How should the nurse respond?**

    1. "It will decompress his stomach and will stop the vomiting."
    2. "It will give the ability to provide him with nutrition."
    3. "It will remove the bacteria from his stomach and make him feel better."
    4. "It will decrease his abdominal pain."

13. **As the nurse is placing the NG tube, Lincoln begins to gag and vomit. What action should the nurse take?**

    1. Continue to insert the tube.
    2. Secure and connect the tube to suction.
    3. Quickly advance the tube into the stomach.
    4. Remove the tube and begin suctioning if needed.

14. **A few hours after the tube is placed, Lincoln feels nauseated. The nurse confirms that the suctioning is working and irrigates the tube with 30 mL of tap water as ordered, but the irrigating fluid does not return. What should the nurse do next?**

    1. Notify the physician.
    2. Auscultate for bowel sounds.
    3. Reposition the tube then confirm placement.
    4. Remove the tube and replace it with a new one.

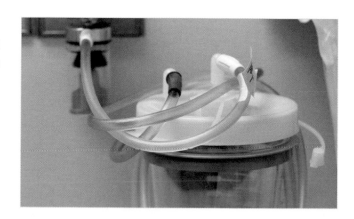

15. A student nurse caring for Mr. Stark performs an abdominal assessment. It is noted that 300 mL of green bile fluid has been removed via low intermittent suction in the last 2 hours. The student reports to the nurse that the bowel sounds have returned to normal upon auscultation. What should the nurse say to the student?

1. "Great! Let's remove the NG tube."
2. "That doesn't make sense to me; let's listen together."
3. "It sounds like his obstruction has cleared."
4. "That is probably from the pain medicine we gave him."

16. The nurse is determining the 24-hour total for the gastric output. How should the nurse report this information based on the intake/output record? _____ mL.

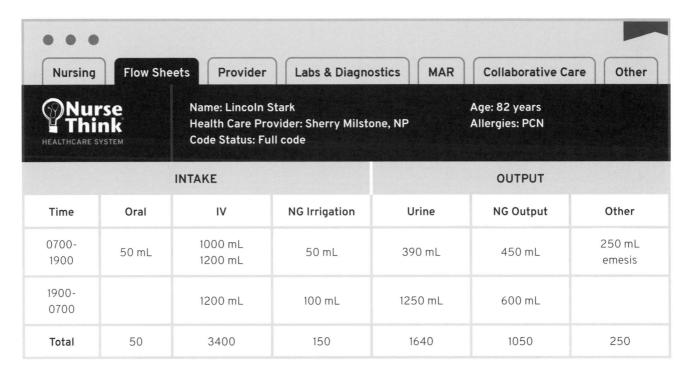

Nursing	Flow Sheets	Provider	Labs & Diagnostics	MAR	Collaborative Care	Other

Nurse Think HEALTHCARE SYSTEM

Name: Lincoln Stark
Health Care Provider: Sherry Milstone, NP
Code Status: Full code

Age: 82 years
Allergies: PCN

	INTAKE			OUTPUT		
Time	Oral	IV	NG Irrigation	Urine	NG Output	Other
0700-1900	50 mL	1000 mL 1200 mL	50 mL	390 mL	450 mL	250 mL emesis
1900-0700		1200 mL	100 mL	1250 mL	600 mL	
Total	50	3400	150	1640	1050	250

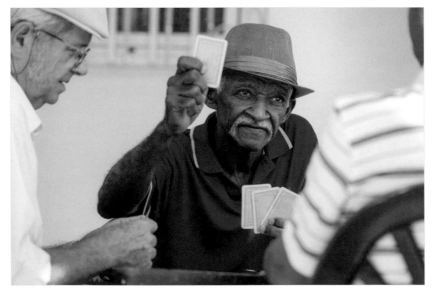

17. After reviewing the 24-hour intake and output record, what hypotheses can be made about each of the following?

   1. Is the bowel obstruction improving? How do you know?

   _____

   2. Is the dehydration improving? How do you know?

   _____

   3. Is the urine output adequate? How do you know?

   _____

   4. Is the NG tube is functioning properly? How do you know?

   _____

18. After two days, Lincoln's bowel obstruction improves, and the NG tube is removed. As he drinks his first clear liquid meal, he feels some nausea. What action should the nurse take?

   1. Make him NPO again.
   2. Replace the NG tube to low intermittent suction.
   3. Advance him to a full liquid diet.
   4. Complete a focused abdominal assessment.

19. Lincoln's nausea passed quickly, and the nurse is determining when to advance his diet. Which assessment changes indicate the need to advance the diet? Select all that apply.

   1. Increased hunger.
   2. Active bowel sounds x 4 quadrants.
   3. Nausea after meals.
   4. Passing flatus with ambulation.
   5. Decreased serum protein levels.

20. It is determined that Lincoln's obstruction was caused by intestinal scaring from his diverticulosis. He is encouraged to maintain healthy bowel habits. What should the nurse include in discharge teaching? Select all that apply.

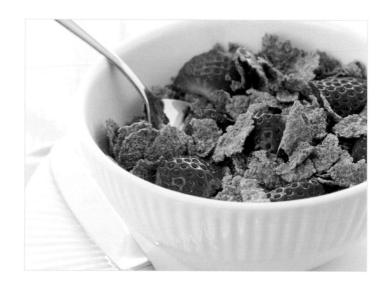

   1. Walk with the assistance of your walker daily.
   2. Increase the number of fresh fruits and vegetables in your diet.
   3. Drink six 8 oz glasses of water each day.
   4. Take your stool softener as prescribed.
   5. Begin daily fiber tablets.

Go To Clinical Case

While caring for this client, be sure to review the concept maps in chapters 3 and 4.

Case 2: Infection and Liver Impairment

Related Concepts: Coping
Threaded Topics: Substance Abuse & Recovery, Organ Donation,
Growth and Development, Macro/Microsystems, Scope of Practice

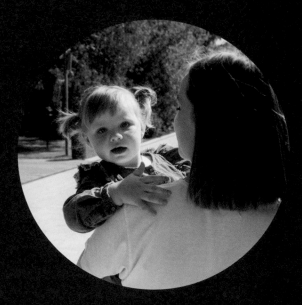

Joylie Herd is a 3-year-old born to a drug-addicted mother. At birth, she contracted hepatitis B from her mother who unknowingly had the virus. Joylie has lacked preventative healthcare, including routine immunizations. She attends an unlicensed daycare while her mother, Jill, a single parent, works at the local supermarket as a cashier. The daycare recently had an outbreak of hepatitis A and is under investigation. Jill has been clean and sober for six months. Jill is proud of her sobriety and the fact that she and Joylie now live in an apartment rather than the shelter.

Joylie is brought into the clinic by her mother for flu-like symptoms including poor appetite and a "tummy ache." She's been running a low-grade temperature. Jill says "she hasn't been her usual active self and is napping a lot."

1. **The nurse begins the assessment. What subjective information should the nurse ask Jill about Joylie? Select all that apply.**
   1. Health history.
   2. Length and severity of current symptoms.
   3. Interactions with her father.
   4. Developmental milestones.
   5. Normal dietary intake.
   6. Immunization record.

2. **What priority safety information should the nurse collect?**
   1. Blood pressure.
   2. Focused abdominal assessment.
   3. Mother-daughter interactions.
   4. Cleanliness of the child.

   Review the CDC's guide on developmental milestones.

   www.cdc.gov/ncbddd/actearly/milestones/index.html

   →

3. **Upon physical assessment, the nurse palpates an enlarged liver. What hypothesis can the nurse make from this finding?**
   1. This is a normal finding in a 3-year-old.
   2. This could be secondary to a respiratory viral infection.
   3. Joylie will likely have a clotting disorder.
   4. The finding is abnormal and requires additional testing.

4. **Because of the enlarged liver, the health care provider orders some additional tests. Which serum labs should the nurse anticipate? Select all that apply.**
   1. AST, ALT, GGT.
   2. Complete blood cell count.
   3. Metabolic panel.
   4. Arterial blood gasses.
   5. Amylase and lipase.

● ● ●

| Nursing | Flow Sheets | Provider | Labs & Diagnostics | MAR | Collaborative Care | Other |

Nurse Think
HEALTHCARE SYSTEM

Name: Joylie Herd
Health Care Provider: Bob Laney, MD
Code Status: Full code

Age: 3 years
Allergies: NKDA

LABORATORY REPORT

Lab	Normal	Mar. 12		
WBC	4,000-10,000 µ/L	6.2		
Hemoglobin	12 -17.0 g/dL	**10.0 L**		
Hematocrit (%)	36 - 51%	**35 L**		
RBC	4.2 – 5.9 cells/L	**3.9 L**		
Platelets	150,000 to 350,000 µL	172,000		
Calcium	9 – 10.5 mq/dL	**7.9 L**		
Chloride	98 - 106 mEq/L	99		
Magnesium	1.5 - 2.4 mEq/L	2.4		
Phosphorus	3.0 - 4.5 mg/dL	4.3		
Potassium	3.5 - 5.0 mEq/L	**3.2 L**		
Sodium	136 - 145 mEq/L	**149 H**		
Glucose, fasting	70 – 100 mg/dL	79		
BUN	8 – 20 mg/dL	**26 H**		
Creatinine	0.7-1.3 mg/dL	0.9		
Total Protein	6 - 7.8 g/dL	**5.8 L**		
Albumin	3.5 - 5.0 g/dL	**3.0 L**		
CPK	30 - 170 U/L	57		
LDH	60 - 100 U/L	**295 H**		
AST	0 - 35 U/L	**68 H**		
ALT	0 - 35 U/L	**69 H**		
GGT	9 - 48 U/L	**58 H**		
Total Bilirubin	0.3 - 1.2 mg/dL	**2.9 H**		

5. After evaluating the lab report, the nurse performs a more thorough assessment. What additional findings should be anticipated?

1. A high temperature.
2. Dark pink mucous membranes.
3. Jaundice of the sclera.
4. A lack of edema.

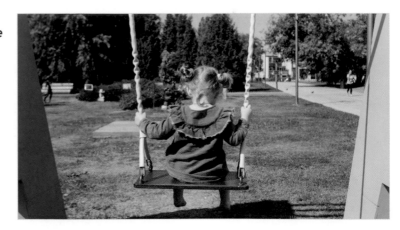

6. **NurseThink® Prioritization Power!**

   Reflect on Joylie's assessment findings and identify the **Top 3 Priority** concerns.

   1. _____

   2. _____

   3. _____

7. Joylie is admitted to the pediatric unit for additional tests. The nurse working that day is precepting a newly graduated licensed practical nurse (LPN) and an experienced unlicensed assistive personnel (UAP). For each of the admission tasks on the left, determine the most appropriate delegation for each skill.

_____ 1. Gather thermometer and blood pressure equipment.	A. Admitting RN
_____ 2. Start an IV.	B. LPN
_____ 3. Request toddler pull-up diapers from central supply.	C. UAP
_____ 4. Obtain health history from the parent.	D. None of these
_____ 5. Perform a head-to-toe assessment.	
_____ 6. Obtain a pull-out bed for the parent.	
_____ 7. Call Provider for admitting prescriptions.	
_____ 8. Obtain admission vital signs, weight and height.	
_____ 9. Monitor other clients on the unit and report concerns.	
_____ 10. Review of immunization record, noting immunization needs.	

Nurse Think
HEALTHCARE SYSTEM

Name: Joylie Herd
Health Care Provider: Bob Laney, MD
Code Status: Full code

Age: 3 years
Allergies: NKDA

GROWTH & DEVELOPMENT ASSESSMENT

Chronical Age: 3 years 2 months 15 days

Personal - Social	> Copies others, especially adults and older children. > Gets excited when with other children. > Shows independent behavior (doing what she has been told not to).
Fine Motor - Adaptive	> Makes or copies straight lines and circles.
Speech	> Points to things or pictures when they are named. > Knows names of familiar people and body parts. > Says sentences with 2 to 4 words. > Follows simple instructions. > Repeats words overheard in conversation. > Points to things in a book.
Gross Motor	> Stands on tiptoe. > Kicks a ball. > Begins to run. > Climbs onto and down from furniture without help. > Walks up and down stairs holding on.
Self-Care	> Helps to pick out clothes. > Needs assistance with buttons and snaps when dressing self.
Growth	> 75% for height. > 50% for weight.

8. **The nurse documents Joylie's developmental assessment with the help of Jill. What hypothesis can the nurse make based on this information?**

    1. She is age-appropriate for development.
    2. She is below age level for development.
    3. She is above age level of development.
    4. This information can not determine the developmental level.

The provider writes these admitting prescriptions.

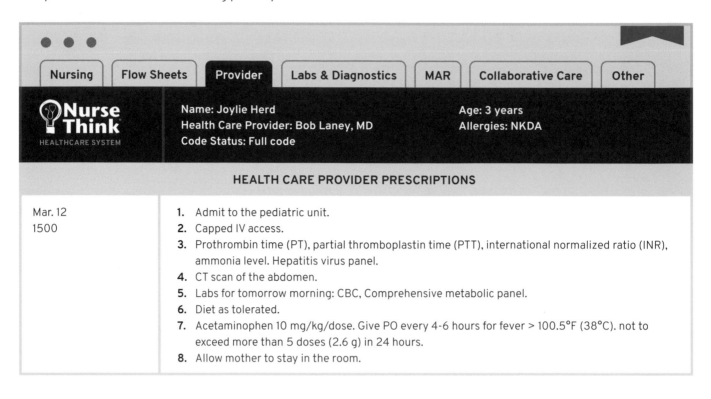

| Nursing | Flow Sheets | **Provider** | Labs & Diagnostics | MAR | Collaborative Care | Other |

NurseThink HEALTHCARE SYSTEM

Name: Joylie Herd
Health Care Provider: Bob Laney, MD
Code Status: Full code

Age: 3 years
Allergies: NKDA

HEALTH CARE PROVIDER PRESCRIPTIONS

Mar. 12
1500

1. Admit to the pediatric unit.
2. Capped IV access.
3. Prothrombin time (PT), partial thromboplastin time (PTT), international normalized ratio (INR), ammonia level. Hepatitis virus panel.
4. CT scan of the abdomen.
5. Labs for tomorrow morning: CBC, Comprehensive metabolic panel.
6. Diet as tolerated.
7. Acetaminophen 10 mg/kg/dose. Give PO every 4-6 hours for fever > 100.5°F (38°C). not to exceed more than 5 doses (2.6 g) in 24 hours.
8. Allow mother to stay in the room.

---

9. The nurse reviews the prescriptions. Which item should be questioned? Why?

_____

The additional labs are drawn and placed in the EHR. The nurse reviews them.

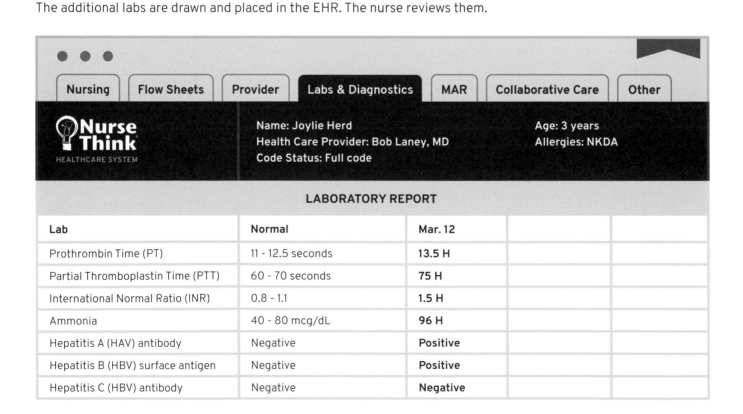

| Nursing | Flow Sheets | Provider | **Labs & Diagnostics** | MAR | Collaborative Care | Other |

NurseThink HEALTHCARE SYSTEM

Name: Joylie Herd
Health Care Provider: Bob Laney, MD
Code Status: Full code

Age: 3 years
Allergies: NKDA

LABORATORY REPORT

Lab	Normal	Mar. 12		
Prothrombin Time (PT)	11 - 12.5 seconds	13.5 H		
Partial Thromboplastin Time (PTT)	60 - 70 seconds	75 H		
International Normal Ratio (INR)	0.8 - 1.1	1.5 H		
Ammonia	40 - 80 mcg/dL	96 H		
Hepatitis A (HAV) antibody	Negative	Positive		
Hepatitis B (HBV) surface antigen	Negative	Positive		
Hepatitis C (HBV) antibody	Negative	Negative		

The nurse receives a verbal report from the radiologist that Joylie's CT scan shows that she has fibrosis of the liver. The nurse speaks with the admitting pediatrician, Dr. Laney who requests a gastrointestinal pediatrician be consulted and that Joylie is transferred to the children's hospital across town.

10. **THIN Thinking Time!**

Reflect on the cues and data about Joylie and apply **THIN Thinking** to prioritizing the concerns.

T – _____

H – _____

I – _____

N – _____

T - Top 3
H - Help Quick
I - Identify Risk to Safety
N - Nursing Process

Scan to access the 10-Minute-Mentor on THIN Thinking. →

NurseThink.com/THINThinking

11. **As the nurse prepares for Joylie's transfer, Dr. Laney speaks with Jill. She is openly distraught and crying. When the nurse enters the room, Jill says "It's all my fault that my little angel is sick." How should the nurse respond?**

1. "It's hard to know how this happened, and it's not your fault."
2. "Joylie acquired this at birth, and it could not be prevented."
3. "I know you are concerned, but we need to get Joylie transferred and we'll talk soon."
4. "What makes you think that?"

12. **Jill has many questions for the nurse. She asks "I learned a year ago that I have hepatitis B and could have spread it to Joylie when she was born, but how could Joylie have gotten hepatitis A?" How should the nurse reply?**

1. Hepatitis A is spread by air droplets when someone coughs.
2. Hepatitis A develops when hepatitis B is not treated.
3. Hepatitis A is a virus that is spread from poor hand hygiene after using the bathroom.
4. Hepatitis A develops as a result of a child is not adequately immunized against it.

13. **The nurse prepares an SBAR hand-off report for the accepting hospital. Complete each section of the communication form.**

S – _____

B – _____

A – _____

R – _____

Clinical Hint:
S - Situation
B - Background
A - Assessment
R - Recommendation

14. **Which medical treatment(s) is/are anticipated in the treatment of the fibrosis and liver failure that Joylie is experiencing? Select all that apply.**

1. Lactulose to lower ammonia level.
2. High protein diet increases serum albumin levels.
3. Vitamin K to treat prolonged PT and INR.
4. Eliminate liver toxic medications and treatments.
5. Calamine lotion to reduce jaundice.

15. **The nurse at the children's hospital assumes care of Joylie and admits her to the gastrointestinal unit. Which precaution(s) should the nurse implement upon admission? Select all that apply.**

1. Contact precautions.
2. Universal precautions.
3. Airborne precautions.
4. Neutropenic precautions.
5. Fall precautions.
6. Bleeding precautions.

16. **Joylie is in the hospital for over a week. Circle or highlight the changes in her EHR that indicate an improvement in her condition.**

| Nursing | Flow Sheets | Provider | **Labs & Diagnostics** | MAR | Collaborative Care | Other |

Nurse Think HEALTHCARE SYSTEM

Name: Joylie Herd
Health Care Provider: Bob Laney, MD
Code Status: Full code

Age: 3 years
Allergies: NKDA

LABORATORY REPORT

Lab	Normal	Mar. 12	Mar. 15	Mar. 20
WBC	4,000-10,000 µ/L	6.2	5.4	4.8
Hemoglobin	12 -17.0 g/dL	10.0 L	10.2 L	11.8 L
Hematocrit (%)	36 - 51%	35 L	39	40
RBC	4.2 – 5.9 cells/L	3.9 L	4.0 L	4.0 L
Platelets	150,000 to 350,000 µL	172,000	120,000 L	89,000 L
Total Protein	6 - 7.8 g/dL	5.8 L	5.5 L	5.3 L
Albumin	3.5 - 5. g/dL	3.0 L	2.9 L	2.8 L
LDH	60 - 70 U/L	295 H	301 H	402 H
AST	0 - 35 U/L	68 H	98 H	104 H
ALT	0 - 35 U/L	69 H	205 H	399 H
GGT	9 - 48 U/L	58 H	61 H	78 H
Total Bilirubin	0.3-1.2 mg/dL	2.9 H	3.1 H	3.4 H
Prothrombin Time (PT)	11 - 12.5 seconds	13.5 H	13.9 H	12.8 H
Partial Thromboplastin Time (PTT)	60 - 70 seconds	75 H	72 H	79 H
International Normal Ratio (INR)	0.8 - 1.1	1.5 H	1.7 H	1.3 H
Ammonia	40 - 80 mcg/dL	96 H	100 H	78

17. **The nurse completes a physical exam on Joylie. Which assessment finding(s) is/are related to the changes in the lab report? Select all that apply.**
    1. Fever and signs of infection.
    2. Bruising and bleeding from the IV site.
    3. Pedal and periorbital edema.
    4. Ascites.
    5. Jaundice of the sclera.
    6. Disorientation.

Over the next week, Joylie's condition continues to deteriorate despite aggressive treatment. She is placed on the liver transplant list. A donor comes available, and she receives a donated liver. Her recovery phase is without complications, and she is discharged from the hospital.

18. **NurseThink® Prioritization Power!**
    As Joylie is being discharged on anti-rejection medications after a liver transplant, identify the **Top 3 Priority** discharge teaching points.

    1. _____

    2. _____

    3. _____

19. **Since Joylie has not achieved several milestones for a 3-year-old, which service(s) should the nurse recommend are initiated upon discharge? Select all that apply.**
    1. Physical therapy.
    2. Nutritional therapy.
    3. Occupational therapy.
    4. Speech therapy.
    5. Home care.
    6. Outpatient services.
    7. Chaplain services.

20. **Jill feels that Joylie's recovery has changed her life. She wants to become more involved in the community's Donor Network. How should the nurse respond?**
    1. "I encourage you to contact the organization and see how you might volunteer."
    2. "There's not much that you can do; they require a medical background."
    3. "Are you signed up as a donor?"
    4. "What skills do you have that could be helpful?"

1. Compare the impaired dietary intake of Lincoln Stark and Joylie Herd. How are they the same and how are they different?

   _____

   _____

2. Compare the impaired food breakdown and absorption of Lincoln and Joylie. How are they the same and how are they different?

   _____

   _____

3. Compare the impaired elimination of Lincoln and Joylie. How are they the same and how are they different?

   _____

   _____

4. How does the nutritional impairment impact Lincoln and Joylie's ability to heal and get stronger?

   _____

   _____

5. In what areas of each case study was basic care and comfort utilized?

   _____

   _____

6. What steps in each case did the nurse take that prevented hospital-acquired injury?

   _____

   _____

7. How did the nurse provide culturally sensitive/competent care?

   _____

   _____

8. How will learning about the case of Lincoln Stark and Joylie Herd impact the care you provide for future clients?

   _____

   _____

Fundamental Quiz

1. **The nurse is counseling a client with a poor appetite and weight loss. Which priority intervention should the nurse recommend?**
   1. Eat your favorite foods to get additional calories, no matter what they are.
   2. Consume high protein, high-calorie replacement drinks between meals.
   3. Take a multivitamin daily.
   4. Eat 6 small meals each day.

2. **A nurse is suggesting interventions for a client with chronic constipation. In which order should the nurse make these recommendations? Place them in the order from 1st recommendation to last recommendation.**

   _____, _____, _____, _____, _____.
   1. Docusate.
   2. Enema.
   3. Increased fiber intake.
   4. Bisacodyl.
   5. Prune juice.

3. **A nurse observes this rash while assessing an infant, recognizing that it is a result of urinary incontinence. What intervention should be added to the plan of care?**
   1. Leave the skin open to air as much as possible.
   2. Apply lubricant jelly to the site three times each day.
   3. Obtain a prescription for an antibiotic ointment.
   4. Apply a cortisone cream.

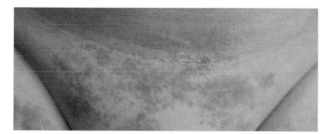

4. **The nurse is caring for a client with a poor appetite, nausea and abdominal distention. What should the nurse anticipate upon auscultation of the abdomen?**
   1. Hyperactivity throughout.
   2. Normal sounds.
   3. Tympanic sounds.
   4. Diminished throughout.

5. **A client is prescribed a diet that can be advanced as tolerated. How does the nurse recognize that the client is ready to be started on regular food? Select all that apply.**
   1. Bowel sounds are present.
   2. Hunger is verbalized.
   3. The client has been NPO for 5 days.
   4. The albumin level is within the normal range.
   5. The health care provider says so.

Advanced Quiz

6. **The nurse is caring for an older adult client with renal insufficiency. Vitals include temperature 99.8°F (37.6°C), heart rate 96, respirations 28, and BP 170/90 (117) mmHg. The client is restless, dyspneic, and anxious. The oxygen saturation drops to 87% when he pulls his oxygen cannula off. Which action should the nurse take after reapplying the oxygen?**
   1. Administer an anti-anxiety medication.
   2. Auscultate the lung sounds.
   3. Check recent labs.
   4. Administer an anti-hypertensive medication.

7. **An older adult female client reports a recent problem with urine hesitancy, decreased force of the flow, a sensation of incomplete emptying of the bladder, and dribbling. Which question should the nurse ask next?**
   1. "Have you had flank pain?"
   2. "Have you experienced abdominal pain?"
   3. "Have you had a daily bowel movement?"
   4. "Have you noticed if it's worse at night?"

8. **A client is admitted with abdominal pain. Based on the information found in the record below, what should the nurse request as "recommendation(s)" for admission orders in the SBAR conversation with the health care provider? Select all that apply.**
   1. Acetaminophen 1000 mg PO every 6 hours PRN pain.
   2. Surgical consultation.
   3. O2 at 2 L/NC PRN.
   4. Regular insulin per sliding scale coverage.
   5. Type and crossmatch for 2 units PRBC.

Nurse's Notes and Labs
Sept. 7 – 0330
Admitted with severe abdominal pain radiating to the back, nausea, vomiting, and a fever. Pain of 8/10. HR 122, Blood Pressure 147/96 (113), Respiration 22, Temp 101.4°F (38.5°C), Sats = 92% on RA. History of diabetes mellitus Type 2, Admits to heavy alcohol use, hypertension and hemorrhoids. Admit to the medical floor.

WBC	Glucose	Hgb	Amylase
14,000 µ/L	322 mg/dL	6.8 g/dL	459 U/L

9. A young, healthy, client with a sudden onset of severe flank and abdominal pain is seen in the emergency department. The client describes the pain as "the worst I've ever had." Intravenous fluids are started, and intravenous pain medication is administered. What is a priority nursing intervention?

    1. Strain all urine.
    2. Give clear liquids only.
    3. Enforce strict bed rest.
    4. Obtain a thorough health history.

10. Circle the client information that supports the nurses decision to give the albumin 25% dose.

Client Information		Resource Information	
Medical Diagnosis	32-year-old with advanced liver disease.	Medication	Albumin 25%
Current Vital Signs	T. 98.7°F (37°C); HR 112 beats; BP 98/62 (74) mmHg; Respirations 24 breaths; Sats 95% RA; Pain free	Indications	Restores plasma volume after burns, hyperbilirubinemia, shock, hypoproteinemia, prevention of cerebral edema, cardiopulmonary bypass procedures, ARDS, nephrotic syndrome
Medical History	ETOH x 16 years; Smokes 2 packs/day x 18 years; peptic ulcer disease; total knee replacement 3 years ago; history of osteoarthritis arthritis.	Contraindications	Hypersensitivity, CHF, severe anemia, renal insufficiency, pulmonary edema
Physical Exam	Oriented x 1; restless and confused; weak, S1S2 heart sounds, fine crackles in lungs, ascites, 3+ pedal edema, urine dark amber.	Interactions	Increase: serum albumin
Lab Tests	Albumin 2.8 g/dL; Na+ 147 mEq/L; K+ 3.2 mEq/L; Ammonia 457; mcg/dL; PT 15.6 seconds; PTT 79 seconds.	Route/dose	Adult: IV 25 g, may repeat in 15-30 min, or 50-75 g of 25% albumin infused at ≤2 ml/min
Meds	Lactulose; Vitamin K	Nursing Concerns	Slowly, to prevent fluid overload; dilute with NS for injection or D5W; 5% is given undiluted; 25% may be given diluted or undiluted; give over 30-60 min, use infusion pump, use large-gauge needle; infusion must be completed within 4 hr.

Hormonal

Neuroendocrine / Glucose Regulation / Metabolism

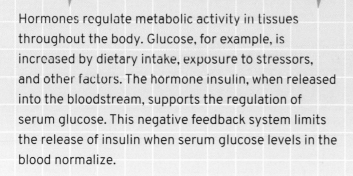

Hormones regulate metabolic activity in tissues throughout the body. Glucose, for example, is increased by dietary intake, exposure to stressors, and other factors. The hormone insulin, when released into the bloodstream, supports the regulation of serum glucose. This negative feedback system limits the release of insulin when serum glucose levels in the blood normalize.

The pituitary gland secretes hormones that act on the adrenal glands, thyroid gland, mammary glands, ovaries, and testes, which in turn produce other hormones. The pituitary gland, often referred to as the 'master gland', helps to control metabolism, growth, sexual maturation, reproduction, blood pressure, and other vital functions and processes within the body. Illness and disease can occur when there is a primary or secondary condition in the pituitary or one of the target organs.

Since the adrenal and thyroid glands each play a fundamental role in metabolism, malfunction can be quite impactful to a person's health and wellness.

Next Gen Clinical Judgment:

> Insulin-dependent (Type I) diabetes occurs when the pancreas no longer secretes adequate insulin to meet the glucose needs of the body. How is Type II diabetes different?

> What hormones are impacted if the pituitary gland is removed?

> What assessment changes are observed if the pituitary gland is removed?

> How does excess cortisol impact glucose regulation?

> What are the 3 hormones released from the adrenal cortex? What hormone is released from the adrenal medulla? List at least one purpose for each hormone.

Go To Clinical Case

While caring for this client, be sure to review the concept maps in chapters 3 and 4.

Case 1: Metabolic Syndrome and Diabetes

Related Concepts: Nutrition, Metabolism
Threaded Topics: Patient Teaching, Medication Calculations

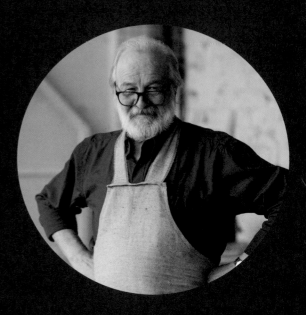

Bart Bunyan is a 62-year-old man from the Pacific Northwest. His hard-working grandparents emigrated from Europe in the early 1900s, establishing a successful woodworking company. Bart has worked for the family business his entire life and now manages the company with over 100 employees. His wife died last year from breast cancer, but his children and grandchildren live nearby and are involved in Bart's life by inviting him to dinner several nights a week. He's had hypertension for 10 years which is controlled with a daily ACE inhibitor and beta blocker. He is 6 foot, 2 inches, weighs 268 pounds (BMI 34.4), is "solid" and is often teased by his family for having a "beer belly." Bart was recently diagnosed with pre-diabetes. He is not surprised by the diagnosis since all three of his siblings have diabetes, as did his mother and her nine siblings.

1. **When evaluating Bart's body mass index (BMI), what hypothesis can be made?**
    1. He is underweight.
    2. He is within a normal weight.
    3. He is overweight.
    4. He is obese.

2. **Which risk factor(s) does Bart have that contribute(s) to the diagnosis of pre-diabetes? Select all that apply.**
    1. Hypertension.
    2. Stress.
    3. BMI.
    4. Family history.
    5. Current medications.

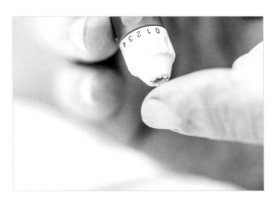

3. **Which lab report confirms Bart's diagnosis of pre-diabetes?**
    1. Hemoglobin A1C of 6.5%.
    2. Fasting glucose of 145 mg/dL.
    3. Amylase level of 92 U/L.
    4. A 1-hour glucose tolerance test of 256 mg/dL.

Bart's practitioner prescribes daily glucose monitoring and a consultation with a diabetic nurse educator for glucose monitoring, diet, and exercise teaching. Bart is encouraged to make lifestyle changes without the introduction of medications, reevaluating the hemoglobin A1C in 3 months.

4. **Jennifer, the diabetic nurse educator, meets with Bart for the first visit. What question(s) should she ask? Select all that apply.**

    1. "How do you feel about this new diagnosis?"
    2. "Can someone check your blood glucose for you?"
    3. "What do you eat in a typical day?"
    4. "How do you feel about taking medication?"
    5. "Do you perform any daily exercise?"

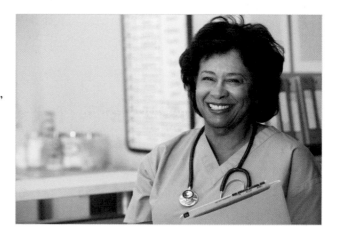

Jennifer documents the one-hour visit with Bart.

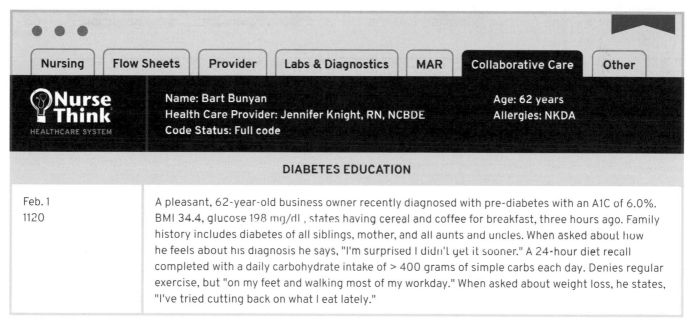

Feb. 1 1120	A pleasant, 62-year-old business owner recently diagnosed with pre-diabetes with an A1C of 6.0%. BMI 34.4, glucose 198 mg/dl , states having cereal and coffee for breakfast, three hours ago. Family history includes diabetes of all siblings, mother, and all aunts and uncles. When asked about how he feels about his diagnosis he says, "I'm surprised I didn't get it sooner." A 24-hour diet recall completed with a daily carbohydrate intake of > 400 grams of simple carbs each day. Denies regular exercise, but "on my feet and walking most of my workday." When asked about weight loss, he states, "I've tried cutting back on what I eat lately."

5. **NurseThink® Prioritization Power!**

    Evaluate the information within the diabetes education note and pick the **Top 3 Priority** teaching concerns.

    1. _____

    2. _____

    3. _____

24-hours Dietary Recall
Breakfast – cereal with whole milk and sugar. Coffee with 3 creams and 3 teaspoons of sugar.
Lunch – pasta with meat sauce, 2 slices of garlic bread, small salad, a slice of peach pie.
Dinner - tortilla chips with salsa, three tacos, refried beans, Mexican rice, margarita, fried ice cream.
Snacks – 3 cookies, a bag of popcorn.

Next Gen Clinical Judgment: Download an app on your phone that calculates carbohydrates. Place Bart's 24-hour dietary recall into the app and determine how many grams of carbohydrates he consumed in the last 24 hours.

6. During the visit, Bart says to Jennifer, "I'm not sure why this is so important, medications can correct the problem, so why does it matter what I eat?" How should the nurse respond?

_____

7. Bart says to Jennifer "the health care provider said that I have metabolic syndrome. Can you tell me what that is?" How should Jennifer respond?
   1. "It is a condition that impairs your ability to maintain a normal metabolic rate; causing added weight around the belly."
   2. "It is a syndrome that occurs with pre-diabetes and cannot be avoided."
   3. "It is another name for pre-diabetes, and you shouldn't be concerned."
   4. "It is several conditions including hypertension and diabetes that place you at a higher risk for heart disease."

8. Jennifer evaluates that Bart has several teaching needs and will need to return for additional visits to reinforce understanding. How should Jennifer prioritize these pre-diabetic teaching points?

	Priority for this visit	Designate for future visits	Not a priority
Accurate use of the blood glucose monitor.			
Difference between Types I and II diabetes.			
Daily logs for glucose readings.			
Limiting daily carbohydrates to 200 g/day.			
Importance of monitoring kidney function.			
Taking medication as prescribed.			
Insulin injection site rotation.			
Daily foot inspection and care.			
Importance of annual eye exams.			
Walking 30 minutes each day.			
Sick day rules.			

Bart has a difficult time adhering to his lifestyle change. His A1C continues to climb over the next 6 months to 7.4%, and Bart is placed on metformin 500 mg twice a day by mouth.

9. Review the oral hyperglycemic medications in the chart and match the medicines on the left to its appropriate drug classification on the right. Each drug class can be used more than once.

_____Glipizide	A. Sulfonylureas
_____Dapagliflozin	B. Biguanides
_____Sitagliptin	C. Thiazolidinediones
_____Metformin	D. Incretin Mimetics
_____Liraglutide	E. DPP-4 inhibitors
_____Glimepiride	F. Sodium-glucose cotransport inhibitors
_____Rosiglitazone	
_____Glyburide	

10. During a follow-up visit with the diabetic nurse educator, Bart brings his glucose record below. What conclusions can Jennifer make? Select all that apply.

   1. Activity helps to lower his glucose levels.

   2. Bart should eliminate his bedtime snack.

   3. He is compliant with checking a fasting glucose level each day.

   4. The stress of illness caused is glucose levels to rise.

   5. Bart's diabetes is well controlled.

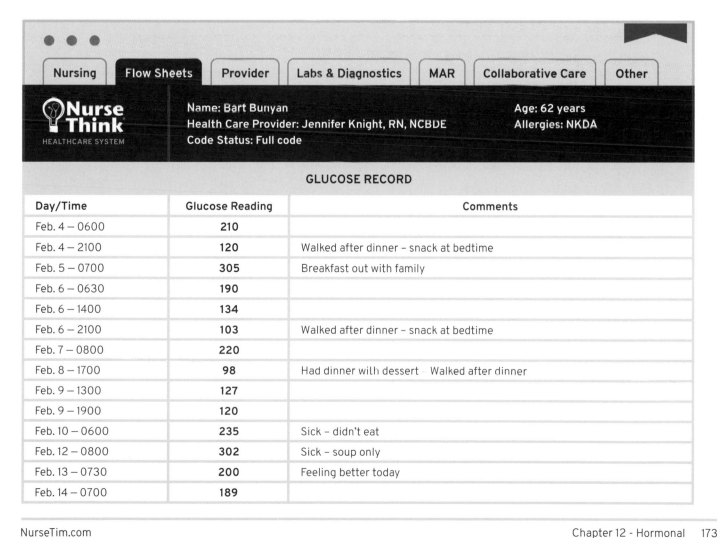

Nursing | **Flow Sheets** | **Provider** | **Labs & Diagnostics** | **MAR** | **Collaborative Care** | **Other**

NurseThink
HEALTHCARE SYSTEM

Name: Bart Bunyan
Health Care Provider: Jennifer Knight, RN, NCBDE
Code Status: Full code

Age: 62 years
Allergies: NKDA

GLUCOSE RECORD

Day/Time	Glucose Reading	Comments
Feb. 4 – 0600	210	
Feb. 4 – 2100	120	Walked after dinner – snack at bedtime
Feb. 5 – 0700	305	Breakfast out with family
Feb. 6 – 0630	190	
Feb. 6 – 1400	134	
Feb. 6 – 2100	103	Walked after dinner – snack at bedtime
Feb. 7 – 0800	220	
Feb. 8 – 1700	98	Had dinner with dessert - Walked after dinner
Feb. 9 – 1300	127	
Feb. 9 – 1900	120	
Feb. 10 – 0600	235	Sick – didn't eat
Feb. 12 – 0800	302	Sick – soup only
Feb. 13 – 0730	200	Feeling better today
Feb. 14 – 0700	189	

11. **NurseThink® Prioritization Power!**

Evaluate the information within the glucose record and pick the **Top 3 Priority** teaching needs.

1. _____

2. _____

3. _____

Bart poorly manages is diabetes over the next few years. One day his daughter finds him on the floor at home, semi-conscious. He is barely arousable and mumbling incoherently. She calls 911. Upon arrival at his home, paramedics document these findings.

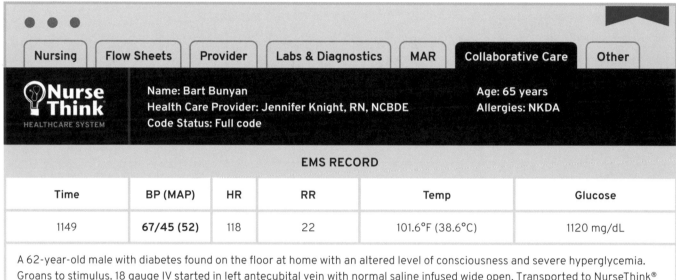

| Nursing | Flow Sheets | Provider | Labs & Diagnostics | MAR | Collaborative Care | Other |

NurseThink HEALTHCARE SYSTEM

Name: Bart Bunyan
Health Care Provider: Jennifer Knight, RN, NCBDE
Code Status: Full code

Age: 65 years
Allergies: NKDA

EMS RECORD

Time	BP (MAP)	HR	RR	Temp	Glucose
1149	67/45 (52)	118	22	101.6°F (38.6°C)	1120 mg/dL

A 62-year-old male with diabetes found on the floor at home with an altered level of consciousness and severe hyperglycemia. Groans to stimulus. 18 gauge IV started in left antecubital vein with normal saline infused wide open. Transported to NurseThink® Emergency Department.

12. **What could be the cause of Bart's hyperosmolar, hyperglycemic, nonketotic syndrome (HHNS)?**

1. Excess food intake.
2. Lack of exercise.
3. Inadequate medication.
4. Infection.

13. **THIN Thinking Time!**

As the emergency department nurse, reflect on the cues and data about Bart and apply **THIN Thinking** to prioritizing care.

T – _____

H – _____

I – _____

N – _____

T - Top 3
H - Help Quick
I - Identify Risk to Safety
N - Nursing Process

Scan to access the 10-Minute-Mentor → *on THIN Thinking.*

NurseThink.com/THINThinking

Emergency room prescriptions are received.

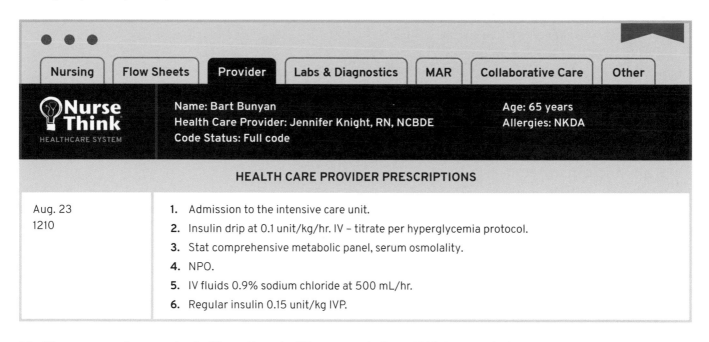

	HEALTH CARE PROVIDER PRESCRIPTIONS
Aug. 23 1210	1. Admission to the intensive care unit. 2. Insulin drip at 0.1 unit/kg/hr. IV – titrate per hyperglycemia protocol. 3. Stat comprehensive metabolic panel, serum osmolality. 4. NPO. 5. IV fluids 0.9% sodium chloride at 500 mL/hr. 6. Regular insulin 0.15 unit/kg IVP.

Name: Bart Bunyan
Health Care Provider: Jennifer Knight, RN, NCBDE
Code Status: Full code
Age: 65 years
Allergies: NKDA

14. **The nurse reviews and prioritizes the admitting prescriptions. Which prescriptions should the nurse perform first, second, and third?**

    1. _____

    2. _____

    3. _____

15. **The nurse calculates for the insulin delivery reviewing the medications on hand.**

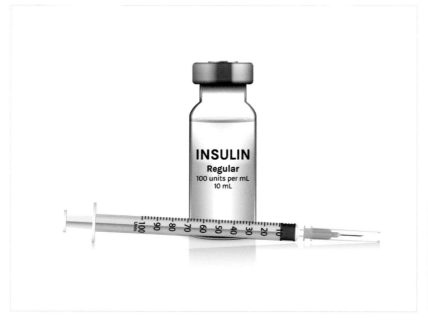

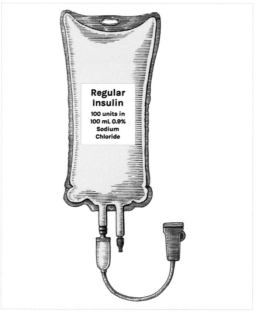

1. How much regular insulin should the nurse deliver IV push? _____ units.

2. At what rate should the nurse begin the insulin infusion via IV pump? _____ mL/hr.

16. **What is the first indication that Bart's condition is improving?**
    1. His glucose begins to decrease.
    2. His mean arterial pressure is > 65 mmHg.
    3. He denies pain and discomfort.
    4. He becomes afebrile.

17. **The nurse is titrating the insulin per protocol. Which assessment(s) indicate that the insulin drip can be removed? Select all that apply.**
    1. Blood pressure is stable.
    2. Urine output is adequate.
    3. Client is alert and oriented.
    4. Glucose is < 200 mg/dL.
    5. Client is hungry.

18. **Because of the poorly controlled blood glucose levels, Bart is discharged home on insulin injections. The nurse reinforces the symptoms of high and low glucose levels. Match the symptom on the left to the appropriate glucose level on the right.**

	Hyperglycemia	Hypoglycemia	Not Related to Glucose Level
Diaphoresis			
Polyphagia			
Tremors			
Confusion			
Bradypnea			
Dry mouth			
Abdominal cramping			
Irritability			
Headache			
Polyuria			
Hypothermia			
Dizziness			
Polydipsia			

19. **What is most important for the nurse to instruct in order to prevent this situation from happening again?**
    1. Decrease calorie intake daily.
    2. Increase daily activity.
    3. Don't miss taking medications.
    4. Check glucose more frequently when you are ill.

20. **Now that Bart is insulin dependent if he develops complications, will he experience hyperosmolar, hyperglycemic, nonketotic syndrome (HHNS) or diabetic ketoacidosis (DKA)?**
    1. HHNS
    2. DKA

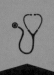

Go To Clinical Case

While caring for this client, be sure to review the concept maps in chapters 3 and 4.

Case 2: Pituitary Tumor with Removal

Related Concepts: Adaptation: Coping & Stress, Homeostasis: Fluid & Electrolytes
Threaded Topics: Complimentary Therapy, Pre/Postoperative Care, Advanced Directives, Medication Error-near Miss, HIPAA

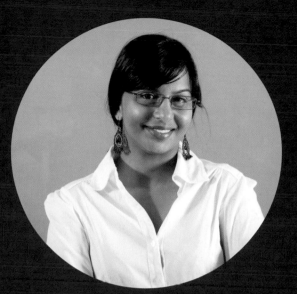

Prisha Patel is a 24-year-old school teacher. She graduated from the university last year and began her dream teaching job in an inner-city, low-income 3rd-grade classroom. She's healthy, maintaining a strict vegetarian diet and runs two miles each day. Her roommate and best friend, Rhonda is a registered nurse, working at a large medical center. Prisha begins to experience headaches. She assumes that they are related to the stress of her job, but when she finds them occurring more frequently, she seeks the advice of her roommate.

1. Prisha describes her headaches as recurring daily with constant throbbing pain. The oral Ibuprofen 400 mg that she's been taking every six-hours makes little difference in the discomfort. The headaches often keep her awake at night. What should Prisha's roommate, Rhonda recommend?

    1. Increasing the dose of ibuprofen to 600 mg every six hours.
    2. Alternating the ibuprofen with acetaminophen.
    3. Implement stress-relieving meditation each day.
    4. To make an appointment with a health care provider.

2. Prisha visits her naturalist practitioner describing the symptoms. She is diagnosed with migraine headaches from stress and hormonal changes and prescribed herbal supplements and acupuncture. What should be included in Prisha's teaching?

    1. She should not take ibuprofen while taking herbal supplements.
    2. The herbal treatments should be completed before acupuncture is started.
    3. The acupuncture treatments will require multiple sessions for best effect.
    4. The herbal supplements can cause nausea and vomiting.

After a week of the naturopathic treatments, Prisha begins to have visual disturbances. Her roommate convinces her to see a practitioner of Western medicine who orders a computed tomography (CT) scan of her brain.

3. **The provider records Prisha's symptoms in the electronic record. Match the medical term on the left with the appropriate symptom on the right.**

_____ Polyuria	A. Weight loss
_____ Hemianopia	B. Double vision
_____ Diplopia	C. No menstrual periods for 3 months
_____ Hypoglycemia	D. Frequent urination
_____ Amenorrhea	E. Loss of peripheral vision
_____ Diaphoresis	F. Low blood glucose
_____ Cachexia	G. Low number of red blood cells
_____ Anemia	H. Excess sweating

Prisha learns that she has a pituitary adenoma tumor, a benign growth on her pituitary gland. Because of her visual disturbances and headaches, it is recommended that she have her pituitary gland removed surgically using the transsphenoidal approach.

4. **Leaving the office that day, the nurse notices that Prisha is visibly upset and crying while scheduling the surgery. What should the nurse say?**
   1. "You'll be all right; this surgery is done all of the time."
   2. "Would it be better if you called us back later to schedule the surgery?"
   3. "Is there someone I can call to be with you?"
   4. "I'm sure you are afraid and overwhelmed; what questions can I answer for you?"

5. **Prisha's parents call Rhonda from India later that day and ask "What is going on with Prisha? She seems distracted each time we speak with her. Is everything all right?" How should Rhonda respond? Select all that apply.**
   1. "She'll be all right, but she needs surgery."
   2. "I wouldn't worry, Prisha is a strong person."
   3. "She got some bad news today, you should call her."
   4. "Nothing, why do you ask?"
   5. "If you are concerned, you should ask her."

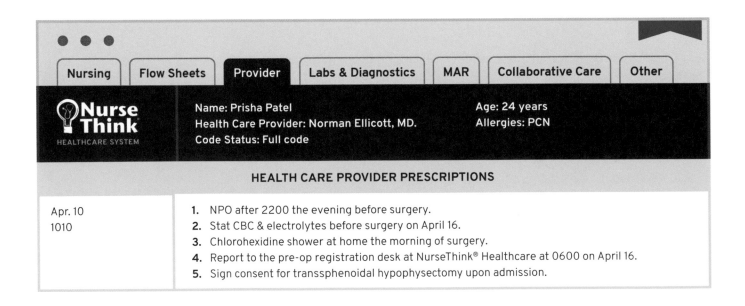

6. Prisha does not understand the information in the preoperative instructions. Mark if the explanation by the nurse is correct or incorrect. In the last column, correct the inaccurate statements made by the nurse.

	Correct	Incorrect	Corrected Statement
"You can brush your teeth the morning of surgery but don't swallow any water."			
"You can have a glass of water at midnight, on April 15, but nothing after that."			
"You need to get blood work done today."			
"You will use a special antibacterial solution and scrub your body in the shower before you come for surgery."			
"The surgical approach will be through your nose."			

7. It is the night before surgery. Prisha is anxious and cannot sleep. What should Rhonda suggest?

   1. Taking one of Rhonda's sleeping pills.
   2. Watching some television or reading a book to relax.
   3. Drinking a glass of hot tea.
   4. Taking a warm bath.

8. As Prisha is completing paperwork the morning of surgery, she is asked if she has advanced directives. She does not but asks if Rhonda can be her health care proxy since her family is outside of the country. How should the nurse respond?

   1. "No, the health care proxy must be family."
   2. "You don't need to designate anyone if you choose."
   3. "Yes, you can choose whomever you feel comfortable assigning."
   4. "It's best to ask Rhonda first to confirm that she is willing and able."

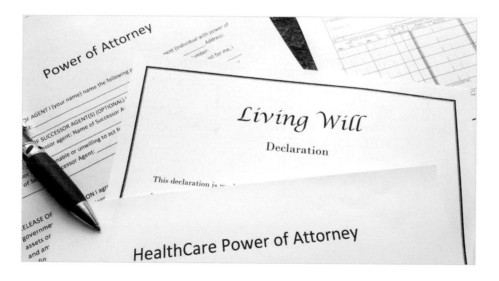

9. Prisha's surgery is successful. She comes to the post-anesthesia care unit (PACU) with a dressing under her nose and one on the right thigh. A new nurse in the PACU asks her mentor why there is a dressing on the thigh. How should the nurse respond?

    1. "That is the graft site that was used to cover the holes made in the skull."
    2. "They take a muscle flap and use it to fill the location where the tumor was removed."
    3. "There is probably a burn on her thigh from the surgical equipment."
    4. "I'm not sure; maybe she came in with it."

10. The post-anesthesia care unit calls the nurse to give the report. Prisha is stable. They'd like to know which room she will be going to. The charge nurse evaluates the room choices on the unit. Which is the best bed placement for Prisha? Check the best option.

Room 545 ☐	Room 546 ☐	Room 547 ☐
Bed 1: Open **Bed 2:** 44-year-old female with asthma and every 2 hours SVNs	**Bed 1:** 74-year-old man with a fracture, in traction. **Bed 2:** 76-year-old man with a head injury from a fall.	**Bed 1:** 37-year-old female on neutropenic precautions. **Bed 2:** Open
Room 548 ☐	**Room 549** ☐	**Room 550 – 4 Bed Ward** ☐
Bed 1: 53-year-old woman with pneumonia – lots of visitors **Bed 2:** Open	**Bed 1:** 36-year-old woman post-appendectomy. **Bed 2:** Open	**Bed 1:** 29-year-old female with newly diagnosed diabetes. **Bed 2:** 48-year-old female to be discharged this afternoon. **Bed 3:** Open **Bed 4:** 70-year-old female with an MRSA infection.
Room 551 ☐	**Room 552** ☐	
Bed 1: Open **Bed 2:** Open	**Bed 1:** Open **Bed 2:** 17-year-old girl newly diagnosed with Crohn's disease.	

11. **NurseThink® Prioritization Power!**

    Prisha is transferred to the medical-surgical care unit. Determine the **Top 3 Priority** assessments for the nurse to make in the first few hours after surgery.

    1. _____

    2. _____

    3. _____

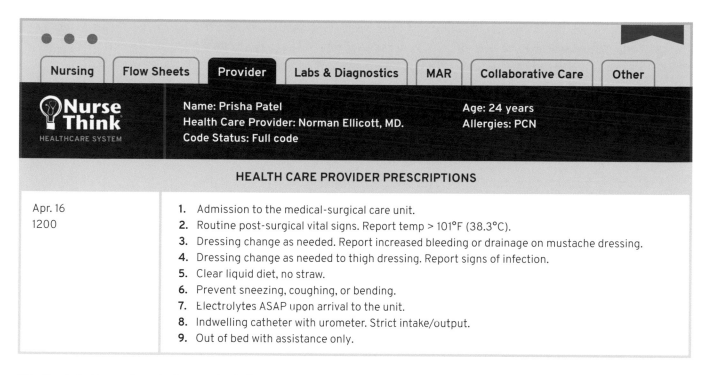

HEALTH CARE PROVIDER PRESCRIPTIONS

Apr. 16	
1200	1. Admission to the medical-surgical care unit.
	2. Routine post-surgical vital signs. Report temp > 101°F (38.3°C).
	3. Dressing change as needed. Report increased bleeding or drainage on mustache dressing.
	4. Dressing change as needed to thigh dressing. Report signs of infection.
	5. Clear liquid diet, no straw.
	6. Prevent sneezing, coughing, or bending.
	7. Electrolytes ASAP upon arrival to the unit.
	8. Indwelling catheter with urometer. Strict intake/output.
	9. Out of bed with assistance only.

12. **Explain the rationale for each of these prescriptions and why they are a specific concern for Prisha.**

1. Report temperature. _____

2. Report increased drainage on mustache dressing. _____

3. No straw. _____

4. Prevent sneezing, coughing, or bending. _____

5. Electrolytes ASAP. _____

6. Strict intake/output. _____

7. Out of bed with assistance only._____

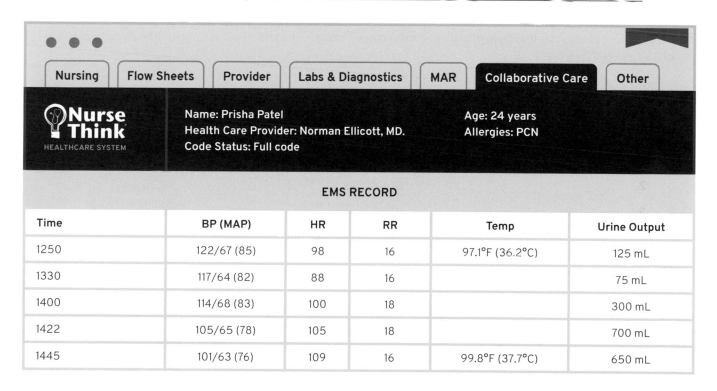

EMS RECORD

Time	BP (MAP)	HR	RR	Temp	Urine Output
1250	122/67 (85)	98	16	97.1°F (36.2°C)	125 mL
1330	117/64 (82)	88	16		75 mL
1400	114/68 (83)	100	18		300 mL
1422	105/65 (78)	105	18		700 mL
1445	101/63 (76)	109	16	99.8°F (37.7°C)	650 mL

13. **THIN Thinking Time!**

    As the nurse, reflect on the cues and data about Prisha's postoperative situation and apply **THIN Thinking** to prioritizing care.

    T – _____

    H – _____

    I – _____

    N – _____

    T - Top 3
    H - Help Quick
    I - Identify Risk to Safety
    N - Nursing Process

    Scan to access the 10-Minute-Mentor on THIN Thinking.

    NurseThink.com/THINThinking

14. The nurse recognizes that a call needs to be placed to the provider about Prisha's changing condition. What additional data should the nurse gather before making the phone call?

    _____

    _____

15. A call is placed to the health care provider. Complete the communication form.

    S – _____

    B – _____

    A – _____

    R – _____

    Clinical Hint:
    S - Situation
    B - Background
    A - Assessment
    R - Recommendation

16. The nurse receives a prescription to administer desmopressin 2 mcg intravenous, NOW and in 12 hours. The nurse obtains the vial below from the medication dispensing machine. How much medication should the nurse administer?

    Answer: _____

17. The nurse recognizes that the pharmacy has incorrectly stocked the medication dispensing machine. How should the nurse handle the situation? Select all that apply.

    1. Notify the charge nurse.
    2. Rearrange the medication to its proper location.
    3. Place a sign on the machine to alert others of the error.
    4. Complete a near-miss report.
    5. Contact the pharmacy.
    6. Document the situation in the client's record.

    Dexamethasone
    4mg/mL

18. **After delivering the correct dose of desmopressin, how will the nurse know if the medicine has been effective?**

    1. The temperature will decrease.
    2. The blood pressure will rise.
    3. The heart rate will decrease.
    4. The urine output will decrease.

19. **The nurse is providing discharge instructions to Prisha. Complete the chart, identifying if the instructions are appropriate or not appropriate for her surgical procedure.**

	Appropriate	Not-Appropriate
Do not bend or lift objects.		
Only drink liquids until your follow-up appointment.		
Follow up with the surgeon in 2 weeks.		
Monitor your weight daily.		
You may develop diarrhea from the medication.		
Report if you have a continuous drip of sinus drainage.		
You may have more pain from your graft site.		
Avoid driving for 6 months.		
You have an increased risk of seizures.		

20. **Given that Prisha has had surgery of her pituitary gland, which symptoms would be vital for her to report to her endocrinologist? Select all that apply.**

    1. Weight change.
    2. Dizziness upon rising.
    3. Sleeplessness.
    4. Constipation.
    5. Moodiness and irritability.

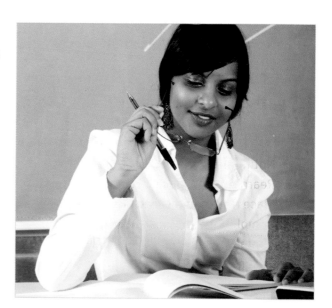

Conceptual Debriefing & Case Reflection

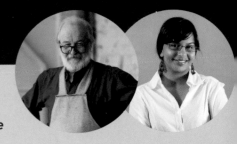

1. Compare the endocrine imbalance of Bart Bunyan and Prisha Patel. How are they the same and how are they different?

    _____

    _____

2. Identify the symptoms of hypo and hyper hormone release in both Bart and Prisha. How are they the same and how are they different?

    _____

    _____

3. In what areas of each case study was basic care and comfort utilized?

    _____

    _____

4. What steps in each case did the nurse take that prevented hospital-acquired injury?

    _____

    _____

5. What techniques of therapeutic communication did the nurse use in each case?

    _____

    _____

6. How did the nurse provide culturally sensitive/competent care?

    _____

    _____

7. How will learning about the case of Bart and Prisha impact the care you provide for future clients?

    _____

    _____

Fundamental Quiz

1. The nurse is caring for a client with a recent diagnosis of hypertension, hyperglycemia, and depression. The nurse notices that the client's arms are covered with bruises and skin tears. What additional information should the nurse gather?

   1. Determine the types of soaps the client is using.
   2. Ask if the client has been injured.
   3. Observe skin on the rest of the body.
   4. Review of medications the client is taking.

2. A client with excess pituitary secretion is experiencing sleeplessness, anxiousness, and weight loss. What should the nurse encourage? Select all that apply.

   1. A soothing bath at bedtime.
   2. Increased physical activity throughout the day.
   3. Frequent, high-protein snacks.
   4. Reevaluation of serum hormone levels.
   5. Slow, deep breathing, and relaxation techniques.

3. The nurse is caring for a client who is NPO and scheduled for a CT scan at 10 am. The client is insulin dependent and has both rapid and long-acting insulin prescribed before breakfast daily. The morning glucose level is 187 mg/dL. Anticipating that the client will be able to eat after the scan, what should the nurse do about the morning insulin prescription?

   1. Hold both the rapid and long-acting insulin.
   2. Hold the rapid-acting and delivery the long-acting insulin.
   3. Hold the long-acting and deliver the rapid-acting insulin.
   4. Deliver both insulins.

4. A client with adrenal insufficiency becomes dizzy after arising from the chair. What should be the nurse next action?

   1. Assess the blood pressure.
   2. Determine the level of consciousness.
   3. Assist the client back to the chair.
   4. Hold the client until the feeling passes.

5. A client with pre-diabetes tells the nurse that she has to get up to the restroom several times a night to urinate. What is the nurse's priority action?

   1. Assess the blood glucose level.
   2. Obtain a urine sample for infection.
   3. Ask if the client's been drinking liquids before bedtime.
   4. Ask what "several times" means.

Advanced Quiz

6. A client in a hypermetabolic state from hormone imbalance is experiencing diaphoresis, palpitations, and tachycardia with irregular beats. What should the nurse request when notifying the health care provider?

   1. Oxygen 2 L/NC.
   2. A beta-blocker.
   3. A 12-lead EKG.
   4. Cardiac enzymes.

7. The nurse is admitting a client with insulin dependent diabetes mellitus with a leg wound, a temperature of 100.9°F, heart rate of 115 beats/minute, blood pressure of 100/60 (73) mmHg, respiratory rate of 30 breaths per minute, oxygen saturation 98%. The serum glucose is 480 mg/dL. Which nursing action would be a priority?

   1. Increase oral fluids to more than a liter per day.
   2. Question the physician's order for subcutaneous insulin.
   3. Apply oxygen at 2 L/NC.
   4. Administer acetaminophen (Tylenol) 650 mg orally.

8. An insulin infusion is prescribed for a client weighing 155 pounds to begin at 0.2 units/kg/hour. Available is a premixed bag of 100 units of regular insulin in 100 mL of NS. A new graduate RN has calculated the infusion pump setting as 11 mL/hour and asked for dosage confirmation. How should the new grad's RN mentor respond?

   1. Advise the new grad to recalculate the infusion rate.
   2. Suggest that the new grad obtain a pump and begin the infusion as calculated.
   3. Suggest the new grad calls the pharmacy to confirm the calculations.
   4. Allow the new grad to independently administer the infusion using his/her own best judgment.

9. A nurse is emergently called to a homebound neighbor's house. The neighbor is found unconscious and has a history of insulin-dependent diabetes. After determining that no functioning glucometer is available, what should the nurse do next?

   1. Activate EMS to transport the client to a medical facility.
   2. Administer 10 units of regular insulin subcutaneously.
   3. Arouse the client to drink 4-6 ounces of orange juice.
   4. Administer glucagon 1 mg subcutaneously.

10. The charge nurse on the medical-surgical unit is making client assignments for the shift. Which client will be most appropriate to assign to an LPN?

    1. A client that is 3 days post-op transsphenoidal hypophysectomy.
    2. A client with insulin-dependent diabetes and glucose of 49, treated with 6 ounces' orange juice 5 minutes ago.
    3. A client with adrenal insufficiency who just received a call that her mother died suddenly.
    4. A client with uncontrolled diabetes and decreased renal function.

Scan QR Code to access the
10-Minute-Mentor
NurseThink.com/casestudy-book

CHAPTER

13

Movement

Mobility / Sensory / Nerve Conduction

People often take for granted the ability to move their body until they are unable to do so easily or pain-free. Mobility refers to purposeful physical movement. It is complex and includes three main components: 1) gross movements (moving the arms and legs when walking), 2) fine movements (picking up a pencil or some peanuts), and 3) the coordination of muscular efforts. Mobility requires the synchronization of both the musculoskeletal and nervous systems. It also relies on adequate cognition, oxygenation, and perfusion to make the muscles and nerves function properly. Mobility takes energy and strength along with a stable skeletal, joint and neuromuscular system. Without each of these factors, mobility is impaired.

Next Gen Clinical Judgment:

> What is the difference between the loss of gross and fine motor movement? Compare and contrast.

> How does nerve conduction and sensation impact movement?

> How does oxygenation and perfusion impair mobility?

> List sensory losses and how it impacts movement.

_____

_____

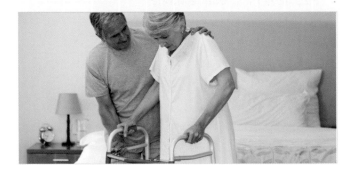

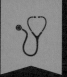

Go To Clinical Case

While caring for this client, be sure to review the concept maps in chapters 3 and 4.

Case 1: Movement Disorder with Fall Injury

Related Concepts: Comfort, Mobility, Elimination
Threaded Topics: Safety, Client Teaching, Older Adult, Interdisciplinary
Team, Socialization, Tremors, Coordination, and Balance

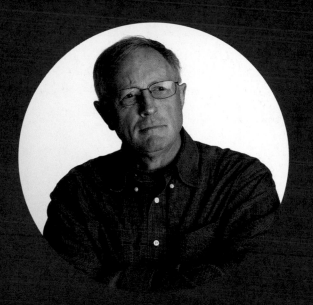

Gary Jansek is a 70-year-old who has lived with Parkinson's Disease for decades. He was a well-respected bank president when diagnosed at the age of 45. When diagnosed, it was expected that Gary would require full-time care within 10 years. After the prognosis and months of depression, his lifestyle changed. He retired early and focused on staying active. He and his wife moved to a community near his adult children. They were able to golf and swim every day, socialize with other couples, eat healthier, and focus on each other. The relaxing lifestyle slowed the progression of his symptoms. Gary and Judy believe that this lifestyle is why Gary is still able to function somewhat independently.

1. **How did Gary's lifestyle changes slow the progression of symptoms? Select all that apply.**
   1. Healthier eating allows for better absorption of medications.
   2. Physical activity builds muscle strength and coordination.
   3. Socialization improves depression.
   4. The reduction of stress decreases the need for dopamine.
   5. Retiring provides for financial security.

Gary is beginning to fall several times a week. He sometimes feels that his feet "stick to the floor" and when he cannot get moving, he falls forward. At other times he becomes very dizzy when standing and loses his balance. He and Judy make an appointment with the provider to discuss their concerns.

2. **The nurse completes an assessment, which finding is most concerning?**
   1. Large hematoma on the right hip.
   2. Tremors of the fingers and hands, right worse than left.
   3. Hunched stature.
   4. Shuffling gait.

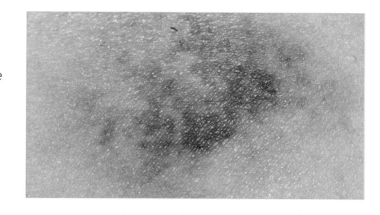

3. Mark in the boxes whether the findings are related or not related to Gary's current situation and disease.

	Finding	Related	Not Related
Medical History: Parkinson's disease (25 years), hypotension, constipation, diverticulitis, cataracts.	Hypotension		
	Constipation		
Surgical History: Deep brain stimulator placed five years ago.	Hypoproteinemia		
Vital Signs: 97.8°F (36.5°C); pulse 99 and irregular; respiratory rate 20; 97/55 (69).	Irregular pulse		
Labs: Hemoglobin 10.2 g/dL; K+ 3.4 mEq/L; Na+ 146 mEq/L; Albumin 3.1 g/dL.	Anemia		
Weight: BMI 18.	Weakened grips and pushes		
Physical Assessment: Right hip hematoma, 6-inch diameter, raised and hard — weakened grips and pushes.	Hematoma		
	Cataracts		
Medications: Levodopa/Carbidopa 25-100 mg TID and PRN; Selegiline 5 mg BID; Benztropine 1 mg daily.	Hypokalemia		
	Dry mouth		

Next Gen Clinical Judgment:

Compare the movement differences of each of these disorders:

Parkinson's disease:

_____

_____

Multiple sclerosis:

_____

_____

Myasthenia gravis:

_____

_____

Guillain–Barré syndrome:

_____

_____

Amyotrophic lateral sclerosis:

_____

_____

4. The nurse is unfamiliar with Gary's medications and accesses resources to learn more. Highlight the areas of the information that is most concerning to his current situation.

Levodopa/Carbidopa	Selegiline	Benztropine
Classification: Dopamine agonist. Antiparkinsonian agent. **Dose and Administration:** 25 mg carbidopa/100 mg levodopa 3 times a day; may increase till effect is achieved (max = 8 tablets/day) **Side effects:** Involuntary movements, dizziness, blurred vision, mydriasis, nausea, dry mouth, melanoma, anemia, leukopenia. **Precautions:** Contraindicated in glaucoma, MAOI therapy. Use cautiously with a history of cardiac, psychiatric, or ulcer disease. **Assessment:** Parkinsonian and extrapyramidal symptoms, lab abnormalities, blood pressure monitoring during dose change.	**Classification:** Monoamine Oxidase Type B Inhibitor (MAOI). Antiparkinsonian agent. **Dose and Administration:** 5 mg twice a day with food. **Side effects:** Confusion, dizziness, fainting, melanoma, nausea, dry mouth. **Precautions:** Do not give with meperidine, opioid analgesics, SSRI or tricyclic antidepressants. The side effect can be life-threatening. **Assessment:** Parkinsonian symptoms, blood pressure.	**Classification:** Anticholinergic. Antiparkinsonian agent. **Dose and Administration:** 1-2 mg/day in 1-2 divided doses. **Side effects:** Confusion, depression, dizziness, arrhythmias, hypotension, constipation, dry mouth, urinary retention. **Precautions:** Contraindicated in angle-closure glaucoma and with tardive dyskinesias. Use cautiously with cardiac dysrhythmias. **Assessment:** Parkinsonian and extrapyramidal symptoms, bowel function, monitor constipation, measure intake and output, orthostatic hypotension.

5. **NurseThink® Prioritization Power!**

   Evaluate the information in the case above and pick the **Top 3 Priority** concerns or cues.

   1. _____

   2. _____

   3. _____

An x-ray of Gary's hip shows no fracture. The hematoma resulted from soft tissue injury sustained on Gary's most recent fall, which occurred yesterday. The health care provider adjusts Gary's medication dosage to minimize his hypotension. A stool softener was added to the medication regimen to help with constipation from Gary's daily benztropine intake. The nurse prepares Gary's discharge paperwork.

6. **What should the nurse include in the discharge teaching? Select all that apply.**
   1. Rest the hip.
   2. Apply an ice pack to the hematoma.
   3. Exercise the affected extremity.
   4. Elevate the right lower extremity.
   5. Apply heat to the hematoma.

7. **Judy is concerned about Gary falling and asks the nurse about some strategies that can be used to minimize Gary's risk of having more falls. What strategies does the nurse suggest? Select all that apply.**
   1. Shuffle the feet when walking.
   2. Consider walking over imaginary lines on the floor.
   3. Don't walk without someone's assistance.
   4. Take medications as prescribed and on time.
   5. Avoid distractions when walking.

It has been four days since Gary sustained the fall with the hematoma. Judy started using heat on the site after 48 hours, and Gary elevates the extremity. However, he reports more pain at the site, and Judy observed that the hematoma has not changed. She calls the provider. They ask Gary to return to the office. After examining the hematoma, the provider determines that an incision and drainage of the hematoma needs to occur and prepares Gary for the minor procedure. The hematoma is drained, and Gary is discharged.

8. **NurseThink® Prioritization Power!**
   What is the **Top 3 Priority** post-procedure discharge teaching that the nurse must reinforce with Judy and Gary?

   1. _____
   2. _____
   3. _____

Gary's hematoma resolves. They return to socializing with friends and family, even though Judy notes that Gary is "not himself." He moves slower, has more tremors, and wants to watch rather than participate when they go golfing and swimming. Judy notices that Gary has trouble with simple tasks like buttoning his shirt, shaving, and mobility in the shower. Gary still wants to be independent in these tasks. Judy calls the healthcare provider's office to ask about assistive devices that might help Gary accomplish these tasks easier.

9. **Based on Judy's assessment information what should the nurse recommend as the Top 3 Priority interventions?**

   1. _____
   2. _____
   3. _____

Judy comes home one day from grocery shopping and finds Gary on the floor. He is conscious but reporting pain to the left hip. He is brought to the emergency department via ambulance.

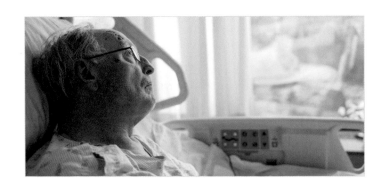

10. An x-ray of Gary's left hip shows a fracture, and he is scheduled for an open reduction and internal fixation (ORIF) surgery in 4 hours. As the nurse plans Gary's postoperative care what are the most important intervention(s) to ensure that Gary's hip fracture heals without complications? Select all that apply.

   1. Perform neurovascular assessments to the affected extremity.
   2. Encourage early and aggressive ambulation.
   3. Maintain proper alignment of the extremity.
   4. Provide nutritional support high in protein.
   5. Assessment of the incision site.

11. The nurse checks on Gary's wife who is sitting in the waiting room, waiting for Gary's surgery to be done. She tells the nurse, "My brother was in the hospital for seven days last year and got a really bad infection in his wound that he got in the hospital. I am worried about Gary getting an infection while he's here." What is the best response by the nurse?

   _____

   _____

Gary is back from surgery. The nurse has performed an initial assessment and Gary is stable and resting in bed with his wife and son at his bedside. His wife is worried that this fracture will now exacerbate Gary's Parkinson's disease, considering his movement and tremors have been more poorly controlled. The nurse assures her that physical and occupational therapists will work with Gary for his hip fracture but that the exercises they do will also help the mobility issues from his Parkinson's disease.

12. The nurse transcribes prescriptions from the surgeon. Highlight the prescriptions that the nurse should question and explain why.

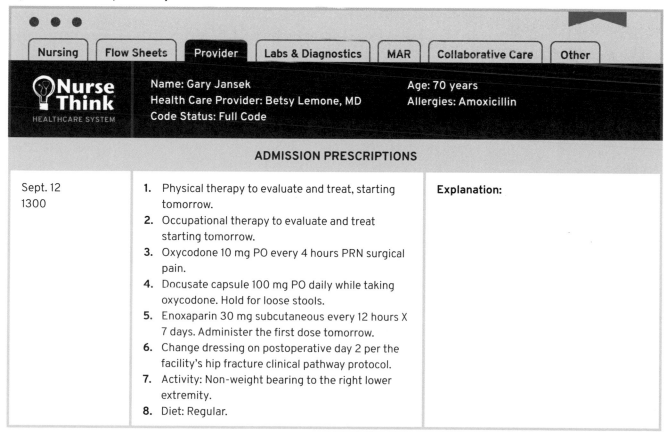

Nursing	Flow Sheets	Provider	Labs & Diagnostics	MAR	Collaborative Care	Other

Nurse Think HEALTHCARE SYSTEM

Name: Gary Jansek
Health Care Provider: Betsy Lemone, MD
Code Status: Full Code

Age: 70 years
Allergies: Amoxicillin

ADMISSION PRESCRIPTIONS

Sept. 12 1300	1. Physical therapy to evaluate and treat, starting tomorrow. 2. Occupational therapy to evaluate and treat starting tomorrow. 3. Oxycodone 10 mg PO every 4 hours PRN surgical pain. 4. Docusate capsule 100 mg PO daily while taking oxycodone. Hold for loose stools. 5. Enoxaparin 30 mg subcutaneous every 12 hours X 7 days. Administer the first dose tomorrow. 6. Change dressing on postoperative day 2 per the facility's hip fracture clinical pathway protocol. 7. Activity: Non-weight bearing to the right lower extremity. 8. Diet: Regular.	Explanation:

13. A new nurse is precepting with Gary's primary nurse and is administering the first dose of enoxaparin to Gary. Examine the image of the nurse administering the enoxaparin to the client. Which observation(s) cause(s) the preceptor to intervene and determine that the new nurse needs additional teaching on the administration of this medication? Select all that apply.

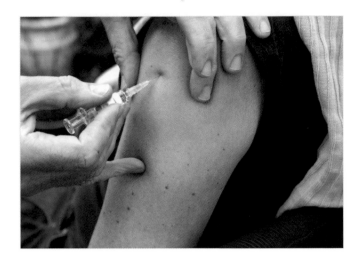

1. The nurse should not pinch the skin.
2. The location of the injection is incorrect.
3. The nurse is not wearing gloves.
4. The client should be lying flat.
5. A larger needle is required.

14. On postoperative day one, the physical and occupational therapists are working with Gary for the first time. At the end of physical therapy, Gary and his wife reported to the nurse that they believe the physical therapist "pushed Gary too hard" today. What activity might have caused this concern?

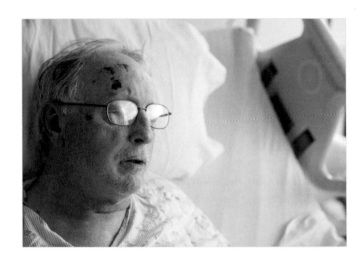

1. Transferred out of bed and sat at the side of the bed.
2. Ambulated 350 feet to the nurses' station using a crutch.
3. Transferred out of bed and sat in a chair for 15 minutes.
4. Ambulated to the bathroom using non-weight bearing to affected extremity.

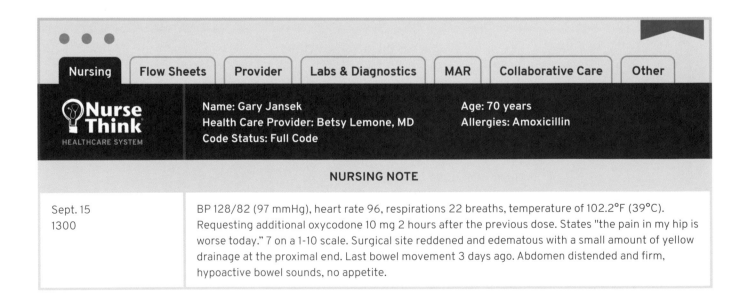

| Nursing | Flow Sheets | Provider | Labs & Diagnostics | MAR | Collaborative Care | Other |

NurseThink
HEALTHCARE SYSTEM

Name: Gary Jansek
Health Care Provider: Betsy Lemone, MD
Code Status: Full Code

Age: 70 years
Allergies: Amoxicillin

NURSING NOTE

| Sept. 15 1300 | BP 128/82 (97 mmHg), heart rate 96, respirations 22 breaths, temperature of 102.2°F (39°C). Requesting additional oxycodone 10 mg 2 hours after the previous dose. States "the pain in my hip is worse today." 7 on a 1-10 scale. Surgical site reddened and edematous with a small amount of yellow drainage at the proximal end. Last bowel movement 3 days ago. Abdomen distended and firm, hypoactive bowel sounds, no appetite. |

15. Thin Thinking Time!

Use the nurse's assessment, and apply **THIN Thinking.**

T – _____

H – _____

I – _____

N – _____

T - Top 3
H - Help Quick
I - Identify Risk to Safety
N - Nursing Process

Scan to access the 10-Minute-Mentor → on THIN Thinking.

NurseThink.com/THINThinking

16. The nurse contacts the provider with SBAR communication. Complete the report.

S – _____

B – _____

A – _____

R – _____

Clinical Hint:
S - Situation
B - Background
A - Assessment
R - Recommendation

17. The nurse receives these verbal orders from the provider. Mark each as appropriate or inappropriate and explain why.

Verbal Order	Appropriate	Inappropriate	Why?
Wound culture for culture and sensitivity after the first antibiotic dose.			
Cephalexin 500 mg Intravenous every 12 hours x 7 days			
Bisacodyl 10 mg by mouth daily for constipation.			
Fleets enema PR daily PRN for impaction.			

The prescriber adjusts the prescriptions and Gary is now doing well with only a few days left of the antibiotic therapy. He responded to the bisacodyl with a large formed bowel movement later day.

A few days later, Gary's physical therapist progresses him from non-weight bearing status to toe-touch, and he is progressing well and looking forward to being discharged to a skilled nursing facility for sub-acute rehabilitation to continue his therapy, before going home.

The day before discharge, the physical therapist is finishing a session with Gary when Gary reports shortness of breath. The therapist calls the nurse to the room. Read the nurse's notes in the chart below.

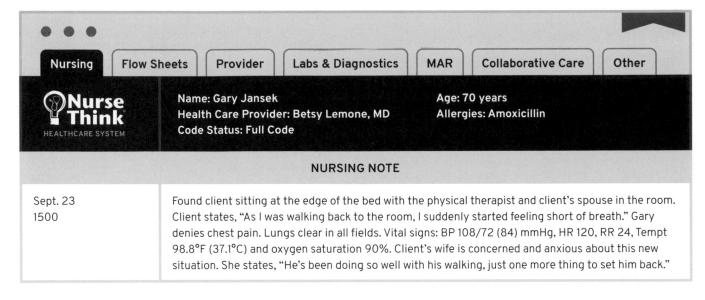

Name: Gary Jansek
Health Care Provider: Betsy Lemone, MD
Code Status: Full Code

Age: 70 years
Allergies: Amoxicillin

NURSING NOTE

Sept. 23 1500	Found client sitting at the edge of the bed with the physical therapist and client's spouse in the room. Client states, "As I was walking back to the room, I suddenly started feeling short of breath." Gary denies chest pain. Lungs clear in all fields. Vital signs: BP 108/72 (84) mmHg, HR 120, RR 24, Tempt 98.8°F (37.1°C) and oxygen saturation 90%. Client's wife is concerned and anxious about this new situation. She states, "He's been doing so well with his walking, just one more thing to set him back."

18. **In order of priority, what actions should the nurse take?**

    _____, _____, _____, _____.

    1. Calm the client's wife to decrease her anxiety.
    2. Place a call to the health care provider.
    3. Assist client back to bed.
    4. Apply oxygen to the client at 2 L/minute via nasal cannula.
    5. Elevate the head of the bed.

19. **A pulmonary embolism is suspected, and the nurse receives STAT labs for D-dimer level and CT angiography. The CT angiography is negative, and the D-dimer level is 0.3 µ/mL. What conclusions can the nurse draw from these results?**

    1. Gary has a pulmonary embolism.
    2. Gary does not have a pulmonary embolism.
    3. Gary has a deep vein thrombosis.
    4. Gary has both a deep vein thrombosis and a pulmonary embolism.

In preparation for discharge, the occupational and physical therapists have taught Gary and his family several safe positioning strategies for Gary to use at home to improve mobility and prevent complications of hip surgery.

20. **What teaching by the physical therapist on safe positioning on the toilet, will the nurse reinforce with Gary? Place the actions in the correct order.**

    _____, _____, _____, _____, _____.

    1. Use a bedside commode with a raised toilet seat.
    2. Place the weight on the unaffected leg, while extending the affected leg out in front.
    3. Grasp the grab bars on the toilet (if your bathroom has grab bars).
    4. Take steps backward toward the toilet until it is felt at the back of the legs.
    5. Sit down on the toilet and scoot back if needed.

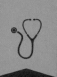
Case 2: Movement: Impaired Nerve and Sensory Function

Related Concepts: Sensation, Protection, Comfort, Elimination
Threaded Topics: Leadership, Delegation, Medication Error, Skin Integrity, Communication, Scope of Practice, Team Nursing, Adverse Events, Quality Improvement

Jeremiah Goldfinch is a 62-year-old client who is riding his horse when the horse becomes spooked and throws him off, spiraling him to the ground. Jeremiah feels a sudden pain in his back and numbness and tingling of his lower extremities. He calls for help and is taken to the emergency department where it is revealed he has suffered an L1-L2 vertebral fracture with spinal nerve damage. He is treated in the acute care setting with effective spinal immobilization and medications until he is stable and ready for transfer to the NurseThink® Rehabilitation Facility.

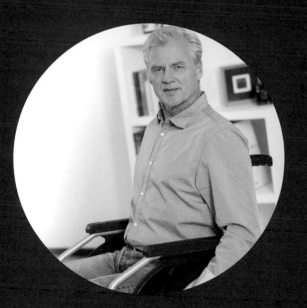

Jeremiah's spinal injury results in sensory deficits and motor loss below the level of damage with varying control of his legs and pelvis. The providers feel that he will eventually return home having a good sitting balance with full independent use of a wheelchair. He may be able to ambulate short distances with leg braces.

1. **NurseThink® Prioritization Power!**

   Evaluate the information in the case and choose the **Top 3 Priority** concerns or cues.

   1. _____

   2. _____

   3. _____

2. **Based on the priority concerns what action should the nurse perform first?**

   1. Assess his ability to move his extremities.
   2. Maintain spinal precautions with immobilization.
   3. Assess his distal responses to pinprick and vibration.
   4. Discuss the signs and symptoms of risks the client may have.

3. Review this image and the area(s) of the body that impact sensation. Based on Jeremiah's injury, what should the nurse anticipate as deficits? Mark the areas on the image.

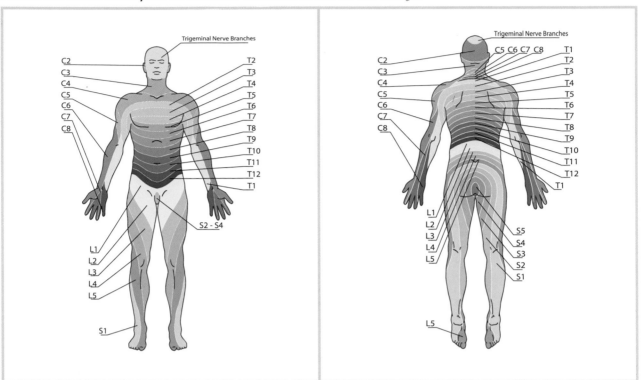

4. The nurse reviews Jeremiah's prescribed medications. Determine the specifics of each of the medications. For each shaded box in the table fill in the correct answer.

Medication	Reason Prescribed	Dose, Route, Frequency	Drug Class	Patient Teaching
Enoxaparin		130 mg, subcutaneous, daily		
Baclofen		10 mg, oral, four times daily		May cause drowsiness, dizziness. Do not drink alcoholic beverages or operate heavy machinery, do not suddenly discontinue
Sertraline		50 mg, oral, daily		
Bisacodyl		One suppository, rectal, timed daily		
Acetaminophen		650 mg, oral, every 6 to 8 hours as needed		

5. **The nurse develops the plan of care for Jeremiah's stay in rehabilitation. Which action is a priority for the prevention of complications?**
   1. Implement fall precautions.
   2. Administer prescribed low dose anticoagulation.
   3. Perform active lower extremity range of motion exercises.
   4. Refer to physical and occupational therapy for assistance.

After gathering a history and performing a head-to-toe assessment, the nurse determines that because of Jeremiah's SCI, he has loss of motor and sensory function below the level of injury. He currently has been prescribed a lumbar brace and foot drop splints.

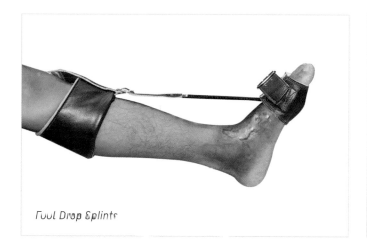

Foot Drop Splints

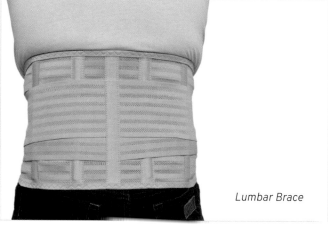

Lumbar Brace

6. **The nurse assesses deep tendon reflexes by using a reflex hammer. What should the nurse expect to evaluate by performing this type of assessment?**
   1. How intact the peripheral nerves are.
   2. How the motor neurons and fibers are reacting.
   3. How fast the impulse will move through the nerve.
   4. The amount of electrical activity produced by skeletal muscles.

7. **Connect the deep tendon reflex tested with the appropriate spinal root involved. Circle those that should be assessed on Jeremiah according to his condition.**

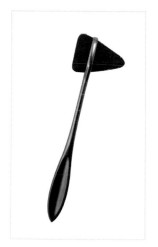

___ Achilles Tendon	A. C5, C6
___ Biceps	B. C6
___ Patellar	C. C7
___ Brachioradialis	D. L4
___ Triceps	E. S1

After the shift assessment, the nurse documents vital signs and plans to complete subsequent focused assessments, focusing in on the parts of the nervous system affected by Jeremiah's condition. It is determined that Jeremiah has lost function of bowel and bladder and is on a bowel and bladder training program. He learns initiate timed urinary catheterization and rectal suppositories.

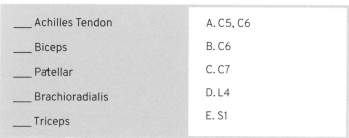

NurseThink
HEALTHCARE SYSTEM

Name: Jeremiah Goldfinch
Health Care Provider: Bob Bratte, MD
Code Status: Full code

Age: 62 years
Allergies: NKDA

	BP (MAP)	HR	RR	Sats	Temp	Pain Level (1-10)	Weight
May 15 0800	130/78 (95)	72	14	96% Room Air	100°F (37.8°C)	0	186 lbs. (84.4 kg)

REHABILITATION NOTE

The client is alert and oriented x 3, self-directing and non-ambulatory. Can transfer with assistance and stand via pivot using full leg braces. Limited gross motor present of bilateral lower extremities. Limited light and deep touch sensation to bilateral anterior and posterior legs absent. Can determine warm and cool sensations to right leg only. Can maneuver wheelchair independently using upper extremities. Lumbar brace intact and bilateral foot drop splints applied. Skin pink, warm, without evidence of breakdown to dependent areas. Last timed bowel movement and urinary catheterization at 2400 hours. Discussed timed urinary catheterization and rectal suppository and the need for intervention. Client verbalizes understanding and readiness to intervene.

The nurse helps to facilitate urinary catheterization and timed rectal suppository. After return demonstration and intervention, it is determined that Jeremiah utilizes the catheter properly while maintaining aseptic technique. However, the nurse notes the urine appears slightly bloody, dark, and cloudy with a foul odor.

8. **NurseThink® Prioritization Power!**

   Evaluate the information within the nurse's assessment and vital sign record and pick the **Top 3 Priority** assessment findings.

   1. _____

   2. _____

   3. _____

9. The nurse gathers information and begins to prepare an SBAR telephone conversation for the provider. Complete each section of the SBAR communication.

   S – _____

   B – _____

   A – _____

   R – _____

   Clinical Hint:
   S - Situation
   B - Background
   A - Assessment
   R - Recommendation

The provider prescribes a urinalysis with culture and sensitivity, a complete blood count (CBC), an international normalized ratio (INR) and IV antibiotics. The provider assumes that the prescriptions will be implemented now. The new nurse plans to obtain urine on the next catheterization scheduled and enters the labs to be drawn on the next lab day, 2 days from now.

10. **Identify two communication mistakes from the information provided that followed the SBAR report:**

    1. _____

    2. _____

11. **Jeremiah is instructed on wearing the lumbar brace at all times to reduce motion of the spine until healing is complete. Which assessment finding should the nurse report immediately to the health care provider?**

    1. Pain level 2 on a 0 to 10 pain scale.
    2. Skin abrasion has developed at the bottom of the brace near the waist.
    3. The client verbalizes that the brace feels too restrictive.
    4. The skin at the pin sites are red and have purulent drainage.

12. **Considering a hierarchy of rehabilitative needs for Jeremiah, and number from highest to lowest priority:**

    1. ___ Self-care and ADLs
    2. ___ Self-actualization
    3. ___ Maintenance of the physiologic systems
    4. ___ Preparation for living at home

There have been recent staffing changes at the NurseThink® Rehabilitation Facility. Margarita, a seasoned registered nurse, is the lead mentor for three newly hired graduate nurses. The ratio of nurses to client care is 1:15 (1 nurse to every 15 clients). The new nurses each have five clients, and Margarita oversees the care they provide acting as the mentor and resource nurse throughout the shift. The team members form a huddle at the beginning of the shift and determine a plan for the delivery of safe and effective care for the day.

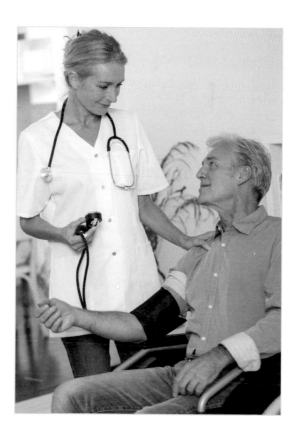

13. **In preparing for the professional nurse's role as a mentor, what best describes the goal of Margarita's leadership position?**

    1. Delivering client and family-centered care.
    2. Disseminating rehabilitation nursing knowledge.
    3. Using supportive technology for improved quality.
    4. Providing client education.

14. Margarita discusses the role of the collaborative team members involved in Jeremiah's rehab care. Connect the NurseThink® Rehabilitation Facility team members with their scope of practice.

____ Case manager	A. Assists the nurses in caring for comfort, hygiene, and mobility needs
____ Dietician	B. Assists in improving strength and coordination, regaining independence of ADLs.
____ Neuropsychologist	C. Coordinates aspects of care that include education, team conferences, communication, insurance companies, and discharge planning.
____ Occupational therapist	D. Helps in regaining strength, balance, coordination, promotes using a wheelchair and manage other activities that enhance mobility.
____ Physical therapist	E. Works closely with the rehab team to respond to physiological and emotional needs; examples include assisting with skin management, bowel/bladder training, and self-care skills as needed.
____ Nursing supervisor	F. Supports and educates the client and family to better able to deal with life changes. Evaluates cognitive, emotional, and intellectual skills; provides supportive psychotherapy.
____ Registered nurse	G. Reviews nutritional needs and provides nutritional education and counseling.
____ Licensed practical nurse	H. Responsible for managing staff, overseeing client care and ensuring adherence to established policies and procedures.
____ Unlicensed assistive personnel	I. Responsible for client care and delivery of medications.

15. Margarita delegates to the new nurse the task of assisting Jeremiah from the wheelchair to the bed. The nurse responds "I understand this is in my job description, but this is the first time I will have done this with a full wheelchair dependent client. Can you show me what to do?" How should Margarita respond?

1. The nurse should find an experienced UAP to demonstrate the task.
2. Margarita should assist the nurse, observe him, and provide feedback.
3. Margarita should complete the task because it is not in the new nurse's job description.
4. Margarita should report and discipline the new nurse for not taking accountability.

16. Which tasks can the nurse safely delegate to the unlicensed assistive personnel (UAP)? Select all that apply.

1. Monitor vital signs and record the results.
2. Collect and assess urine from straight catheterization.
3. Monitor intake and output, and record the results.
4. Assist the client from the wheelchair to the bed.
5. Reposition client and evaluate skin and pressure areas for breakdown.

17. What resource can the new nurse use that will provide information and is considered the determinant for the decision to delegate within the legal scope of delegation rules?

1. The facility's policies and procedural manual.
2. A nurse practice act.
3. The American Nurses Association Code of Ethics.
4. The Joint Commission Patient Care Standards.

Several of the rehabilitation clients require medications. Margarita gathers the new nurses to learn how the team administers several medications to multiple clients each day. The nurses are expecting a standardized medication dispensing system, but instead, there is a cart with wheels and several medications contained within drawers. The nurses push the cart through the hallway to each room, where they administer the medications. The residents do not wear identification, but there is a chart at the door with their name and client identification number.

Nurse's Anne and Kevin are working together. Anne prepares the medications and places them into a cup. She hands the pills to Kevin who then enters the client's room to deliver the medicines.

Kevin enters Jeremiah's room, hands him the medicine cup with a tablet in it, and says "here's your sertraline." Jeremiah swallows the tablet with water. Kevin returns to the medication cart and realizes that there are two identical bottles of sertraline next to each other on the cart. One bottle is labeled "50 mg/tablet", and the other bottle is labeled "100 mg/tablet". He realizes that the wrong tablet was placed into the medication container by Anne and that he administered to Jeremiah. Kevin tells Anne "I think you prepared the wrong tablet that I gave to Mr. Goldfinch. Do you think he'll be okay?" Anne responds, "I think it'll be okay, it's just an antidepressant, and there are limited harmful side effects."

---

18. **THIN Thinking Time!**

Reflect on the scenario and apply THIN Thinking.

T – _____

H – _____

I – _____

N – _____

T - Top 3
H - Help Quick
I - Identify Risk to Safety
N - Nursing Process

Scan to access the 10-Minute-Mentor → *on THIN Thinking.*

NurseThink.com/THINThinking

---

19. **The nurses discuss how the error could have been prevented. What actions should the nurse have taken to avoid the incident? Select all that apply.**

1. Following the rights of medication administration.
2. Compare the medication prescription with the client profile when obtaining it from the medication cart.
3. Validate the medication with the medication administration record before placing it into the medication cup.
4. Verify the medication with the client at the time of administration.
5. The nurse preparing the medications should be the individual administrating it.

Next Gen Clinical Judgment:

Discuss each of these questions with a peer:

> How might communicating with the client at the time of medication administration benefit the situation?

_____

> If Anne believes everything will be okay and Kevin trusts her judgment, should Kevin report the error?

_____

> How should the nurse's document the incident?

_____

> Should Jeremiah be told about the error?

_____

20. Complete the Incident Reporting Form:

Incident Reporting Form

Use this form to report any workplace accident, injury, incident, close call or illness. Return completed form to the Nursing Supervisor or Management.

This is documenting an:

☐ Lost Time/Injury   ☐ First Aid   ☐ Incident   ☐ Close Call   ☐ Observation

Details of the person injured or involved:

Jeremiah Goldfinch, Medical Record # 1234567

Person Completing Report: _____ Date: _____

Person(s) Involved: _____

Event Details: Medication error

Date of Event: _____

Location of Event: NurseThink® Rehabilitation Facility; Floor 2, Room 9

Time of Event: 9:30am

Description of Events (Describe tasks being performed and sequence of events):

_____

_____

_____

*If more space is required please use the back of this sheet

Was event / injury caused by an unsafe act (activity or movement) or an unsafe condition?
Please explain:

_____

_____

_____

To Be Completed Only If Lost Time/Injury Or First Aid Was Required	
Type of injury sustained:	None
Was the medical treatment necessary?	Yes _____ No _____ If yes, name of hospital or physician:

Signature of Employee: _____ Date: _____

Signature of Employee: _____ Date: _____

Signature of Supervisor: _____ Date: _____

Incident Management

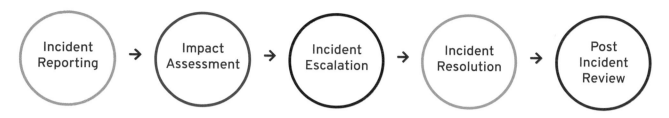

Incident Reporting	→	Impact Assessment	→	Incident Escalation	→	Incident Resolution	→	Post Incident Review

Next Gen Clinical Judgment:

Review the process of incident management and describe the steps that should be followed:

> Incident Reporting _____

> Impact Assessment _____

> Incident Escalation _____

> Incident Resolution _____

> Post Incident Review _____

Although Jeremiah suffers no consequences from receiving the wrong dose of the medication, it led the team to investigate and modify the normal operations of medication administration. The nursing supervisors have collected data which revealed medication errors have been on the rise in the rehabilitation facility. Funding was allocated to promote a safer environment with less risk for errors to occur. They have been working with team members and have implemented the new method for medication administration. The institution completed a follow-up investigation and found a 95% reduction in medication administration, confirming that a positive outcome was achieved.

The Five Rights of Medication Administration

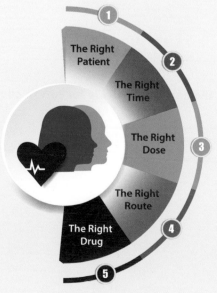

1. Check the name on the order and the patient.
   Use 2 identifiers.
   Ask patient to identify himself/herself.

2. Check the frequency of the ordered medication.
   Check that you are giving the ordered dose at the correct time.
   Confirm when the last dose was given.

3. Check the order.
   Confirm appropriateness of the dose using a current drug reference.
   If necessary, calculate the dose and have another nurse calculate the dose as well.

4. Again, check the order and appropriateness of the route ordered.
   Confirm that the patient can take or receive the medication by the ordered route.

5. Confirm the rationale for the ordered medication.
   What is the patient's history? Why is he/she taking this medication?
   Revisit the reasons for long-term medication use.

The Right Patient
The Right Time
The Right Dose
The Right Route
The Right Drug

Conceptual Debriefing & Case Reflection

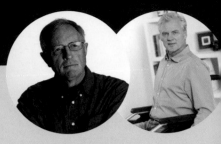

1. Compare the mobility issues of Gary Jansek and Jeremiah Goldfinch. How are they the same and how are they different?

   _____

   _____

2. Differentiate between the mobility, sensory, and neuro conduction issues of both Gary and Jeremiah. How were the conceptual areas the same? How were they different for each of these individuals?

   _____

   _____

3. In what areas of each case study was basic care and comfort utilized?

   _____

   _____

4. What steps in each case did the nurse take that prevented hospital-acquired injury?

   _____

   _____

5. What techniques of therapeutic communication did the nurse use in each case?

   _____

   _____

6. How did the nurse provide culturally sensitive/competent care?

   _____

   _____

7. How will learning about the case of Gary and Jeremiah impact the care you provide for future clients?

   _____

   _____

Fundamental Quiz

1. **The nurse is transferring a client with a mobility disorder from the bed to a wheelchair. What is the most important action by the nurse?**
   1. Applying light pressure under the client's arms when standing up.
   2. Allowing the client to help as much as possible.
   3. Place a foot between the clients to support the weight.
   4. Placing the bed lower than the height of the wheelchair.

2. **The nurse cares for a client who recently sustained a fall with tibial-fibula fracture. A cast was applied two hours ago. The nurse comes into the room and sees the image here. What action by the nurse is the priority?**

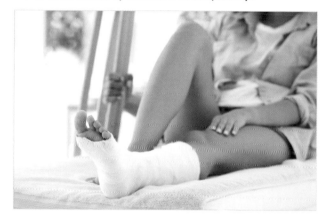

   1. Remove the crutches from the client.
   2. Assess the circulation to the toes.
   3. Apply ice to the ankle.
   4. Elevate the casted leg on pillows.

3. **The nurse is completing an assessment for a client with a femur fracture and a long leg cast. The toes in the affected leg are pale and cool. The client says they feel numb. What should the nurse do next?**
   1. Apply a warm blanket.
   2. Remove the cast.
   3. Assess the pedal pulses.
   4. Notify the practitioner.

4. **A nurse at the clinic is evaluating a client who's been using crutches for a week. The client says "my underarms are sore and the skin is all red and bruised." How should the nurse respond?**
   1. "You are spending too much time using the crutches; you need to be sitting more."
   2. "Maybe the crutches are too small for you; let's take a look."
   3. "You should use your arms to lift yourself off of the crutches so that you don't rest on them."
   4. "I'll get you some additional padding for the crutches to make the armrests softer."

5. **A client with a movement disorder is admitted with fall precautions prescribed. What actions should be included in the plan of care? Select all that apply.**
   1. Identifying the client with a "fall precautions" wristband.
   2. Placing a pad on the floor at the bedside.
   3. Raise all 4 side rails.
   4. Apply non-skid slippers.
   5. Confirm call light is within reach.

Advanced Quiz

6. **The nurse is teaching a client after having an open reduction, internal fixation (ORIF) of the right hip about putting on a pair of shorts. In what order should the client perform these steps?**

   _____, _____, _____, _____, _____, _____, _____, _____.

   1. Put the pants on to the unaffected extremity.
   2. When steady, use both hands to pull pants up around the waist.
   3. Use a reacher to grasp the waist of the pants.
   4. Sit on the side of the bed (can use a chair as well).
   5. Hold the waist of the pants with one hand.
   6. Put the pants on to the affected extremity.
   7. Push self-up to a standing position with the other hand.
   8. Pull the pants up above the knee by using the reacher.

7. **The nurse is caring for an older adult in the intensive care unit who is experiencing sensory overload. Which actions should the nurse take to improve client outcomes? Select all that apply.**
   1. Use a lower tone when communicating with the client.
   2. Coordinate routine visits from the hospital pet therapy program.
   3. Decrease environmental noise.
   4. Open curtains during the day for natural light.
   5. Limit the use of sedatives during the day.

8. **The nurse is caring for the client with this traction. What interventions are a priority? Select all that apply.**

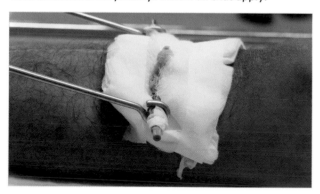

   1. Assess for circulation of distal extremity.
   2. Assess the site for redness and drainage.
   3. Monitor for fever.
   4. Turn the client on to the left and right side each hour.
   5. Keep weight handing freely.

9. The nurse cares for a client recovering from surgical repair of a hip fracture. During the assessment the nurse notes that the client has difficulty lying with the head of the bed lowered. Which assessment(s) support(s) a respiratory concern secondary to the immobility? Select all that apply.

   1. BP = 108/64 (79).
   2. RR 24 BPM.
   3. HR 118 BPM.
   4. Crackles in the bilateral bases.
   5. Pain of 8/10 when coughing.

10. The nurse is ambulating an older adult for the first time since admission. The client says "I'm dizzy and I'm starting to pass out." Place the actions of the nurse in the priority order.

    _____, _____, _____, _____, _____.

    1. Grasp the client's gait belt.
    2. Stay with the client and call for help.
    3. Place feet wide apart with one foot between the client's legs.
    4. Gently slide the client down to the floor.
    5. Pull the weight of the client backward against the nurse.

Comfort

Pain / Tissue Integrity / Fatigue

The American Pain Society (APS) defines pain as an unpleasant sensory and emotional experience associated with actual or potential tissue damage. Pain is one of the most common reasons that individuals seek medical attention and it may be acute or chronic. Because of its potentially debilitating impact on a person's livelihood and quality of life, pain assessment and treatment are complex. Pain is both physical and emotional. Nurses must recognize that a person's pain response is often a result of his/her culture and past experiences with pain and pain management. Pain is subjective, and the nurse needs to treat the individual based on his or her perceived pain response.

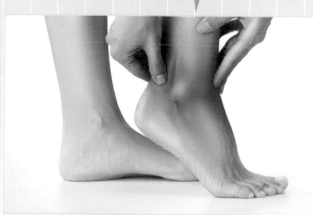

Next Gen Clinical Judgment:

> How does discomfort impact a person's health and well-being?

> Besides pain, what are other ways a person is uncomfortable?

> How can a nurse determine discomfort in a person who is not verbal?

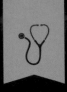

Go To Clinical Case

While caring for this client, be sure to review the concept maps in chapters 3 and 4.

Case 1: Impaired Tissue Integrity and Pain

Related Concepts: Circulation, Protection, Emotion, Nutrition
Threaded Topics: Skin Integrity, Wound Care, Infection, Pain
Management, Safety

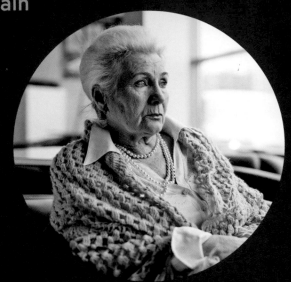

Mattie Smith is an 88-year-old who has lived alone in Florida since the death of her husband three years ago. They were married for 60 years. Mattie has had failing health over the past months, and her son John, who lives out of state, has been concerned about her and asked that she moves out of her home and come to live with him in Tennessee. Mattie and her son have never been close, and she refused his offer. He is visiting her for the holidays and finds her home untidy, with dirty dishes and clothes strewn everywhere. She looks disheveled, lacks proper hygiene, and says there is a lot of pain near her "buttock" area. He recalls that his mother always kept a clean house and had a lot of pride when it came to her appearance. He coaxes her to let him take her to the emergency department, but she refuses.

1. **What information in the case cues John that something is not quite right with his mother?**

   _____

   _____

   _____

John is on the second day of his 4-day visit and notices that his mother rarely moves from one location on the couch where she sits to watch television. Occasionally she will briefly get up to go to the bathroom, get something to eat, or go to bed at night. When she walks, he notices a limp. He questions her about the limp, but Mattie minimizes it, saying "I'm just a little uncomfortable from a sore spot on my right heel." She refuses to let him see her heel. John also observes that her meals consist of cakes, pies, coffee, and soda. He is concerned about Mattie and brings up going to the hospital again. This time, she reluctantly agrees.

Online Videos, Downloads, and Answers—Visit NurseThink.com/casestudy-book

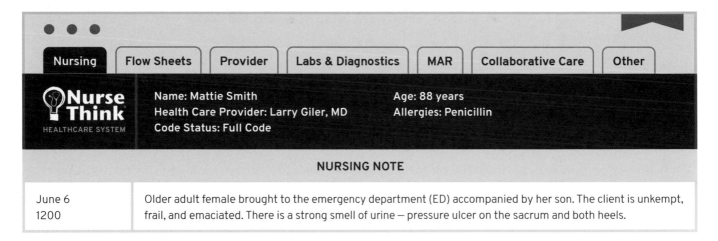

NURSING NOTE

June 6 1200	Older adult female brought to the emergency department (ED) accompanied by her son. The client is unkempt, frail, and emaciated. There is a strong smell of urine — pressure ulcer on the sacrum and both heels.

2. **Along with the pressure ulcers, what information is vital for the emergency department nurse to convey to the floor nurse in the report? Select all that apply.**

   1. Mattie's smell of urine.
   2. Mattie's poor nutrition.
   3. Loss of her spouse.
   4. Mattie's behavior at home.
   5. Mattie's refusal to live with her son.

Mattie is admitted to the medical unit. The floor nurse determines that Mattie is not incontinent but that she has not had a proper bath in a while. The unlicensed assistive personnel (UAP) bathes Mattie and settles her in bed. The nurse transcribes the admission prescriptions in the electronic record.

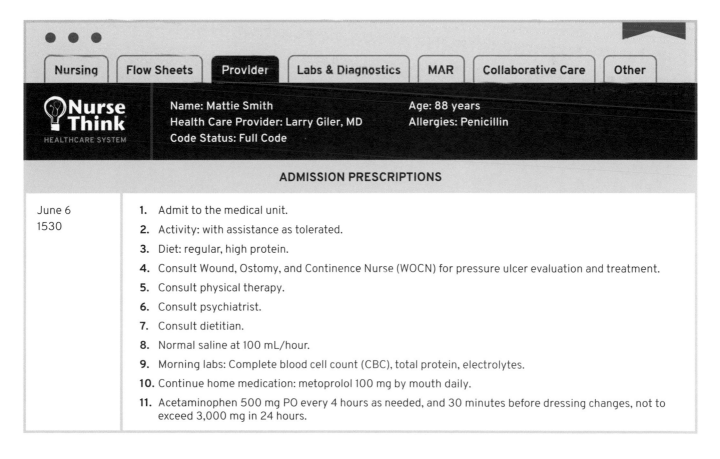

ADMISSION PRESCRIPTIONS

June 6 1530	1. Admit to the medical unit.
	2. Activity: with assistance as tolerated.
	3. Diet: regular, high protein.
	4. Consult Wound, Ostomy, and Continence Nurse (WOCN) for pressure ulcer evaluation and treatment.
	5. Consult physical therapy.
	6. Consult psychiatrist.
	7. Consult dietitian.
	8. Normal saline at 100 mL/hour.
	9. Morning labs: Complete blood cell count (CBC), total protein, electrolytes.
	10. Continue home medication: metoprolol 100 mg by mouth daily.
	11. Acetaminophen 500 mg PO every 4 hours as needed, and 30 minutes before dressing changes, not to exceed 3,000 mg in 24 hours.

3. How should the nurse respond when the client's son asks, "Why does the doctor want a psychiatrist to come see my mom?"

_____

_____

_____

4. The nurse reviews the results of the morning blood work in Mattie's chart. Highlight the lab result that is the highest priority.

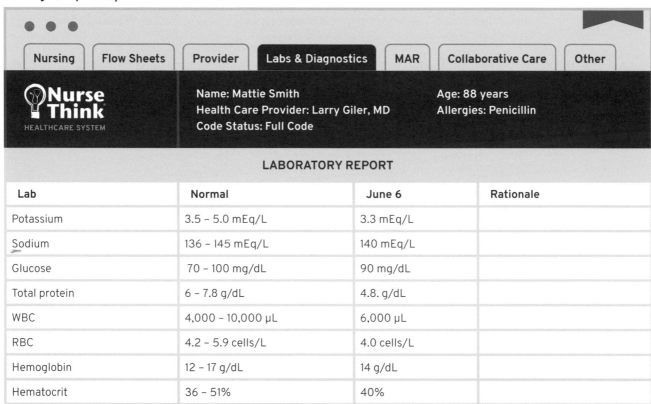

Nursing | Flow Sheets | Provider | **Labs & Diagnostics** | MAR | Collaborative Care | Other

Nurse Think HEALTHCARE SYSTEM

Name: Mattie Smith
Health Care Provider: Larry Giler, MD
Code Status: Full Code

Age: 88 years
Allergies: Penicillin

LABORATORY REPORT

Lab	Normal	June 6	Rationale
Potassium	3.5 – 5.0 mEq/L	3.3 mEq/L	
Sodium	136 – 145 mEq/L	140 mEq/L	
Glucose	70 – 100 mg/dL	90 mg/dL	
Total protein	6 – 7.8 g/dL	4.8. g/dL	
WBC	4,000 – 10,000 µL	6,000 µL	
RBC	4.2 – 5.9 cells/L	4.0 cells/L	
Hemoglobin	12 – 17 g/dL	14 g/dL	
Hematocrit	36 – 51%	40%	

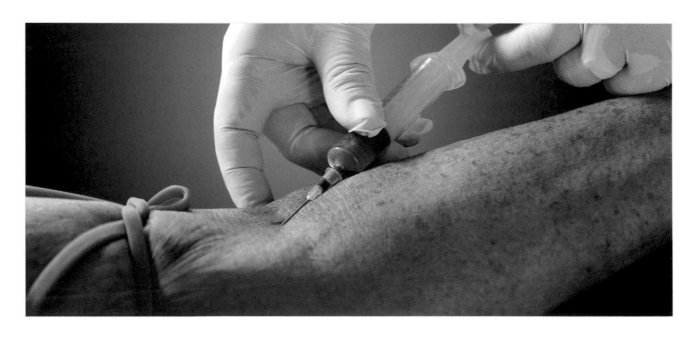

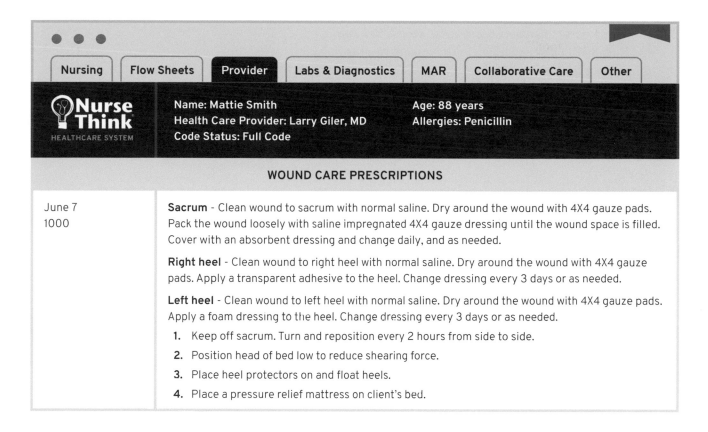

WOUND CARE PRESCRIPTIONS

June 7 1000	**Sacrum** - Clean wound to sacrum with normal saline. Dry around the wound with 4X4 gauze pads. Pack the wound loosely with saline impregnated 4X4 gauze dressing until the wound space is filled. Cover with an absorbent dressing and change daily, and as needed.

Name: Mattie Smith
Health Care Provider: Larry Giler, MD
Code Status: Full Code

Age: 88 years
Allergies: Penicillin

Right heel - Clean wound to right heel with normal saline. Dry around the wound with 4X4 gauze pads. Apply a transparent adhesive to the heel. Change dressing every 3 days or as needed.

Left heel - Clean wound to left heel with normal saline. Dry around the wound with 4X4 gauze pads. Apply a foam dressing to the heel. Change dressing every 3 days or as needed.

1. Keep off sacrum. Turn and reposition every 2 hours from side to side.
2. Position head of bed low to reduce shearing force.
3. Place heel protectors on and float heels.
4. Place a pressure relief mattress on client's bed.

5. **The WOCN examines Mattie's wounds and writes the prescriptions shown in the chart. Which factors are used to explain the differences in wound care prescriptions? Select all that apply.**
   1. Wound size.
   2. Wound depth.
   3. Wound smell.
   4. Wound severity.
   5. Wound location.

6. **What action must the nurse take to prevent possible cross-contamination of the wounds when performing dressing changes?**
   1. The nurse ensures glove changes between all three sites.
   2. The nurse utilizes sterile supplies for dressing changes.
   3. The nurse does not cross the sterile field once set up.
   4. The nurse 'lips' the bottle before pouring.

Mattie moans in pain when the nurse performs the dressing changes, especially the dressing to her sacrum. She rates her pain at 5/10 despite pre-medication.

7. **The nurse prepares an SBAR hand-off report for the accepting hospital. Complete each section of the communication form.**

S – _____

B – _____

A – _____

R – _____

Clinical Hint:
S - Situation
B - Background
A - Assessment
R - Recommendation

8. **The nurse enters Mattie's room to re-assess her pain and finds her in bed as shown in the image. What is most concerning to the nurse?**

    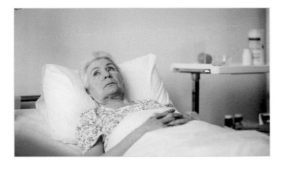

    1. Her appearance of boredom.
    2. That she is on her back.
    3. That she is propped up on two pillows.
    4. That her side rails are down.

9. **The dietitian completes the consultation and determines that Mattie needs a high protein diet with adequate hydration. Which foods should the nurse recommend?**

    1. Pasta, vegetables, and eggs.
    2. Meats, eggs, and cheese.
    3. Tofu, rice, and fruits.
    4. Breads, cereals, and vegetables.

Mattie loves sweet foods and asks her son to bring her cakes and other fresh pastries. She does not like to drink water, favoring coffee and diet sodas instead.

10. **The nurse receives a hand-off report on her assigned patients and is starting to make rounds when she observes that Mattie's son has brought her the breakfast, shown in the image. What teaching points need to be reinforced?**

    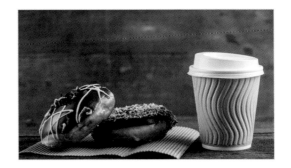

    1. She should not consume that much sugar in one meal.
    2. No caffeine is allowed on her diet.
    3. These items don't have protein needed for healing.
    4. She should not have anything to eat or drink until later.

Physical therapy is working with Mattie, and though she is resistant to work with them, she is starting to be more cooperative. The psychiatrist has also completed the consultation and concluded that Mattie is suffering from depression, triggered by the loss of her husband and living alone.

11. **The psychiatrist prescribes sertraline 200 mg taken orally once daily. The nurse reviews the drug guide before delivering the medication and decides to call the psychiatrist before administering the drug to Mattie. Highlight the cues within the drug guide that caused the nurse to question this prescription.**

Sertraline	
Class: Antidepressant	**Dosage:** Adult/geriatric PO 25-50 mg/day; may increase to a max of 200 mg/day; do not change dose at intervals of < 1 week; administer daily in morning or night.
Action: Inhibits serotonin reuptake in CNS.	
Uses: Major depressive disorder, obsessive-compulsive disorder, posttraumatic stress disorder, panic disorder, social anxiety disorder, premenstrual dysphoric disorder.	**Side effects:** seizures, neuroleptic malignant-syndrome-like reaction, serotonin syndrome, suicidal ideations, hepatitis, diarrhea, nausea, SIADH, palpitations.
Contraindications: Hypersensitivity to this product or SSRIs.	**Black Box Warning:** Mental status, mood. Sensorium, suicidal tendencies, depression, panic attacks.
Precautions: Pregnancy, breastfeeding, geriatric patients, renal/hepatic disease, epilepsy, recent MI, latex sensitivity.	
Interactions: Altered lithium levels, MAOIs, SSRIs.	

12. **Mattie's wounds are healing very slowly. On day 10 of admission, she reports more pain to her sacrum and is refusing to get out of bed. When the nurse performs the dressing change, the nurse observes this. The wound has thick, purulent drainage and is malodorous. It is 10 cm x 5 cm in size. How should the nurse proceed?**

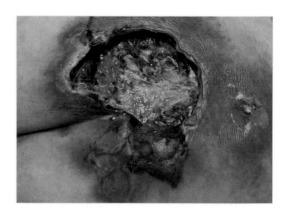

1. Document the findings.
2. Dress as per WOCN prescriptions.
3. Contact the WOCN to re-evaluate the prescription.
4. Culture the wound.

13. **Based on what is known about Mattie's case and her course of hospitalization, place an X in the table to indicate assessment factors that contributed directly, indirectly, or did not contribute to Mattie's poor wound healing.**

Factors	Contributed directly	Contributed indirectly	Did not contribute
Laying on her back			
Eating pies and cakes			
Resistant to mobility			
Keeping an untidy house			
Depression			
Poor hydration			

14. **NurseThink® Prioritization Power!**

Based on Mattie's wound what are the **Top 3 Priority** concerns?

1. _____

2. _____

3. _____

The WOCN determines that Mattie's sacral wound must be debrided since it is infected. The wound is debrided the next day, and new wound care prescriptions are received. Mattie is started on an intravenous antibiotic every 8 hours.

15. **How will the nurse know that the antibiotic is effective? Select all that apply.**
    1. The client no longer reports pain with dressing changes.
    2. The yellow and black slough is no longer present in the wound bed.
    3. The wound drainage changes from thick yellow to serous.
    4. The wound size decreases from 10 cm to 8 cm.
    5. The wound is no longer malodorous.

16. **The night nurse is rounding on Mattie when her son complains about the nurse from the day shift, stating, "Mom is still hurting from today, that nurse is no good!" Review the documentation in Mattie's chart, written by the day shift nurse. What error in care may have contributed to Mattie's discomfort?**

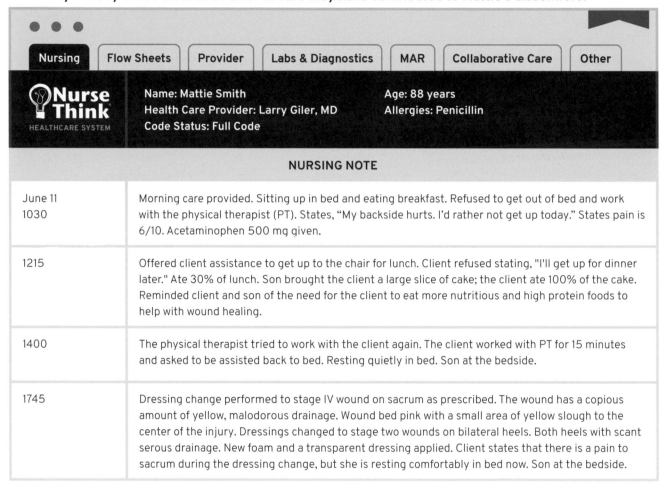

| Nursing | Flow Sheets | Provider | Labs & Diagnostics | MAR | Collaborative Care | Other |

Nurse Think HEALTHCARE SYSTEM

Name: Mattie Smith
Health Care Provider: Larry Giler, MD
Code Status: Full Code

Age: 88 years
Allergies: Penicillin

NURSING NOTE

June 11 1030	Morning care provided. Sitting up in bed and eating breakfast. Refused to get out of bed and work with the physical therapist (PT). States, "My backside hurts. I'd rather not get up today." States pain is 6/10. Acetaminophen 500 mg given.
1215	Offered client assistance to get up to the chair for lunch. Client refused stating, "I'll get up for dinner later." Ate 30% of lunch. Son brought the client a large slice of cake; the client ate 100% of the cake. Reminded client and son of the need for the client to eat more nutritious and high protein foods to help with wound healing.
1400	The physical therapist tried to work with the client again. The client worked with PT for 15 minutes and asked to be assisted back to bed. Resting quietly in bed. Son at the bedside.
1745	Dressing change performed to stage IV wound on sacrum as prescribed. The wound has a copious amount of yellow, malodorous drainage. Wound bed pink with a small area of yellow slough to the center of the injury. Dressings changed to stage two wounds on bilateral heels. Both heels with scant serous drainage. New foam and a transparent dressing applied. Client states that there is a pain to sacrum during the dressing change, but she is resting comfortably in bed now. Son at the bedside.

1. Spent too long up in the chair.
2. Physical therapy sessions too aggressive.
3. Wound care performed too aggressively.
4. Failed to pre-medicate before wound care.

Mattie's wounds are showing signs of healing. Culture from the wound indicates that the infection is gone, and Mattie no longer needs antibiotics. The antidepressant is starting to be effective, and Mattie is in a more cooperative mood. She has been working with physical therapy and getting stronger. The health care provider tells Mattie and her son that she should not live at home alone again. John decides to move Mattie to Tennessee to live with him, his wife, and children. Though Mattie is saddened to leave her home, she agrees. John has many questions about Mattie's care.

17. **Prioritize the discharge teaching by placing an X in the appropriate column and offer the rationale for your decision.**

	Priority	Not a priority	Rationale
Home health nurse to do Mattie's dressing changes.			
Mattie should not share a room with any family members.			
Do not allow Mattie to take anymore acetaminophen to prevent her from being addicted.			
Remove loose rugs from the home.			
Place grab bars in Mattie's shower.			
Shop for high protein foods.			
Transport Mattie back to see her home in Florida periodically.			
Monitor Mattie's antidepressant administration.			

Mattie has been living with her son for the past two months, and things are not going well. Mattie is back to her old ways of eating poorly. She gets her granddaughter to buy her sweet treats and only picks at the high protein foods that John's family cooks. The wounds to her heels have healed, but the home health nurse notes that the wound on Mattie's sacrum has a quarter size black area in the center and Mattie still reports pain when the dressing change is done. Mattie is disagreeable and argumentative with John and his wife. She sits on the couch and refuses to get up and walk around, even though John got her a walker to assist her with staying safe when she walks. She says, "I'm not using it." John has decided to place Mattie in a nursing home. Mattie is furious.

---

18. **THIN Thinking Time!**

The home health nurse ponders the information above about Mattie and applies the concept of THIN Thinking.

T – _____

H – _____

I – _____

N – _____

T - Top 3
H - Help Quick
I - Identify Risk to Safety
N - Nursing Process

Scan to access the
10-Minute-Mentor →
on THIN Thinking.

NurseThink.com/THINThinking

19. The charge nurse at the nursing home is determining the best room placement for Mattie. Place an X in the room that is most appropriate for Mattie.

Room 324	Room 325	Room 326
Bed A: 80-year-old female with dementia who wanders. Bed B: Open	Bed A: Open Bed B: 75-year-old female who is confused, bedbound and has multiple pressure ulcers. Bed C: 82-year-old female who is confused and yells all the time.	Bed A: 40-year-old female who was in a motor vehicle accident and is receiving short-term, skilled care. Bed B: Open
Room 327	**Room 328**	**Room 329**
Bed A: 90-year-old male who is bedbound, has a tracheostomy and requires frequent suctioning. Bed B: Open	Bed A: 50-year-old female who has paraplegia. Bed B: 60-year-old female with multiple sclerosis. Bed C: 48-year-old female who is bedbound and non-verbal from injuries sustained in a violent home invasion.	Bed A: 90-year-old female who had a stroke, is quiet, pleasant, ambulates with a walker and likes to sit in the dayroom. Bed B: Open
Room 330	**Room 331**	**Room 332**
Bed A: Open Bed B: 86-year-old female with MRSA infected wound to the lower extremity.	Bed A: 82-year-old male who is ambulatory. Bed B: Open	Bed A: Open Bed B: 94-year-old female who grumpy and not friendly.

20. Which actions of the admitting nurse in the nursing home will help to alleviate Mattie's stress as she moves to her new home? Select all that apply.

1. Encourage Mattie to fill her room with familiar personal items.
2. Introduce her to some of the other residents.
3. Let her tour the facility.
4. Show her the schedule of meals and activities.
5. Let her know she will have the freedom to come and go as she pleases.

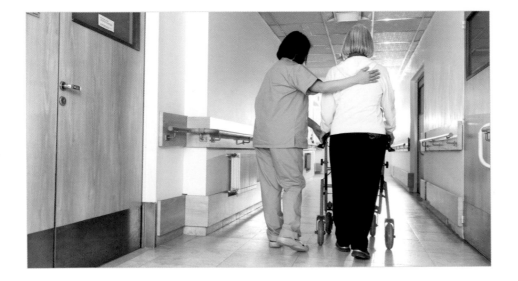

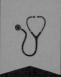

Case 2: Acute Pain

Related Concepts: Circulation, Protection, Emotion
Threaded Topics: Skin integrity, PCA management, Pharmacology

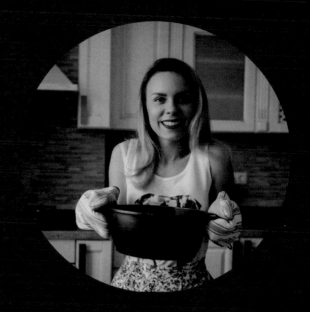

Molly Juniper, a 32-year-old, was cooking at home one evening when she accidentally spilled a pot of boiling water. The water spilled over her left hand causing second degree, partial thickness, scalding burns to her fingers, hand, and an area surrounding the left, anterior forearm, approximating 3% total body surface area (TBSA). The scald burns scattered throughout the hand and fingers and there is a small circumferential burn on the forearm. She is healthy and has no medical history, taking daily vitamins with breakfast. She lives in an apartment with her two children, ages six and nine years and is the primary provider for her family.

Molly's neighbor drove her to the Emergency Department of the local city hospital. The emergency team was notified for assessment and care, and after the initial evaluation, she was transferred to a regional hospital with a Burn Care Center and admitted to a room on the Burn Care floor. The neighbor is currently watching Molly's children until her parents arrive from out of town.

1. **NurseThink® Prioritization Power!**
   Evaluate the information in the case and determine the **Top 3 Priority** concerns or cues.

   1. _____

   2. _____

   3. _____

2. **Based on the priority concerns, which action(s) should the nurse perform? Select all that apply.**

   1. Complete a head to toe assessment.
   2. Evaluate the pain level using a pain scale.
   3. Obtain a full set of vital signs.
   4. Discuss infection control guidelines for the burned client.
   5. Provide emotional support.
   6. Encourage the client to verbalize concerns.

3. **Which of these factors predispose the client to be transferred to the Burn Care Center?**

   1. Current age.
   2. The depth of the burn is partial thickness/second degree.
   3. The burn involves the hands.
   4. The burn is a scald type of injury.

4. **The nurse reviews the agency policy on burn classification. What assumptions can the nurse make, based on this chart about Molly's situation?**

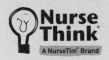

BURN CLASSIFICATIONS

SUPERFICIAL: FIRST DEGREE
Red, dry, painful without blisters, blanches with pressure.

Do not include TBSA % estimate.

Epithelium injured but intact.

Examples: Sunburn or propane flash.

PARTIAL THICKNESS: SECOND DEGREE
Red, blisters, weepy, shiny, blanches with pressure, moderate to severe pain.

Likely to scar.

Epithelium and varying layers of dermis are destroyed.

Example: Scald

FULL THICKNESS: THIRD DEGREE
Red, dry, white, charred, leathery in appearance.

Hair follicle removes easily, diminished pain.

High probability of deformity and scarring.

Epidermis and dermis are destroyed. Extends to subcutaneous layers, muscle, and bones.

Example: Flame

1. The burn will remain dry with minimal pain.
2. The depth of the burn is into the epithelium and will be painful.
3. The burn is considered deep and should not have pain.
4. The hair will not grow back.

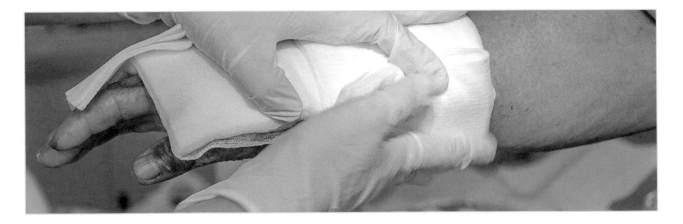

5. The nurse completes a head to toe assessment and documents the findings. Circle or highlight the area on the electronic record that is the highest priority.

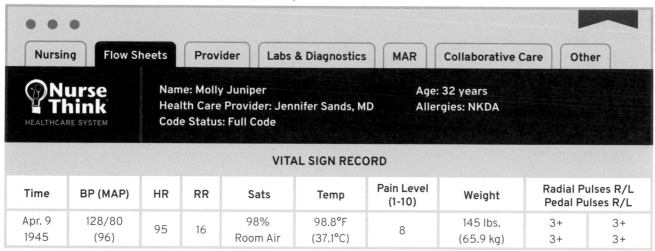

| Nursing | Flow Sheets | Provider | Labs & Diagnostics | MAR | Collaborative Care | Other |

Nurse Think HEALTHCARE SYSTEM

Name: Molly Juniper
Health Care Provider: Jennifer Sands, MD
Code Status: Full Code

Age: 32 years
Allergies: NKDA

VITAL SIGN RECORD

Time	BP (MAP)	HR	RR	Sats	Temp	Pain Level (1-10)	Weight	Radial Pulses R/L Pedal Pulses R/L	
Apr. 9 1945	128/80 (96)	95	16	98% Room Air	98.8°F (37.1°C)	8	145 lbs. (65.9 kg)	3+ 3+	3+ 3+

6. The nurse uses a numerical rating scale (1-10) to assess Molly's pain. Which other pain assessment tool is the next best method to assess Molly's physical pain and psychological distress?
1. Visual Analog Scale (VAS).
2. Pain Thermometer Scoring.
3. Faces Pain Rating Scale.
4. Color Analogue Scale.

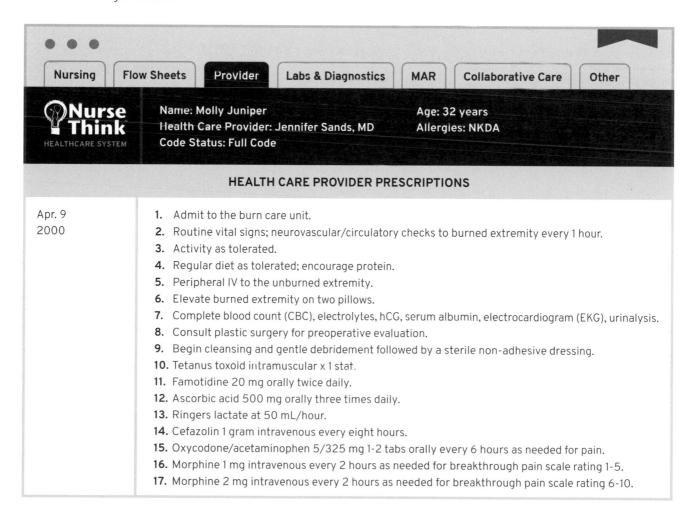

| Nursing | Flow Sheets | Provider | Labs & Diagnostics | MAR | Collaborative Care | Other |

Nurse Think HEALTHCARE SYSTEM

Name: Molly Juniper
Health Care Provider: Jennifer Sands, MD
Code Status: Full Code

Age: 32 years
Allergies: NKDA

HEALTH CARE PROVIDER PRESCRIPTIONS

Apr. 9
2000

1. Admit to the burn care unit.
2. Routine vital signs; neurovascular/circulatory checks to burned extremity every 1 hour.
3. Activity as tolerated.
4. Regular diet as tolerated; encourage protein.
5. Peripheral IV to the unburned extremity.
6. Elevate burned extremity on two pillows.
7. Complete blood count (CBC), electrolytes, hCG, serum albumin, electrocardiogram (EKG), urinalysis.
8. Consult plastic surgery for preoperative evaluation.
9. Begin cleansing and gentle debridement followed by a sterile non-adhesive dressing.
10. Tetanus toxoid intramuscular x 1 stat.
11. Famotidine 20 mg orally twice daily.
12. Ascorbic acid 500 mg orally three times daily.
13. Ringers lactate at 50 mL/hour.
14. Cefazolin 1 gram intravenous every eight hours.
15. Oxycodone/acetaminophen 5/325 mg 1-2 tabs orally every 6 hours as needed for pain.
16. Morphine 1 mg intravenous every 2 hours as needed for breakthrough pain scale rating 1-5.
17. Morphine 2 mg intravenous every 2 hours as needed for breakthrough pain scale rating 6-10.

7. **The nurse develops the plan of care and notes the provider's prescriptions. In what order should the nurse perform the interventions?** _____, _____, _____, _____, _____.

1. Insert peripheral IV and begin Ringers lactate infusion.
2. Elevate the burned extremity.
3. Medicate for pain with oxycodone/acetaminophen.
4. Obtain vital signs and perform neurovascular/circulatory assessment.
5. Provide tetanus toxoid injection.

Several hours have passed, and Molly has required maximum pain medication allotted. Molly remains alert and oriented, her neurovascular assessments remain within normal parameters, with pulses strong and equal, and capillary refill < 3 seconds. Molly verbalizes feeling severely anxious regarding her pain and her concern for how long the neighbor can watch her children. The nurse prepares to call the on-call health care provider (HCP) to discuss Molly's situation.

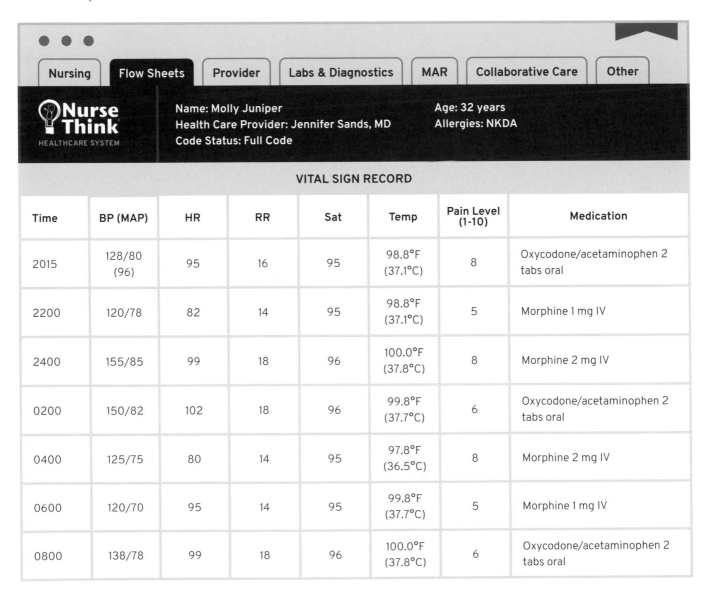

Nursing | **Flow Sheets** | **Provider** | **Labs & Diagnostics** | **MAR** | **Collaborative Care** | **Other**

NurseThink HEALTHCARE SYSTEM

Name: Molly Juniper
Health Care Provider: Jennifer Sands, MD
Code Status: Full Code

Age: 32 years
Allergies: NKDA

VITAL SIGN RECORD

Time	BP (MAP)	HR	RR	Sat	Temp	Pain Level (1-10)	Medication
2015	128/80 (96)	95	16	95	98.8°F (37.1°C)	8	Oxycodone/acetaminophen 2 tabs oral
2200	120/78	82	14	95	98.8°F (37.1°C)	5	Morphine 1 mg IV
2400	155/85	99	18	96	100.0°F (37.8°C)	8	Morphine 2 mg IV
0200	150/82	102	18	96	99.8°F (37.7°C)	6	Oxycodone/acetaminophen 2 tabs oral
0400	125/75	80	14	95	97.8°F (36.5°C)	8	Morphine 2 mg IV
0600	120/70	95	14	95	99.8°F (37.7°C)	5	Morphine 1 mg IV
0800	138/78	99	18	96	100.0°F (37.8°C)	6	Oxycodone/acetaminophen 2 tabs oral

8. **NurseThink® Prioritization Power!**

   Evaluate the information within the nurse's assessment and vital sign record and pick the **Top 3 Priority** assessment concerns.

   1. _____

   2. _____

   3. _____

9. **The nurse gathers information and begins to prepare an SBAR telephone conversation for the HCP. Complete each section of the SBAR communication.**

   S – _____

   B – _____

   A – _____

   R – _____

   Clinical Hint:
   S - Situation
   B - Background
   A - Assessment
   R - Recommendation

The HCP prescribes to discontinue the morphine sulfate and the oxycodone with acetaminophen and to begin hydromorphone via a Patient Controlled Analgesia (PCA). Also prescribed is a social services consultation to assist Molly's home situation of her children. The HCP and the nurse discuss preparing Molly for surgery, which is scheduled for the afternoon.

The HCP changes the pain medication prescription for Molly stating "Let's get her pain better controlled." The prescription reads as follows:

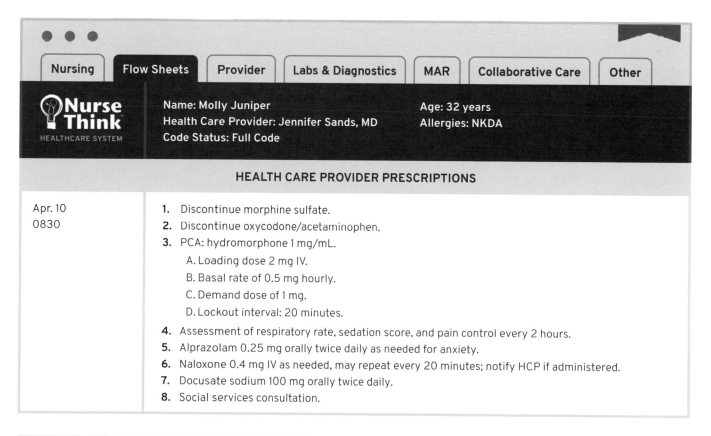

| Nursing | Flow Sheets | Provider | Labs & Diagnostics | MAR | Collaborative Care | Other |

Nurse Think HEALTHCARE SYSTEM

Name: Molly Juniper
Health Care Provider: Jennifer Sands, MD
Code Status: Full Code

Age: 32 years
Allergies: NKDA

HEALTH CARE PROVIDER PRESCRIPTIONS

Apr. 10
0830

1. Discontinue morphine sulfate.
2. Discontinue oxycodone/acetaminophen.
3. PCA: hydromorphone 1 mg/mL.
   A. Loading dose 2 mg IV.
   B. Basal rate of 0.5 mg hourly.
   C. Demand dose of 1 mg.
   D. Lockout interval: 20 minutes.
4. Assessment of respiratory rate, sedation score, and pain control every 2 hours.
5. Alprazolam 0.25 mg orally twice daily as needed for anxiety.
6. Naloxone 0.4 mg IV as needed, may repeat every 20 minutes; notify HCP if administered.
7. Docusate sodium 100 mg orally twice daily.
8. Social services consultation.

10. **Explain each of the prescriptions and its purpose, specific to Molly's care. In other words, why is it being prescribed?**

1. PCA: hydromorphone 1 mg/mL.

   _____

2. Loading dose 2 mg IV.

   _____

3. Basal rate 0.5 mg hourly.

   _____

4. Demand dose 1 mg.

   _____

5. Lockout interval: 20 minutes.

   _____

6. Assessment of respiratory rate, sedation score, and pain control every 2 hours.

   _____

7. Alprazolam 0.25 mg orally twice daily as needed for anxiety.

   _____

8. Naloxone 0.4 mg IV as needed, may repeat every 20 minutes; notify HCP if administered.

   _____

9. Docusate sodium 100 mg orally.

   _____

10. Social services consultation.

    _____

11. **The nurse is reviewing the prescriptions and anticipates the possibility of administering the naloxone. Which description would indicate the proper rationale for the nurse to administer this medication?**
    1. The client has a decrease in alertness; vital signs remain within desired parameters.
    2. The client has a decrease in the level of consciousness and breathing pattern as a result of the alprazolam.
    3. The client has a decrease in the level of consciousness and breathing pattern as a result of the hydromorphone.
    4. The client's pain and anxiety goals are unmet, and there is the need for adjuvant therapy for better control.

12. **The nurse is reviewing the side effects of naloxone. What clinical manifestations can the nurse expect to find after its administration?**
    1. Rapid pulse, nervousness and constipation.
    2. Urticaria, drowsiness and nausea and vomiting.
    3. Increased BP and ventricular arrhythmias.
    4. Respiratory depression, palpitations, and urinary retention.

13. **Acute pain and chronic pain differ in cause, the course of progression, manifestations, and treatment. Fill in the shaded areas in the table to differentiate between acute and chronic pain.**

	Acute Pain	Chronic Pain
Onset		Gradual or sudden
Duration		Greater than 3 months
Severity		
Course of Pain		Does not go away
Anticipated physical and behavioral manifestations		> Flat affect > Decreased physical activity > Fatigue > Withdrawal from social interaction
Goal of treatment	Pain control with eventual elimination	

The nurse receives the hydromorphone medication, PCA machine, and begins to gather equipment for the infusion.

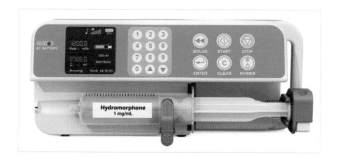

14. **The nurse considers the teaching components and importance in helping Molly have adequate pain control. Before the teaching, what is most important for the nurse to assess?**
   1. How much pain medication the client has received.
   2. The client's readiness and willingness to learn.
   3. When the client is going to be discharged.
   4. At what time the client will be going to surgery.

15. **The nurse is preparing to teach Molly about the PCA machine and important considerations. Which instructions are essential for the nurse to give the client? Select all that apply.**
   1. Emphasize the safety features of the machine.
   2. Plan to teach the client in the preoperative period rather than postoperatively.
   3. How to self-administer the pain medication.
   4. Wait for the nurse's assistance when feeling the need for pain medication.
   5. As the pain lessens, the client can adjust to lower doses and eventually stop the analgesic.

16. THIN Thinking!

The nurse is entering Molly's room with the PCA machine, supplies, and prescribed medication. What are the priority safety measures required before PCA narcotic administration?

T - _____

H - _____

I - _____

N - _____

T - Top 3
H - Help Quick
I - Identify Risk to Safety
N - Nursing Process

Scan to access the 10-Minute-Mentor on THIN Thinking.

NurseThink.com/THINThinking

17. Complete the PCA flow sheet by filling in the shaded areas.

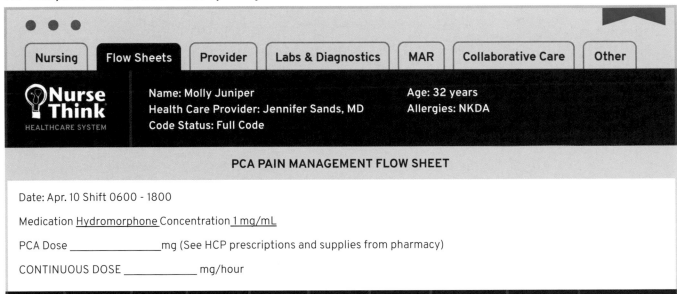

| Nursing | Flow Sheets | Provider | Labs & Diagnostics | MAR | Collaborative Care | Other |

NurseThink HEALTHCARE SYSTEM

Name: Molly Juniper
Health Care Provider: Jennifer Sands, MD
Code Status: Full Code

Age: 32 years
Allergies: NKDA

PCA PAIN MANAGEMENT FLOW SHEET

Date: Apr. 10 Shift 0600 - 1800

Medication <u>Hydromorphone</u> Concentration <u>1 mg/mL</u>

PCA Dose _____ mg (See HCP prescriptions and supplies from pharmacy)

CONTINUOUS DOSE _____ mg/hour

Time	Location of Pain	Pain Rating	Level of arousal	# of demand doses	# delivered	Basal rate	Cumulative Total (mg)	Cumulative Total (mL)	Notes
0930	Fingers Wrist	7	2	0	0	0	2	2	PCA initiated & Loading dose
1030	Fingers Wrist	4	2	2	2	0.5 mg			
1130	Fingers Wrist	5	1	2	2				
1230	Fingers Wrist	5	2	2		0.5 mg	10	10	
1330	Fingers Wrist	3	2	1	1	0.5 mg	11.5	11.5	
1430	Fingers Wrist	2	2	1		0.5 mg			Transferred to surgery @ 1430
Cumulative Shift Totals									

ASSESSMENT PARAMETERS

Level of Arousal Scale				
1	**2**	**3**	**4**	**5**
Awake & Alert Oriented	Normal Sleep Easy to Rouse to Verbal Stimulation	Difficult to Rouse to Verbal Stimulation	Responds Only to Physical Stimulation	Does Not Respond to Verbal or Physical Stimulation

18. **Based upon a review of the PCA flow sheet what can the nurse determine about Molly's use of the PCA machine and medication? Select all that apply.**

   1. The amount of medication she is demanding supersedes the amount delivered.
   2. The level of arousal indicates she is receiving too much medication.
   3. The machine delivers a specific amount of medication each hour regardless of her demands.
   4. The demand for medication was greatest when her pain level was the highest.
   5. The least amount of medication was delivered when her pain rating was at "2".

Molly was transferred to the operating room at 1430 for surgical wound debridement of her fingers and forearm, and placement of an anterior forearm skin graft. The PCA medication is placed into a locked system while she is off the unit.

Several hours later she returns to the burn unit.

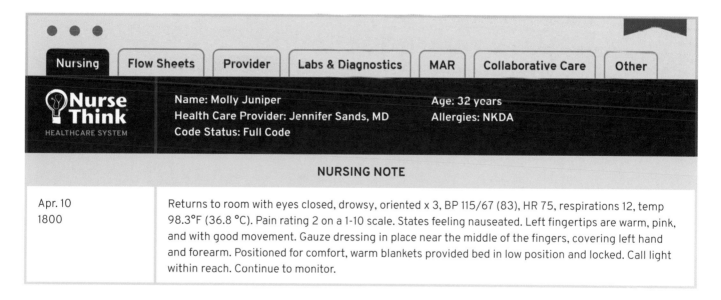

| Nursing | Flow Sheets | Provider | Labs & Diagnostics | MAR | Collaborative Care | Other |

Nurse Think HEALTHCARE SYSTEM

Name: Molly Juniper
Health Care Provider: Jennifer Sands, MD
Code Status: Full Code

Age: 32 years
Allergies: NKDA

NURSING NOTE

Apr. 10 1800	Returns to room with eyes closed, drowsy, oriented x 3, BP 115/67 (83), HR 75, respirations 12, temp 98.3°F (36.8 °C). Pain rating 2 on a 1-10 scale. States feeling nauseated. Left fingertips are warm, pink, and with good movement. Gauze dressing in place near the middle of the fingers, covering left hand and forearm. Positioned for comfort, warm blankets provided bed in low position and locked. Call light within reach. Continue to monitor.

NurseThink
HEALTHCARE SYSTEM

Name: Molly Juniper
Health Care Provider: Jennifer Sands, MD
Code Status: Full Code

Age: 32 years
Allergies: NKDA

HEALTH CARE PROVIDER POST-OPERATIVE PRESCRIPTIONS

Apr. 10
1800

1. Bedrest; assist to the bathroom; ambulate in the morning.

2. Ice chips, advance to regular diet; encourage protein.

3. PCA: hydromorphone 1 mg/mL.

   A. Loading dose 2 mg IV.

   B. Basal rate of 0.5 mg hourly.

   C. Demand dose of 1 mg.

   D. Lockout interval: 20 minutes.

4. Page the healthcare provider for any problems with the patient's level of pain control, the presence of side effects, if 1-hour limit is reached before 1 hour with poor pain relief and/or if sedation score = 3.

5. Assessment of respiratory rate, sedation score, and pain control every 2 hours.

6. Alprazolam 0.25 mg orally twice daily as needed for anxiety.

7. Naloxone 2 mg IV as needed, may repeat every 20 minutes; notify HCP if administered.

8. Ringers Lactate 75 mL/hour.

9. Famotidine 20 mg orally twice daily.

10. Docusate sodium 100 mg orally twice daily.

11. Ascorbic acid 500 mg orally three times daily.

12. Surgical team to be present for the first dressing change in 24 hours.

Molly and the nurse discuss her desires for adequate pain control and identify what an acceptable pain level is. Molly verbalizes a 2 to 3 on the 1 through 10 numerical rating scale as tolerable. Molly has been informed that her parents are arriving from out of town and will care for the children until her discharge.

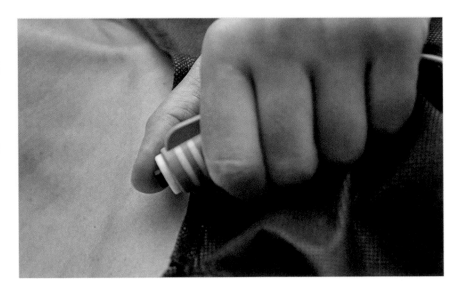

19. Complete the PCA flow sheet by filling in the shaded areas:

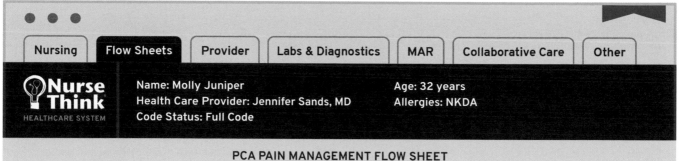

PCA PAIN MANAGEMENT FLOW SHEET

Date: Apr. 10 Shift 1800 - 0600

Medication <u>Hydromorphone</u> Concentration <u>1 mg/mL</u>

PCA Dose _____mg (See HCP prescriptions and supplies from pharmacy)

CONTINUOUS DOSE _____ mg/hour

Time	Location of Pain	Pain Rating	Level of arousal	# of demand doses	# delivered	Basal rate	Cumulative Total (mg)	Cumulative Total (mL)	Notes
1800	Fingers Wrist	2	3	0	0	0	2	2	PCA initiated upon return to surgery; loading dose provided
2000	Fingers Wrist	2	3	0	0	0.5 mg			
2200	Fingers Wrist	6	1	4	2				
0000	Fingers Wrist	4	2	1		0.5 mg	8	8	
0200	Fingers Wrist	2	2	1	1	0.5 mg			
0400	Fingers Wrist	2	3	0		0.5 mg			
0600	Denies	2	3	0	0	0.5 mg			
0800	Denies	2	1	0	0	0.5 mg	13	13	Ate breakfast/ Ambulated
1000	Fingers Wrist	2	2	1	1	0.5 mg			Nonopioid Interventions applied
1200	Denies	1	1	0	0	0.5 mg	16	16	
1400	Fingers Wrist	1	1	1	1	0.5 mg	18	18	
1600	Wrist	3	1	2	2	0.5 mg	21	21	Up to the bathroom
1800	Wrist	2	1	0	0	0.5 mg	22	22	Ambulated
Cumulative Shift Totals									

ASSESSMENT PARAMETERS

		Level of Arousal Scale		
1	**2**	**3**	**4**	**5**
Awake & Alert Oriented	Normal Sleep Easy to Rouse to Verbal Stimulation	Difficult to Rouse to Verbal Stimulation	Responds Only to Physical Stimulation	Does Not Respond to Verbal or Physical Stimulation

20. **Molly's pain ratings have remained acceptable with activity and rest. The next day Molly is started on oral pain medications, and the PCA machine is discontinued. Over the next few days, she requires less frequent oral medications and continues to improve. The nurse is preparing her for discharge, what is essential to include? Complete the discharge instructions form.**

Discharge Instructions	
Discharge	Diet:
	Activity:
	Follow up with Burn Care Center: Wound care
	Pain Management:
	Problems to report to HCP:
	Collaborative Care:
	Medication Instructions: > Daily vitamins > Ascorbic acid > Famotidine > Docusate sodium > Hydrocodone/acetaminophen

A few months later Molly visits the Burn Care Unit and shares that her wounds are healing well and she has spaced out her need for oral pain medications. She verbalizes her use of meditation and guided imagery has helped with her pain levels and coping, and she will be returning to work and her weekend yoga classes when her wounds are healed. She is happy to be back home with her children and ready for her life to resume.

Conceptual Debriefing & Case Reflection

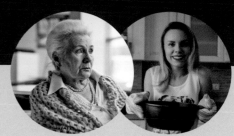

1. Compare the impaired comfort that Mattie Smith experienced with the impaired comfort of Molly Juniper. How are they the same and how are they different?

   _____

   _____

2. What was your single most significant learning moment while completing the case of Mattie Smith? What about Molly Juniper?

   _____

   _____

3. How did the nursing care provided to Mattie Smith and Molly Juniper change the outcome for each of them?

   _____

   _____

4. Identify safety concerns for both Mattie Smith and Molly Juniper for each case.

   _____

   _____

5. In what areas of each case study was basic care and comfort utilized?

   _____

   _____

6. What steps in each case did the nurse take that prevented hospital-acquired injury?

   _____

   _____

7. How did the nurse provide culturally sensitive/competent care?

   _____

   _____

8. How will learning about the case of Mattie Smith and Molly Juniper impact the care you provide for future clients?

   _____

Fundamental Quiz

1. The nurse is caring for a client that is bed-bound and unable to communicate. Which assessment changes indicate that the client may be experiencing discomfort?
   1. Confusion to place and time.
   2. Blood pressure increase over the last two hours.
   3. Socially withdrawn.
   4. Rubbing hands together.

2. The nurse is reviewing the laboratory report for a client expressing pain. Which lab report supports this finding?
   1. Elevated erythrocyte sedimentation rate.
   2. Elevated red blood cell count.
   3. Decreased hemoglobin.
   4. Decreased hematocrit.

3. The nurse is caring for a client experiencing joint pain which ranges on a scale of 4 to 8 on a 1 to 10 scale, depending on the time since pain medication was delivered. What functional abilities may be impaired as a result of this? Select all that apply.
   1. Mobility.
   2. Nutritional status.
   3. Sleep patterns.
   4. Elimination patterns.
   5. Mood and affect.

4. The nurse is caring for a client on bedrest who says they are very uncomfortable and restless on their back and they feel like their "butt is numb." What action should the nurse take first?
   1. Reposition the client on their side.
   2. Medicate with pain medicine.
   3. Assess the skin on the back.
   4. Obtain vital signs.

5. The nurse provides comfort measures to a client before bedtime to facilitate sleep. What actions should the nurse take? Select all that apply.
   1. Position for comfort.
   2. Provide oral care.
   3. Offer a prescribed sleep aid.
   4. Offer a back massage.
   5. Ask what helps the client best sleep.

Advanced Quiz

6. The nurse is caring for a client experiencing pain of 6 on a 1 to 10 scale for post-operative pain. Review the client information and determine the best medication option.

Age: 88 years old **Surgical procedure yesterday:** ORIF right hip	
Client Information	**Medication Record**
Vital Signs: BP (MAP): 90/67 (75) HR: 117 beats per minute RR: 22 breaths per minute Sats: 94% (room air) Temp: 100.9°F (38.3°C) **Abnormal Assessment Findings:** Confused to place, nauseated, abdomen slightly distended.	Morphine Sulfate 4 mg IVP every 4 hours PRN for pain. Oxycodone 5 mg orally, every 6 hours PRN for pain. Ketorolac 30 mg IVP, every 6 hours PRN for pain. Acetaminophen 500 mg orally, every 6 hours PRN pain.

   1. Morphine sulfate.
   2. Oxycodone.
   3. Ketorolac.
   4. Acetaminophen.

7. The nurse is caring for a client using patient-controlled analgesia (PCA) with IV morphine delivered at 1 mg every 10 minutes to control the pain. Several times during the night, the client awakens in severe pain, and it takes more than an hour to regain pain relief. What is the nurse's best action?
   1. Request an order for a bolus dose of morphine to be given when the client awakens with pain.
   2. Request an order adding a continuous low-dose morphine infusion to the PCA regimen at night.
   3. Instruct the client to push the button every 10 minutes for an hour before going to sleep.
   4. Administer a dose of morphine every 1 to 2 hours from the PCA machine while the client is sleeping.

8. The nurse is setting up patient-controlled analgesia (PCA) for morphine delivery. Which action is most important before beginning the medication?

   1. Caution the client to limit the number of times he presses the dosing button.
   2. Instruct the client to administer a dose only when experiencing pain.
   3. Explain that the family should never administer a dose.
   4. Ask another nurse to double-check the setup.

9. The nurse is caring for a client under the care of hospice. Prescribed is 75 mg of oral morphine solution. How many mL should the nurse deliver?

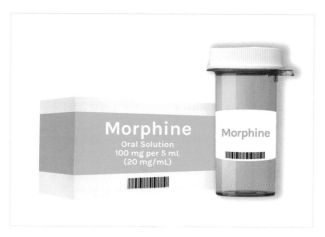

10. The nurse educates a client about alternative therapies for comfort. What options should the nurse discuss? Select all that apply.

    1. Acupuncture.
    2. Hypnosis.
    3. Massage.
    4. Reiki.
    5. Dietary supplements.

Adaptation

Stress / Violence / Coping / Addiction

Adaptation is a person's ability to respond positively to uncomfortable emotional situations or stressors. The ability to adapt is impacted by a lifetime of experiences, both positive and negative, as well as the development of coping mechanisms. Stress from violence and other internal and external physical and psychological stimuli can activate coping mechanisms. Coping skills for most people during the most stressful situations are adaptive. For others, addiction and other harmful behaviors can be the outcome of maladaptive coping. Often during times of illness, a person's ability to adapt is challenged. It is the nurses' role to assess a client's stress levels and coping mechanisms, intervening with therapeutic treatment modalities when indicated.

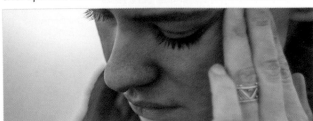

Next Gen Clinical Judgment:

> Compare signs of stress (physical and behavioral) in each age group: infant, toddler, school-aged child, teenage, adult, and older adult.

> Contrast how coping may be different among different races, cultures, religions, and sexes.

> How will coping vary during different phases of life?

> Reflect on this question; does a person develop better coping skills the more they are exposed to stress?

> List as many types of addiction as you can think of. Consider how each will be managed differently.

_____

_____

_____

_____

_____

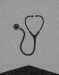

Go To Clinical Case

While caring for this client, be sure to review the concept maps in chapters 3 and 4.

Case 1: Stress, Crisis, and Coping

Related Concepts: Circulation, Comfort, Emotion, Grief, Mood, Anxiety
Threaded Topics: Developmental Level, Culture and Spirituality, Wellness,
Family Dynamics, Self-management, Sleep Disorder

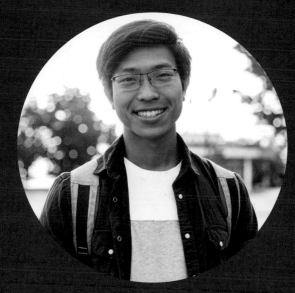

Brandon Kwong is an 18-year-old freshman college student. He was raised on the west coast in a traditional Asian community with his parents and grandparents who immigrated from China. His family owns and runs a small restaurant in a large metropolitan area where Brandon worked 30 to 60 hours a week from age 12 until he left for college. He currently attends a prestigious east coast university on a full scholarship which requires him to maintain a 3.75 grade-point average. He is majoring in biology and chemistry with the hopes of being a neurosurgeon one day, which has always been his grandfather's dream. Brandon feels pressured by his family to be successful. He believes that if he fails, he will disgrace his family. He is excited to be in college but fearful of not maintaining his scholarship.

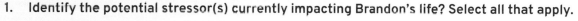

1. **Identify the potential stressor(s) currently impacting Brandon's life? Select all that apply.**

   1. Of Asian descent.

   2. Parents are immigrants.

   3. Worked 30 to 60 hours a week for years.

   4. College student away from home.

   5. Student of a prestigious university.

   6. Pressure from family to be successful.

   7. Goal is to be a neurosurgeon.

   > **Clinical Hint:** Stress may be acute or chronic. Stressors may be internal (ex. fear, or a lack of control) or external (ex. life changes or unpredictable events).

2. **Recognizing that Brandon is transitioning between Erikson's psychosocial level of Identity versus Role Confusion and Intimacy versus Isolation, what factors are important to consider? Select all that apply.**

   1. Brandon is going through an intense exploration of personal values, beliefs, and goals.
   2. Brandon will begin exploring relationships that may lead to a long-term commitment with someone other than his family.
   3. Brandon needs to recognize that he is no longer financially dependent upon his family and become independent from them.
   4. Brandon will explore intimate relationships in the next few years or risk being socially isolated.

Brandon ends his first semester confidently. He was able to obtain a 4.0 grade-point average, although he admits it was difficult and he spent most of his time studying. He is not able to go home over the winter break due to the cost of airfare. Spending four weeks alone on campus over the holiday is difficult for him. He is lonely and misses his family desperately. To keep himself busy he finds himself cleaning and organizing his dorm room, computer files, and bookshelf. As soon as he's completed a job, he feels the need to reorganize it a different way. The repetitive thoughts driving these actions don't seem to leave his mind. They keep him awake at night. Although he sometimes had these types of thoughts in high school, it's never been this severe. He is confident that once classes begin, he will be better.

3. **NurseThink® Prioritization Power!**
   Evaluate the behaviors that Brandon is exhibiting and determine the **Top 3 Priority** assessment findings.

   1. _____

   2. _____

   3. _____

Classes begin, and they are harder than ever. Brandon's obsessive thoughts are poured into his coursework, and he only gets 2-3 hours of sleep each night. His roommate talks him into taking a "break" from his school work and invites him to a party. Brandon wants to fit in with the other college students and experiments with alcohol and marijuana for the first time. He likes how it helps him relax and takes away his repetitive thoughts.

4. **Which statement by Brandon is most concerning about his coping skills?**
   1. "It's good that I'm consumed by my schoolwork, it will help me get better grades."
   2. "College students are social, and I'm just fitting in with my friends."
   3. "Drinking and smoking pot helps me relax and gets rid of my obsessive thoughts."
   4. "I want to be accepted by kids my age, and I'm considering joining a fraternity."

Brandon's roommate begins to see a change in his behavior. He begins drinking and smoking marijuana regularly. Initially, his drinking was contained to the weekends, but lately, he's been using alcohol to help him fall asleep. His grades begin to fall. One of Brandon's professors recognizes the change in his grades and requires him to make an office appointment. When Brandon does not show up for the scheduled appointment, he is referred to campus counseling.

5. **What is important for the nurse to include in the initial assessment at the campus counseling center? Select all that apply.**
   1. Vital signs.
   2. History of mental health issues.
   3. Spiritual and cultural beliefs.
   4. Use of substances.
   5. Identification of coping mechanisms.
   6. Support systems.

   Clinical Hint: Mental health facilities do not routinely perform physical assessments.

| Nursing | Flow Sheets | Provider | Labs & Diagnostics | MAR | Collaborative Care | Other |

Nurse Think HEALTHCARE SYSTEM

Name: Brandon Kwong
Health Care Provider: I. Stiller, MH-FNP
Code Status: Full Code

Age: 19 years
Allergies: NKDA

NURSING NOTE

Feb. 13
1300

Background and Assessment: Freshman male referred to counseling by Professor Hutchinson for a change in behavior, class absences, and falling grades. Student feels it is silly that he must be seen and that he's "doing fine." History includes obsessive thoughts and behaviors at times. He was raised in a strict household in a "traditional" Asian culture. He feels college has not allowed him to practice his traditional customs since "everyone here is different from me." He admits to drinking alcohol and smoking marijuana at parties to fit in but denies abuse of prescription medications or "hard drugs." He identifies his coping mechanism is to work harder which is something he learned growing up. His father often told him that "failure is a result of not working hard enough." He cannot identify a support system or someone that understands him and what he's going through.

---

6. **NurseThink® Prioritization Power!**

Evaluate the Intake Note and determine the **Top 3 Priority** cues that require a follow-up by the nurse.

1. _____

2. _____

3. _____

---

7. **The nurse identifies that Brandon is experiencing several mental health concerns. For each finding, specify whether it is associated with Anxiety (A), Obsessive-Compulsive Disorder (O), Substance Abuse (S), or Cultural Distress (C).**

1. ____ Fear of not maintaining his scholarship.

2. ____ Inability to practice his preferred customs.

3. ____ School work that interrupts sleep.

4. ____ Using alcohol and marijuana to eliminate obsessive thoughts.

5. ____ Missing the close personal connections from the family restaurant.

6. ____ Repetitive thoughts that don't seem to leave his mind.

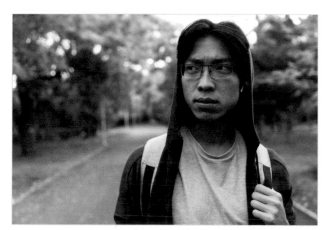

8. **When creating the treatment plan, the nurse works with Brandon to identify actions that would reduce his anxiety. Which action should the nurse recommend?**
    1. Eat three balanced meals a day.
    2. Spend 30 minutes each day in quiet reflection.
    3. Take diphenhydramine 25 mg orally at bedtime to assist with sleep.
    4. Take a 10-minute break for every 4 hours of homework.

9. **The nurse addresses the need for Brandon to gain control over his obsessive thoughts and behaviors. Which action should the nurse suggest?**
    1. Leave the room when an obsessive behavior begins.
    2. Think about something happy when the thoughts overtake his mind.
    3. Have Brandon identify what triggers his obsessive behaviors.
    4. Complete the obsessive behavior quickly, then move on to something else.

10. **The nurse is concerned about Brandon's cultural isolation. Which action should the nurse take first when creating the plan of care to best meet his cultural and spiritual needs?**
    1. Guide him in recognizing what beliefs and rituals are most important to him.
    2. Encourage him to attend a place of worship regularly.
    3. Suggest he finds a cultural, social club on campus that meets his needs.
    4. Recommend he takes 30 minutes each day to focus on the cultural and spiritual preferences.

11. **What is most important for the nurse to obtain from Brandon before he leaves the counseling center after his first appointment?**
    1. A contract that he will not hurt himself.
    2. An appointment to follow-up on this treatment plan.
    3. A verbal commitment that he will not drink or smoke.
    4. An appointment with his preferred spiritual leader.

Brandon returns to his dorm room emotionally exhausted. He feels that the nurse made too big of a deal about his situation and determines that he can control his grades and actions without the nurse's "plan." He knows that to maintain his scholarship, he must comply with the counseling appointments and get his grades up. He feels his instructor betrayed him and did not want his roommate or friends to know about what is going on. He decides it is better if he's alone and begins studying and sleeping in the library.

As the semester progresses, Brandon feels more isolated. He has distanced himself from everyone. One Friday night, 2 weeks before final exams he gets a phone call from home that his grandfather died suddenly while working at the restaurant. He refuses to go home for the family emergency since his grades could slip again. He knows that his grandfather would be most proud if he continues to work hard and be strong.

Later that weekend, Brandon wakes up with severe chest pain and palpitations. His hands are numb and tingling. He is diaphoretic and short of breath. He awakens his roommate, and they call campus emergency medical transport who take him to the emergency department.

12. **As the triage nurse in the emergency department, what is the priority focused assessment?**
    1. Stress and anxiety.
    2. Cultural and spiritual.
    3. Medical history.
    4. Cardiac and respiratory.

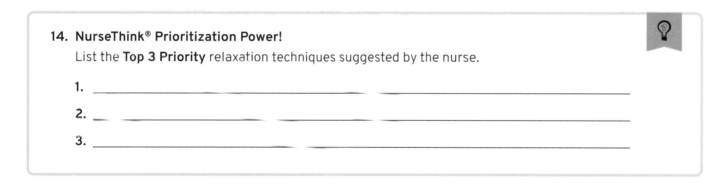

13. **THIN Thinking Time!**

    Reflect on the events that have occurred with Brandon and apply **THIN Thinking** to the nurse's actions.

    T – _____

    H – _____

    I – _____

    N – _____

    T - Top 3
    H - Help Quick
    I - Identify Risk to Safety
    N - Nursing Process

    Scan to access the 10-Minute-Mentor on THIN Thinking. →

    NurseThink.com/THINThinking

After the cardiac workup showed nothing, it is determined that Brandon is having a panic attack. The discharge nurse encourages Brandon to identify techniques that he could use, should he experience another panic attack.

14. **NurseThink® Prioritization Power!**

    List the **Top 3 Priority** relaxation techniques suggested by the nurse.

    1. _____

    2. _____

    3. _____

Upon discharge, Brandon is given these discharge prescriptions.

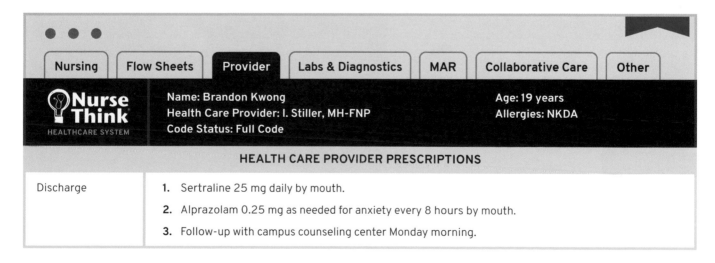

Nursing	Flow Sheets	Provider	Labs & Diagnostics	MAR	Collaborative Care	Other

NurseThink HEALTHCARE SYSTEM

Name: Brandon Kwong
Health Care Provider: I. Stiller, MH-FNP
Code Status: Full Code

Age: 19 years
Allergies: NKDA

HEALTH CARE PROVIDER PRESCRIPTIONS

Discharge	1. Sertraline 25 mg daily by mouth.
	2. Alprazolam 0.25 mg as needed for anxiety every 8 hours by mouth.
	3. Follow-up with campus counseling center Monday morning.

15. NurseThink® Prioritization Power!

Evaluate the discharge instructions and determine the **Top 3 Priority** teaching needs for the new prescription for sertraline.

1. _____
2. _____
3. _____

16. NurseThink® Prioritization Power!

Evaluate the discharge instructions and determine the **Top 3 Priority** teaching needs for the new prescription for alprazolam.

1. _____
2. _____
3. _____

17. **The nurse completes the discharge instructions for Brandon. Which of his statement(s) require further follow-up? Select all that apply.**

1. "I don't expect that medication will make much difference."
2. "I have a friend that takes alprazolam like candy."
3. "My culture does not believe in the use of medications."
4. "Do I have to pay to get these prescriptions filled?"
5. "I'll take both of these medications when I begin to feel stressed."

Brandon returns to campus counseling on Monday as instructed. The concerns identified by the nurse during the initial appointment and recent panic attack include:

> Anxiety leading to panic.
> Obsessive-compulsive disorder.
> Substance abuse as a coping mechanism.
> Cultural and spiritual distress.

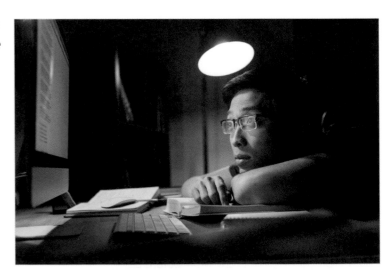

His appointment focuses on the creation of a success plan. With his nurse, Brandon agrees to this success plan.

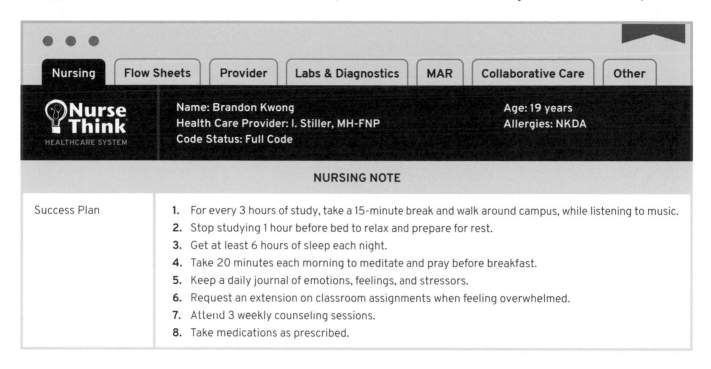

| Nursing | Flow Sheets | Provider | Labs & Diagnostics | MAR | Collaborative Care | Other |

NurseThink
HEALTHCARE SYSTEM

Name: Brandon Kwong
Health Care Provider: I. Stiller, MH-FNP
Code Status: Full Code

Age: 19 years
Allergies: NKDA

NURSING NOTE

Success Plan	1. For every 3 hours of study, take a 15-minute break and walk around campus, while listening to music.
	2. Stop studying 1 hour before bed to relax and prepare for rest.
	3. Get at least 6 hours of sleep each night.
	4. Take 20 minutes each morning to meditate and pray before breakfast.
	5. Keep a daily journal of emotions, feelings, and stressors.
	6. Request an extension on classroom assignments when feeling overwhelmed.
	7. Attend 3 weekly counseling sessions.
	8. Take medications as prescribed.

18. **After analyzing the identified concerns and the success plan determine which statement is true.**
    1. The plan is comprehensive and meets the needs of the identified concerns.
    2. The plan lacks an intervention in dealing with his stress.
    3. The plan does not meet his spiritual needs.
    4. The plan does not address his use of substances.

19. **At Brandon's 1-week follow-up visit he shares his journal with his nurse. Which statement within the journal is most concerning?**
    1. "My professor agreed to let me take my final exam two days later than assigned."
    2. "The alprazolam helps me sleep well each night."
    3. "I'm so sad I cannot be with my family as my grandfather is buried, I cry often."
    4. "I sat on the bench in the park for a while today rather than walking around campus."

20. **As the semester comes to an end, Brandon plans to return home for the summer. Which recommendation(s) should the nurse make to support his coping progress? Select all that apply.**
    1. Continue daily relaxation techniques.
    2. Find an OCD community support group at home.
    3. Continue to journal daily.
    4. See a counselor if he has difficulty adapting.
    5. Continue to take the alprazolam daily.

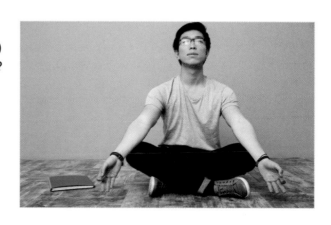

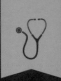
Case 2: Substance Abuse and Addiction

Related Concepts: Comfort: Pain, Mobility, Emotion: Mood, Anxiety
Threaded Topics: Family Dynamics, Legal Issues, Role Development,
Communication

Marge Sanderson is a 43-year-old registered nurse who
works 36 hours a week on a neuro-trauma rehabilitation
unit as the charge nurse in a large metropolitan hospital.
She has been married for 20 years and has three
teenaged children. She has worked on this unit for 10
years and loves the close relationships she has with
her colleagues. While working one busy day, Marge
developed sudden lower back pain that is radiating
down her legs after helping to move a client in bed. She
can hardly stand up after the event and goes home early
from her shift.

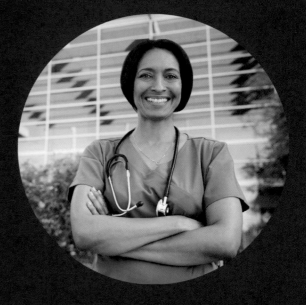

1. **What comfort measure(s) should Marge choose to help minimize the pain for this acute injury? Select all that apply.**

    1. Imagery and relaxation.

    2. Back strengthening exercises.

    3. Heat and/or Ice.

    4. Massage to the back.

    5. Proper use of body mechanics.

    > **Clinical Hint:** Comfort measures should be integrated prior to, and during the medical treatment plan.

2. **After two weeks, the pain does not improve with comfort measures and over-the-counter pain medication, so Marge makes an appointment with her primary health care provider. What prescription(s) should Marge anticipate? Select all that apply.**

    1. CT scan of the back.

    2. Outpatient physical therapy.

    3. Surgery.

    4. Stronger pain medicine.

    5. Referral to a pain specialist.

    6. Light duty activities.

3. **NurseThink® Prioritization Power!**

   Marge is prescribed acetaminophen with oxycodone as needed for pain. What are the **Top 3 Priorities** for education?

   1. _____

   2. _____

   3. _____

The CT scan report returns and Marge learns she has a herniated disc and is referred to a surgeon. Because of the surgeon's busy schedule, she is not able to obtain an appointment for 6 weeks. She continues to use the acetaminophen with oxycodone every 4 hours, which is becoming less helpful at relieving the excruciating pain. She continues to work on "light duty" since she wants to save her paid time off for after surgery.

4. **As a registered nurse taking prescribed narcotic pain medicine, which statement is true about the legal responsibility Marge has to her patients, employer, and state licensing board?**

   1. Marge is required to tell everyone that she is taking a prescribed narcotic.
   2. Marge should disclose to her manager that she is taking a prescribed narcotic for pain.
   3. Marge is not able to take any narcotics during the shift at work.
   4. Marge must notify the state licensing board of her prescription.

As the surgery gets closer, Marge is no longer able to function at work on light duty. She cannot sleep at night because of the pain and spends most of her days and nights in the recliner chair. She is taking the maximum dose of prescribed medication, and her surgeon refuses to increase the dose. She returns to her primary care physician who agrees to increase the dosage of pain medicine.

Marge has a discectomy of the lumbar spine. The surgical procedure was complicated, requiring more extensive work than expected. Marge awoke from surgery crying and screaming in pain.

5. **What is the priority assessment before the delivery of pain medication for Marge?**

   1. Client's perception of pain on a 1-10 scale.
   2. Assessment of surgical site.
   3. Vital signs.
   4. Location of pain.

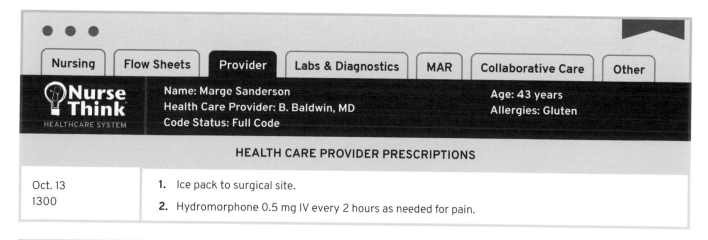

| Nursing | Flow Sheets | Provider | Labs & Diagnostics | MAR | Collaborative Care | Other |

Nurse Think HEALTHCARE SYSTEM

Name: Marge Sanderson
Health Care Provider: B. Baldwin, MD
Code Status: Full Code

Age: 43 years
Allergies: Gluten

HEALTH CARE PROVIDER PRESCRIPTIONS

| Oct. 13 1300 | 1. Ice pack to surgical site. |
| | 2. Hydromorphone 0.5 mg IV every 2 hours as needed for pain. |

6. **After reviewing the order for hydromorphone, what should the nurse consider?**
   1. Hydromorphone is contraindicated for someone who has recently been taking oxycodone.
   2. The hydromorphone dose is too low for someone who has previously been taking opioids.
   3. Hydromorphone at that dosage will cause respiratory depression and arrest.
   4. Delivery of postoperative opioids will cause addiction.

Marge continues to use the maximum dose of ordered intravenous pain medication throughout the hospital stay. The day before discharge, her provider switches her to oral hydromorphone 5 mg every 4 hours and adds ketorolac 30 mg IV every 6 hours to decrease the discomfort.

7. **Marge is upset about the change and knows the oral hydromorphone will not be as effective in relieving her "horrific" pain. How should the nurse respond?**
   1. "I'm sure you are hurting a lot; your surgery was extensive. Tell me why you don't think the oral medication will work as well?"
   2. "You know you cannot go home on IV pain meds, so there is not another option if you want to go home."
   3. "It probably won't work as well since it's oral, we can increase the dose if it's not effective."
   4. "Ketorolac is a strong medication and will relieve your pain."

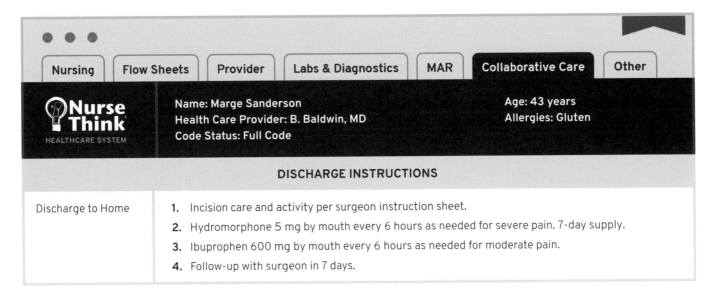

| | Nursing | Flow Sheets | Provider | Labs & Diagnostics | MAR | Collaborative Care | Other |

NurseThink HEALTHCARE SYSTEM

Name: Marge Sanderson
Health Care Provider: B. Baldwin, MD
Code Status: Full Code

Age: 43 years
Allergies: Gluten

DISCHARGE INSTRUCTIONS

Discharge to Home	1. Incision care and activity per surgeon instruction sheet.
	2. Hydromorphone 5 mg by mouth every 6 hours as needed for severe pain. 7-day supply.
	3. Ibuprophen 600 mg by mouth every 6 hours as needed for moderate pain.
	4. Follow-up with surgeon in 7 days.

After discharge, Marge's need and desire for the hydromorphone continues. She feels she is unable to function until she gets the dose and "feels good" for about 3 hours after taking the pill. Rather than monitoring the time since her last medication, she takes it when she feels she needs it. After 4 days her medication is gone. She contacts the surgeon's office and is given a 3-day supply.

At the postoperative appointment, the surgeon feels her recovery is progressing as expected. He notes that her pupils are pinpoint and that she occasionally misspeaks. Her husband is at the appointment and voices concern about her need for pain medication a week after surgery. He says "I'd have thought the pain would be gone after surgery." The surgeon refuses to renew her hydromorphone prescription, voicing concern about dependency. He tells Marge that she needs to use ibuprofen for pain and return in 5 weeks.

Marge is upset about the decision and contacts her primary care provider saying she spilled her medications into the toilet by accident and she needed a refill. Her primary provider refuses to refill, referring her back to the surgeon. She is angry at her husband and blames him for her inability to get a refill from the surgeon. She tells him "you just don't understand the pain I'm having!"

8. **NurseThink® Prioritization Power!**

What are the **Top 3 Priority** assessment findings that support addiction?

1. _____

2. _____

3. _____

Marge is out of pain medication and is feeling desperate. While her husband is at work, she convinces her 17-year-old son to drive her to the emergency department because the pain is so severe. In the emergency department, she has a CT scan of the back which shows nothing outside of what is anticipated given the surgical procedure she had 12 days prior. She is treated with ketorolac intravenously and discharged. Feeling bad for his mother, her son suggests she talk to his friend Greg from school, who can get her something to help her feel better.

Marge returns to work 5 weeks later. Her 'pain' is controlled with the combination of opioid drugs she's able to obtain from Greg. Her family is not aware that she is continuing to take narcotics, they believe she is "back to her old self." The financial strain of buying drugs from Greg is concerning for Marge, but she knows she can "stop any time."

9. **Which behavioral change(s) would indicate to Marge's co-workers that she is experiencing substance use disorder? Select all that apply.**

   1. Change in job performance.
   2. Frequent trips to the bathroom.
   3. Making frequent errors.
   4. Excessive amount of helpfulness.
   5. Arriving late to the shift.

10. **Which physiological change(s) would indicate to Marge's co-workers that she is experiencing substance use disorder? Select all that apply.**

    1. Clumsy or uncoordinated actions.
    2. Increase or decrease in appetite.
    3. Runny nose or bloodshot eyes.
    4. Distracted easily.
    5. Unusual breath, body, or clothing odors.

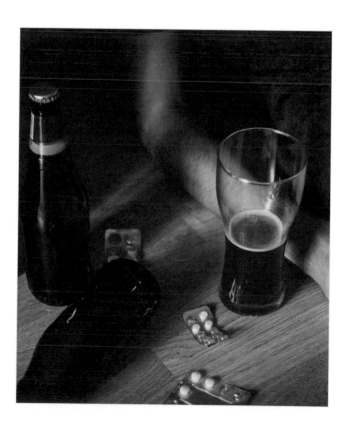

11. **Which psychological and emotional change(s) would indicate to Marge's co-workers that she is experiencing substance use disorder? Select all that apply.**

   1. Spending more time with old friends.
   2. Acting unusually anxious.
   3. Exhibiting outbursts of anger for no reason.
   4. Appearing sleepy.
   5. Undergoing personality changes.

12. **One of Marge's co-workers, Juan sees her place a narcotic vial into her pocket rather than wasting it with a co-signature. He approaches her asking about it, and she laughs saying, "I was going to get someone to co-sign the waste later." What should be Juan's next action?**

   1. Nothing, Marge is his charge nurse.
   2. Watch to see if it is done later.
   3. Offer to observe the waste and co-sign now.
   4. Report the incident to the supervisor.

13. **Because of the incident, Marge's supervisor begins to watch her more closely. She recognizes several symptoms of substance use disorder at work. Place the actions in the order in which the manager should complete them. _____, _____, _____, _____, _____.**

   1. Arrange for Marge to have a ride home.
   2. Notify the state board of nursing.
   3. Ask Marge if she is using substances.
   4. Perform a for-cause drug screen per agency policy.
   5. Remove Marge from the patient care area.

Marge's urine drug screen is positive for opiates without a prescription, and she is reported to the board of nursing. She is not able to practice nursing until she completes three, randomly ordered negative drug screens over the next month. She must also attend Narcotics Anonymous meetings weekly. The situation creates a significant amount of stress on her family and marriage both emotionally and financially.

14. **What free community resource(s) is/are available to Marge's husband and children to deal with this life change? Select all that apply.**

   1. Narcotics Anonymous.
   2. Nar-Anon family groups.
   3. Private counseling.
   4. Clergy at their place of worship.
   5. Alcoholics Anonymous.

   Next Gen Clinical Judgment: Compare and contrast these community resources and determine when each would be appropriately referred.
   > Narcotics Anonymous
   > Nar-Anon
   > Alcoholics Anonymous

15. **Marge tries to stop using the opioids but finds heroin is now her drug of choice. Her family is concerned she will accidentally hurt or kill herself. Which statement would lead her family to believe she may be in danger?**

   1. "I'm so disappointed with my life choices; I'll never be able to face my co-workers again."
   2. "I have to use more and more heroin to feel better."
   3. "I don't need you to tell me how to be happy; I'll be fine without you."
   4. "It's not my fault this happened; the doctors should have known and stopped it sooner."

16. **Marge's friends and family convince her to go into an inpatient acute detoxification unit for withdrawal from heroin. Which statement is true about heroin?**

   1. It is quickly removed from the body and withdrawal symptoms resolve in 24 hours.
   2. Medical supervision of withdrawal is suggested but not required.
   3. Withdrawal symptoms begin within 2-3 days of the last dose.
   4. Symptoms of withdrawal are worse the longer that heroin is used.

17. **Which symptom(s) can Marge anticipate as she withdraws from heroin? Select all that apply.**

   1. Nausea.
   2. Tremors.
   3. Sweating.
   4. Nervousness.
   5. Flaccid muscles.

   Clinical Hint: The types and severity of the physical and emotional symptoms of withdrawing from addictive substances will vary, based on the substance and the individual.

18. **Marge's medical treatment plan includes the use of longer-acting opioids, partial opioid antagonists and low dose opioid antagonists. Which statement(s) about these drug categories is/are accurate? Select all that apply.**

   1. Medication management cannot be successful without supportive counseling.
   2. Longer-acting opioids like methadone help control drug cravings.
   3. Partial opioid antagonists like buprenorphine remain active longer so dosing can be weaned.
   4. Partial agonists do not create the same "high" making them less likely to be abused.
   5. Opioid antagonists bind to opioid receptor sites and "block" other opioids from activation.

19. **As the nurse is discharging Marge, she asks about how often she should attend the community support group meetings. What should the nurse recommend?**

   1. "Only go when you feel you need it."
   2. "Daily is sufficient."
   3. "Once a week is adequate."
   4. "Go several times a day, if needed."

20. **Marge has been able to stay clean and sober for several months with daily support group meetings. She contacts the state board of nursing about returning to work. What is likely the outcome?**

   1. She will have to re-take the NCLEX-RN® examination.
   2. She may be able to work, depending on the status of her license.
   3. She will be able to work part-time only.
   4. She will only be able to work in non-patient care areas.

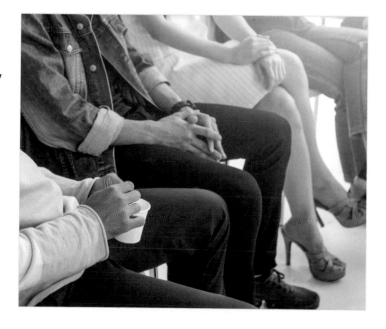

Conceptual Debriefing & Case Reflection

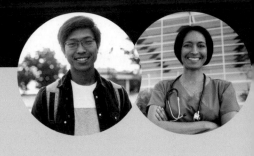

1. Compare the impaired adaptation that Brandon Kwong experienced with the impaired adaptation of Marge Sanderson. How are they the same and how are they different?

_____

_____

2. What was your single greatest learning moment while completing the case of Brandon Kwong? What about Marge Sanderson?

_____

_____

3. How did the nursing care provided to Brandon Kwong and Marge Sanderson change the outcome for each of them?

_____

_____

4. Identify safety concerns for both Brandon Kwong and Marge Sanderson for each case.

_____

_____

5. In what areas of each case study was basic care and comfort utilized?

_____

_____

6. What steps in each case did the nurse take that prevented hospital-acquired injury?

_____

_____

7. How did the nurse provide culturally sensitive/competent care?

_____

_____

8. How will learning about the case of Brandon Kwong and Marge Sanderson impact the care you provide for future clients?

_____

Fundamental Quiz

1. The nurse is teaching a group of pre-teen girls about life balance and proper nutrition during times of stress. Which statement by the nurse should be included?

   1. "During times of stress, it is easy to make unhealthy food choices. It is important to balance the unhealthy food choices with adding more exercise."
   2. "Exercising strenuously several times a day can help to release the stress you feel. Since you will be consuming more calories, you must eat more."
   3. "To maintain a healthy lifestyle during times of stress, it is important to continue to eat healthily and exercise regularly."
   4. "Exercising routinely and making healthy food choices will eliminate stress."

2. An older adult who lives alone comes to the clinic. He smells of body odor and is unkempt. He tells the nurse, "I've had a hard time functioning since my wife passed away." How should the nurse respond?

   1. "Tell me more about your wife?"
   2. "Was your wife sick for a while before she died?"
   3. "How long have you been alone?"
   4. "What things have become more difficult for you?"

3. As a nurse is preparing medications for a younger client with a new diagnosis of an incurable, chronic illness, the client tells the nurse, "I just cannot handle taking all of these medications every day, I feel like an old person." What should be the nurse's next action?

   1. Stop preparing the medications and pull up a chair beside the bed.
   2. Ask the client to prepare the medications.
   3. Ask the client if they know why the medications are important.
   4. Pause the medication preparation and ask the client to share more.

4. The nurse is admitting a client who does not speak the same language. When assessing the client's normal level of self-care, what actions should the nurse take?

   1. Smell for body odor and cleanliness of hair, nails, and teeth.
   2. Observe what the client is capable of doing independently when given hygiene supplies.
   3. Ask a family member how independent the client is at home.
   4. Obtain an interpreter to assist with translation.

5. A recovering alcoholic is working through a 12-step program. How will the nurse determine if the client is moving toward recovery by changing behavior?

   1. The client is attending daily recovery meetings.
   2. The client states they are no longer drinking alcohol.
   3. They are talking to family and repairing broken relationships.
   4. They read their recovery material each day.

Advanced Quiz

6. A client in a locked inpatient facility has a knife in his hand and is threatening to hurt himself. What should be the nurse's next action?

   1. Ask the client to "calm down" and give you the knife.
   2. Ask the client why they would want to hurt himself.
   3. Approach the client and gently remove the knife from his hand.
   4. Call security.

7. During a clinic visit, a teen shares with the nurse that at night she gets out of bed several dozen times to be sure her bedroom door is locked. How should the nurse respond?

   1. "It sounds to me like you are having obsessive-compulsive thoughts. Are there other things you do this with?"
   2. "Sometimes victims of rape and violence will do that. Have you ever had that happen to you?"
   3. "Do you feel unsafe?"
   4. "Why would you do that?"

8. Upon assessment of a pre-teen, the nurse identifies that the client has a body mass index (BMI) of 15 kg/m², and teeth enamel corrosion. What should the nurse do? Select all that apply.

   1. Place the pre-teen on a daily calorie count.
   2. Obtain a 24-hour food recall assessment.
   3. Ask the parents if they are ever concerned about their child's eating.
   4. Ask the pre-teen how they feel about their weight.
   5. Ask the pre-teen how often he/she brushes his/her teeth.

9. A woman in her late 20s shares with the nurse that she feels like such a failure because she's been married and divorced three times and has a child from each marriage. How should the nurse respond?

   1. "Tell me why that makes you feel like a failure?"
   2. "Tell me more about your children, how old are they?"
   3. "It's hard to find the right life partner."
   4. "You are still young; I'm sure you'll find the right person."

10. A military veteran is in the clinic for anxiety related to post-traumatic stress disorder. What should the nurse include in the plan of care? Select all that apply.

    1. Development of a professional relationship based on trust.
    2. Provide an environment that is therapeutic for the client.
    3. Assist in the identification of anxiety triggers.
    4. Administer sedative medication if the client becomes stressed.
    5. Recognize therapeutic stress-relieving options.

Emotion

Mood / Anxiety / Grief

Emotion is a state of mind related to thoughts, feelings, perceptions, and environmental surroundings. Emotions describe feelings associated with different life events, including stressors and everyday occurrences such as the death of a loved one or final exams. Everyone perceives situations differently and reacts uniquely, causing a wide range of emotions from happiness to sadness. Experiencing a range of emotions is a typical human response. However, for some people, emotion regulation can be burdensome due to an underlying psychiatric condition. It is the nurse's responsibility to assess a client's emotional state through a comprehensive assessment that includes mood and affect intervening with appropriate therapeutic modalities when indicated. The term mood is used by nurses to help describe the client's current emotions. Affect is a term used by the nurse to describe how the client appears or how the person reacts when describing the mood.

Next Gen Clinical Judgment:

> Describe emotions in terms of mood and affect.

> List as many terms for emotions, including mood and affect that you know.

> List some examples of positive and negative events that can cause changes in emotion.

> How do emotions vary during different life events?

> How can someone's mood be directly affected by grief?

> Some people can't regulate their mood. List as many examples as you can describing when this could occur.

_____

_____

_____

_____

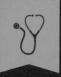
Case 1: Anxiety and Grief

Related Concepts: Adaptation: Coping
Threaded Topics: Wellness, Family dynamics, Self-management, Safe
medication administration, Teaching, Non-pharmacological therapies

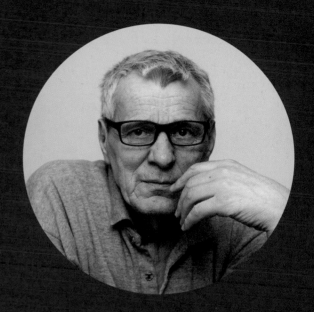

Peter Allen is a 60-year-old man. He has worked as a government clerk for the past 40 years. About four months ago, his supervisor suggested that he consider retirement rather than being laid off, as his department was cutting back. He is a private person who has always lived with his mother, a woman who just one month ago was diagnosed with Parkinson's disease. He has just two friends, both of whom are from work, and avoids social interaction. He describes himself as "always sensitive to what others think of me." He presents today with feelings of anxiety, restlessness, and irritability which has been increasing over the last four months. Peter makes poor eye contact during the visit and is restless. He looks scared and is timid when asked questions.

1. The nurse reviews Peter's statements to identify potential stressor(s) that are currently impacting Peter's life and emotional state. Which factors should the nurse consider? Select all that apply.

   1. Forced retirement.
   2. Lack of friends.
   3. Mother's recent diagnosis.
   4. Worked as a government clerk for 40 years.
   5. Lives with his mother.

2. Considering Peter's situation and presentation, what should be the nurse's next action?

   1. Assess the anxiety and restlessness that Peter mentioned.
   2. Refer to a mental health clinician.
   3. Admit to the mental health unit.
   4. Nothing, this appears to be normal behavior for him.

3. What would be the appropriate way for the nurse to chart congruent affect and mood for Peter?

   1. Labile and sad.
   2. Irritable and anxious.
   3. Flat and angry.
   4. Constricted and euphoric.

Peter says that his anxiety and restlessness began when his boss told him he needed to retire to avoid being laid off from work. Along with these symptoms, he also reports difficulty falling asleep with mild insomnia and early morning awakening. He has been having feelings of guilt about his problems in performing at work and always worries about his future. He reports a loss of energy and difficulty concentrating. His appetite is decreased, and he has lost 5 pounds over the past three months on his already small body frame.

4. **NurseThink® Prioritization Power!**
   Evaluate the behaviors that Mr. Allen is exhibiting and determine the **Top 3 Priority** cues.

   1. _____

   2. _____

   3. _____

5. **The nurse is assessing Peter's level of anxiety. Which statement provides the best indication?**
   1. "I feel so tired all the time. I don't know what to do or where to go for help."
   2. "I have never felt this way before; I would rate my anxiety as an 8 on a 10-point scale."
   3. "My anxiety is so bad right now, that I can't sleep or eat, and I am just not doing well at work."
   4. "I have so many stressors in my life right now that I can't just concentrate on anything."

6. **For each of the nurse's comments to Peter listed in the box, mark if it is therapeutic or non-therapeutic to the conversation.**

Nurse's statement	Therapeutic	Non-therapeutic
"Have you considered looking for another job?"		
"What does your mother think about you retiring?"		
"It sounds like you are going through a lot right now."		
"Do you enjoy your job?"		
"What are your greatest fears about the future?"		
"Who do you feel is most supportive in your life?"		
"Do you go to church?"		

7. **The nurse reviews the symptoms of generalized anxiety disorder. Check the items on this list that are associated with this. Then check the items that Peter is exhibiting.**

	Symptoms of Anxiety Disorder	Symptoms that Peter is exhibiting
Excessive anxiety or worry almost all the time.		
Worrying about different situations.		
The worrying is difficult to control and leads to impairment in functioning.		
Increased socialization.		
Feelings of restlessness.		
Obsessive thoughts.		
Inability to concentrate.		
Irritability.		
Hyperactivity.		
Insomnia.		
Suicidal thoughts.		
Depressed mood.		
Easily fatigued or tired.		
Panic attacks.		

Upon further assessment, Peter's medical history reveals arthritis and hypertension. He is worried about both of these conditions worsening as he gets older. He also voices concern that he will not be able to care for his mother as she progresses with her Parkinson's disease.

8. **The nurse is concerned that Peter is experiencing an acute stress reaction related to grief and brought on by anticipatory grief. List the five stages of grief. Determine which stage you feel Peter is currently experiencing.**

    1. _____
    2. _____
    3. _____
    4. _____
    5. _____

Peter agrees to see a healthcare provider, and the nurse makes a referral to the mental health clinic for further follow-up and treatment.

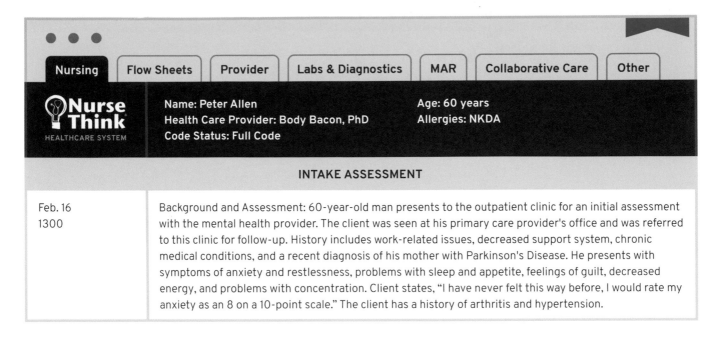

| Nursing | Flow Sheets | Provider | Labs & Diagnostics | MAR | Collaborative Care | Other |

NurseThink HEALTHCARE SYSTEM

Name: Peter Allen
Health Care Provider: Body Bacon, PhD
Code Status: Full Code

Age: 60 years
Allergies: NKDA

INTAKE ASSESSMENT

| Feb. 16 1300 | Background and Assessment: 60-year-old man presents to the outpatient clinic for an initial assessment with the mental health provider. The client was seen at his primary care provider's office and was referred to this clinic for follow-up. History includes work-related issues, decreased support system, chronic medical conditions, and a recent diagnosis of his mother with Parkinson's Disease. He presents with symptoms of anxiety and restlessness, problems with sleep and appetite, feelings of guilt, decreased energy, and problems with concentration. Client states, "I have never felt this way before, I would rate my anxiety as an 8 on a 10-point scale." The client has a history of arthritis and hypertension. |

9. **NurseThink® Prioritization Power!**

Evaluate the Intake Note and determine the **Top 3 Priority** findings or cues that require a follow-up by the nurse.

1. _____

2. _____

3. _____

10. **What priority nursing assessment is missing from the above intake note? Select all that apply.**
    1. Suicidality.
    2. Depression.
    3. Psychosis.
    4. Panic Attacks.
    5. Hyperactivity.

11. **When planning care for the client, the nurse works with Peter to identify actions to help decrease his anxiety. Which statement made by Peter shows that he understands how to manage his anxiety?**
    1. "When I feel anxious, I'll just take lorazepam."
    2. "I should avoid all situations that make me anxious."
    3. "Once my meds start working, I won't be anxious anymore."
    4. "I need to make sure to take time for myself, at least 30 minutes every day."

12. **The nurse is concerned about Peter's lack of social support with his mother's recent diagnosis. Which action should the nurse take first when creating the plan of care to meet his social support needs best?**
    1. Encourage him to attend support groups for caregivers.
    2. Suggest he finds a support group for family caregivers.
    3. Guide him in recognizing his personal preferences for social support.
    4. Give him the pamphlet with local support groups in his area.

After meeting with the mental health provider, Peter is given the following prescriptions and follow-up plan.

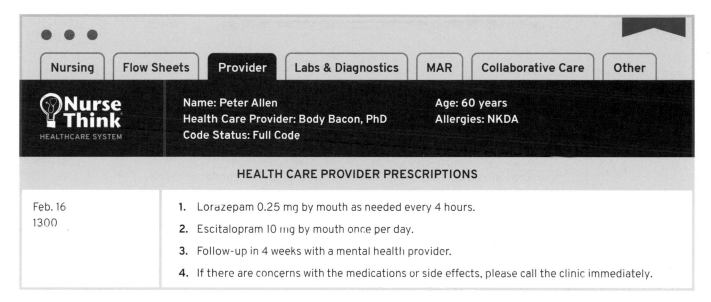

| Nursing | Flow Sheets | Provider | Labs & Diagnostics | MAR | Collaborative Care | Other |

NurseThink
HEALTHCARE SYSTEM

Name: Peter Allen
Health Care Provider: Body Bacon, PhD
Code Status: Full Code

Age: 60 years
Allergies: NKDA

HEALTH CARE PROVIDER PRESCRIPTIONS

Feb. 16 1300	1. Lorazepam 0.25 mg by mouth as needed every 4 hours.
	2. Escitalopram 10 mg by mouth once per day.
	3. Follow-up in 4 weeks with a mental health provider.
	4. If there are concerns with the medications or side effects, please call the clinic immediately.

13. **As the nurse plans for discharge instructions, what teaching is priority regarding lorazepam?**
    1. It should not be taken with antidepressant medications as this could cause excessive sedation.
    2. It is used as the temporary bridge when initiating treatment with an antidepressant being used for anxiety.
    3. It does not require tapering upon discontinuation, and there is no concern for tolerance or withdrawal symptoms.
    4. It can be used safely in all clients and works well in the treatment of generalized anxiety disorder.

14. **NurseThink® Prioritization Power!**
    Evaluate the new prescriptions and determine the **Top 3 Priority** teaching needs for the prescription for lorazepam.

    1. _____

    2. _____

    3. _____

Clinical Hint: Identify the medication by it's ending.
Benzodiazepines (Anti-anxiety - Anticonvulsive - Sedative) = -pam, -lam.
Phenothiazines (Anti-psychotic - Anti-emetic - Sedative) = -zine.

15. **NurseThink® Prioritization Power!**

Evaluate the new prescriptions and determine the **Top 3 Priority** teaching needs for the prescription for escitalopram.

1. _____

2. _____

3. _____

16. **The nurse is reviewing the medications with Peter. Which of his statement(s) require further follow-up? Select all that apply.**

1. "I can't wait to feel better next week when these meds start working."
2. "I am fine with taking lorazepam because I know I won't become addicted."
3. "I will take these medications only when I am feeling anxious."
4. "I know that this will take time, and I need to wait for the escitalopram to start working."
5. "My aunt took escitalopram when she had her anxiety issues, and it worked for her."

Peter returns to the mental health provider for his four-week follow-up. He states that he has been taking the medication as prescribed without any significant side effects. However, he is still having "a lot" of anxiety about his mother's diagnosis. He does not know how to move forward knowing that her condition will worsen and he'll lose her. The nurse decides to use some motivational interviewing techniques to help Peter see the importance of caregiver resources for him to take care of his mother.

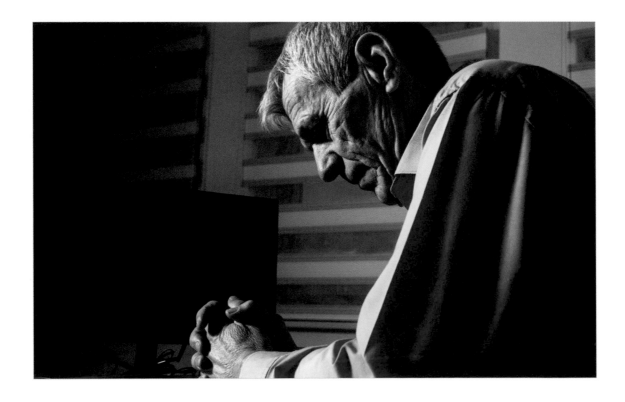

17. **Select the statements that the nurse could use to assess Peter's readiness for change when using motivational interviewing techniques. Select all that apply.**

    1. "Let me suggest some things that might be helpful for you."
    2. "Why do you think you're feeling this way now?"
    3. "Could I have your permission to discuss the behavior and elicits pros and cons?"
    4. "I'd like to ask your perception of the importance of change on a scale of 1-10."
    5. "I'd like to ask your perception of the confidence to change on a scale of 1-10."

18. **Peter asks to discuss nonpharmacological measures to help with his anxiety. Which teaching would be most helpful to him regarding anxiety reduction?**

    1. Explain how Peter should avoid anxiety in his life.
    2. Teach Peter how to eliminate anxiety from his life.
    3. Demonstrate alternative methods of anxiety reduction that he might try.
    4. Suggest to Peter what herbal remedies may be taken that will reduce anxiety.

19. **Mindfulness is an effective nonpharmacologic treatment method for anxiety. What are the basic principles of mindfulness related to anxiety? Select all that apply.**

    1. Self-intention.
    2. Focused attention.
    3. Virtue.
    4. Physical health.
    5. Judgment.
    6. Attitude.

> **Next Gen Clinical Judgment:**
> Commit to practicing mindfulness for one full week. See if it changes your perception on life and reduces your anxiety.

Peter agrees to see a counselor in a one-on-one setting. He doesn't feel that he will be comfortable in a support group type setting. His medications are working, but he is still experiencing anxiety. He is willing to try alternative therapies but was also agreeable when the mental health provider increased his dose of escitalopram to 20 mg by mouth once per day. The nurse recommends a counselor that specializes in cognitive behavioral therapy.

20. **Peter asks what cognitive behavioral therapy is. How should the nurse respond?**

    1. This type of therapy highlights the role of risk and protective factors in anxiety.
    2. This type of therapy works on identifying and changing automatic thoughts surrounding the anxiety.
    3. This type of therapy links the dual roles of nature and nurture in the development of anxiety.
    4. This type of therapy identifies the family as a whole contributing to the client's anxiety.

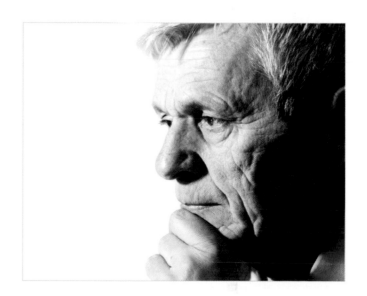

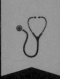

Go To Clinical Case

While caring for this client, be sure to review the concept maps in chapters 3 and 4.

Case 2: Bipolar Disorder with Depression

Related Concepts: Adaptation: Coping
Threaded Topics: Wellness, Self-management, Medication management, Suicide attempt

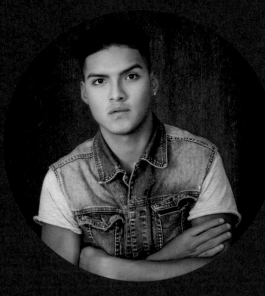

Luis Chaves is a 22-year-old who migrated to Miami at the age of 2 years with his parents. He is unemployed and lives with his sister. He is actively involved with an intercity gang and depressed. Today he intentionally overdosed with paroxetine, zolpidem, oxycodone, and alcohol. He goes to his sisters apartment to say goodbye after taking the drugs and alcohol and confesses to overdosing. His sister immediately calls 911 as he became unconscious. On the way to the emergency department Luis was treated with naloxone, which produces a rapid improvement in his level of consciousness. He becomes agitated and starts yelling that he "doesn't want to live anymore."

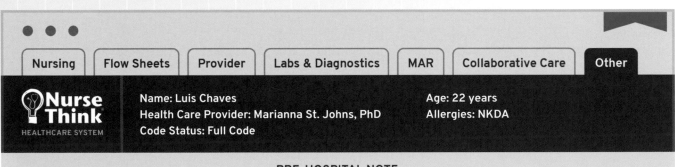

Nursing	Flow Sheets	Provider	Labs & Diagnostics	MAR	Collaborative Care	Other

Name: Luis Chaves
Health Care Provider: Marianna St. Johns, PhD
Code Status: Full Code
Age: 22 years
Allergies: NKDA

PRE-HOSPITAL NOTE

Oct. 26 2300	Paramedics responded to the residence at 2204. Upon arrival to the scene found a 22-year-old male unconscious. Sister reports that the client stated overdosing with paroxetine, zolpidem, oxycodone, ibuprofen, and alcohol. Patent airway and breathing spontaneously at 8 respirations per minute, pulse 60 beats per minute, blood pressure 90/58 (69) mmHg. Naloxone administered during transport and client's consciousness level increased. Begin yelling "I don't want to live anymore." Respirations 20 breaths per minute, pulse 90 beats per minute, blood pressure 148/98 (115). Handoff report to the emergency department nurse.

Go to the National Suicide Prevention Lifeline website and learn 3 new things. →

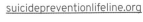
suicidepreventionlifeline.org

1. **NurseThink® Prioritization Power!**

   The nurse receives the high handoff from emergency medical personnel that brought Luis into the emergency department. What are the 3 priority concerns or cues?

   1. _____

   2. _____

   3. _____

2. **As the triage nurse in the emergency department, what is the priority focused assessment?**
   1. Cultural preferences.
   2. Respiratory status.
   3. Suicide risk.
   4. Substance use history.

3. **The client responded to naloxone on the way to the emergency department. Which substance(s) would not react to naloxone? Select all that apply.**
   1. Paroxetine.
   2. Zolpidem.
   3. Oxycodone.
   4. Ibuprofen.
   5. Alcohol.

Luis is stabilized in the emergency department. He reports feeling "desperate" over being estranged from his 4-year-old son and the negative consequences of his current life decisions. He goes on to discuss conflicts that he has with his mother, his inability to find employment, the recent death of several close friends murdered in gang violence, and feelings of self-loathing, helplessness, hopelessness, and depression. Luis shares that his biological father is an alcoholic and has a drug abuse problem. However, the client denies that he has any problems with alcohol because he "just doesn't like the taste," and only drinks one to two times per month. He also doesn't take drugs because he doesn't "like the way they make me feel." Luis states that his family history is positive for depression, schizophrenia, and bipolar disorder. At age 14 he tried to commit suicide for the first time and has made three attempts since then with a previous psychiatric admission. He says "I wish I hadn't gone to my sister and told her what I did; then this would be over." Client denies current suicidal ideation.

4. **What is the best predictor of a suicide attempt?**
   1. A family history of suicide attempts.
   2. Previous suicide attempts.
   3. Stating suicidal intent.
   4. Having a friend who had a suicide completion.

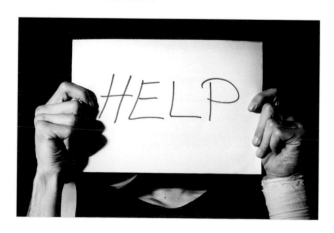

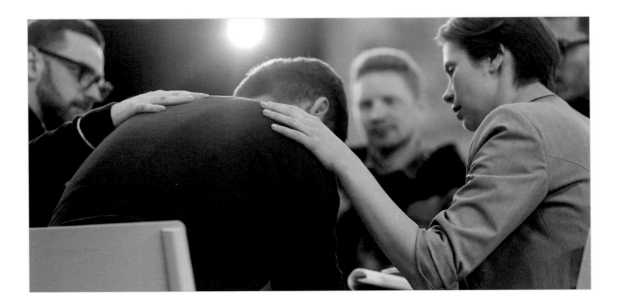

5. The nurse reviews suicide risk factors and mentally compares them Luis's situation. Mark each box appropriately.

	Suicide Risk Factors	Factors that place Luis at a Higher Risk for Suicide
Defined plan, means, and intent.		
Previous attempts.		
A family history of alcohol use.		
A family history of suicide.		
Being in a committed relationship.		
Lack of social support system.		
The recent loss of a close relationship.		
Male gender.		
Employment status.		
Mental Illness.		

Luis denies chronic illnesses in his family besides his mother having bone marrow cancer. He is currently taking oxycodone for leg pain. Three months ago, he was climbing a spiked fence when he slipped, and his leg was caught on one of the spikes, where he was left dangling. He now walks with a slight limp but states that it only hurts if he tries to walk without the limp.

6. **THIN Thinking Time!**

   Reflect on the information the nurse has gathered about Luis and apply **THIN Thinking.**

   T – _____

   H – _____

   I – _____

   N – _____

   T - Top 3
   H - Help Quick
   I - Identify Risk to Safety
   N - Nursing Process

   Scan to access the
   10-Minute-Mentor →
   on THIN Thinking.

   NurseThink.com/THINThinking

7. **The nurse continues the assessment. What question(s) should the nurse ask? Select all that apply.**

   1. "What medications are you currently prescribed besides oxycodone?"
   2. "Tell me about any illicit drugs you have taken in the past."
   3. "How do you feel about your attempt being unsuccessful?"
   4. "What is your relationship like with your sister?"
   5. "Tell me more about your family history of mental illness."
   6. "How has your mood been lately?"

8. **What are the criteria for a diagnosis of major depressive disorder? Select all that apply.**

   1. Depressed mood.
   2. Lack of interest in activities that used to be enjoyable.
   3. Manic mood.
   4. Change in appetite.
   5. Fatigue or loss of energy.
   6. Feelings of elation.
   7. Feelings of worthlessness.
   8. Inability to concentrate.
   9. Thoughts of death.
   10. Increase in a goal-focused activity.

   Use the National Institute of Mental Health to help answer this question.

   www.nimh.nih.gov/health/topics/
   depression/index.shtml

   →

9. **The nurse discovered that Luis takes paroxetine for a major depressive disorder. Which statement is correct about this medication?**

   1. Paroxetine is a monoamine oxidase inhibitor that works by blocking the breakdown of tyramine, a precursor to dopamine.
   2. Paroxetine is a tricyclic antidepressant that works by altering norepinephrine and serotonin levels at the synapse.
   3. Paroxetine is a selective serotonin reuptake inhibitor that works by helps serotonin get to the synapses where it is needed.
   4. Paroxetine is a heterocyclic that works by inhibiting neuronal uptake of norepinephrine and dopamine.

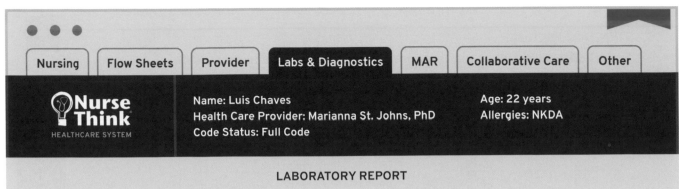

LABORATORY REPORT

Lab	Normal	Admit
WBC	4,000 - 10,000 µL	5.6
Hemoglobin	12.0 - 17.0 g/dL	11.2 L
Hematocrit (%)	36 - 51%	32 L
RBC	4.2 - 5.9 cells/L	4.0 L
Platelets	150,000 to 350,000 µL	156,000
Calcium	9 - 10.5 mg/dL	9.0
Chloride	98 - 106 mEq/L	103
Magnesium	1.5 - 2.4 mEq/L	1.4 L
Phosphorus	3.0 - 4.5 mg/dL	4.5 H
Potassium	3.5 - 5.0 mEq/L	3.4 L
Sodium	136 - 145 mEq/L	136
Glucose, fasting	70 – 100 mg/dL	104 H
BUN	8 - 20 mg/dL	25 H
Creatinine	0.7- 1.3 mg/dL	1.3
CPK	30 - 170 U/L	63
LDH	60 - 100 U/L	156 H
AST	0 - 35 U/L	38 H
ALT	0 - 35 U/L	31
GGT	9-48 U/L	23
Thyroid Stimulating Hormone	0.5 – 5 mU/L	5.4 H

10. **The nurse reviews the lab report completed in the Emergency Department. Which labs could be a result of his current symptoms?**

    1. Liver function.
    2. Kidney function.
    3. Metabolic function.
    4. Thyroid function.

Luis was medically cleared from the emergency department and transferred to the psychiatric inpatient unit.

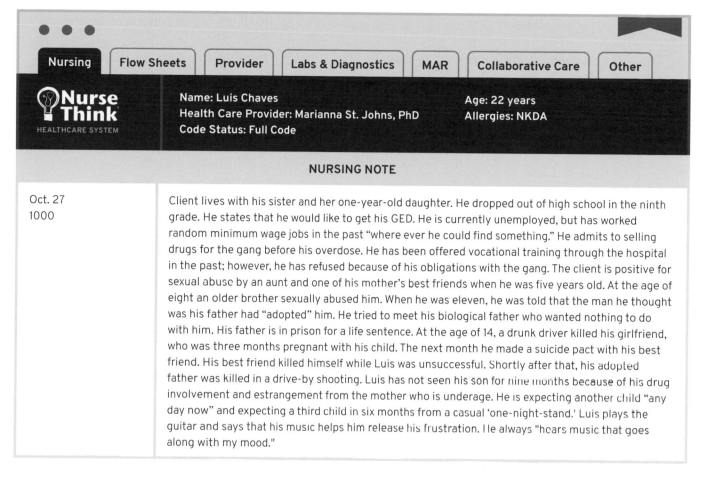

Nursing | Flow Sheets | Provider | Labs & Diagnostics | MAR | Collaborative Care | Other

Nurse Think
HEALTHCARE SYSTEM

Name: Luis Chaves
Health Care Provider: Marianna St. Johns, PhD
Code Status: Full Code

Age: 22 years
Allergies: NKDA

NURSING NOTE

| Oct. 27 1000 | Client lives with his sister and her one-year-old daughter. He dropped out of high school in the ninth grade. He states that he would like to get his GED. He is currently unemployed, but has worked random minimum wage jobs in the past "where ever he could find something." He admits to selling drugs for the gang before his overdose. He has been offered vocational training through the hospital in the past; however, he has refused because of his obligations with the gang. The client is positive for sexual abuse by an aunt and one of his mother's best friends when he was five years old. At the age of eight an older brother sexually abused him. When he was eleven, he was told that the man he thought was his father had "adopted" him. He tried to meet his biological father who wanted nothing to do with him. His father is in prison for a life sentence. At the age of 14, a drunk driver killed his girlfriend, who was three months pregnant with his child. The next month he made a suicide pact with his best friend. His best friend killed himself while Luis was unsuccessful. Shortly after that, his adopted father was killed in a drive-by shooting. Luis has not seen his son for nine months because of his drug involvement and estrangement from the mother who is underage. He is expecting another child "any day now" and expecting a third child in six months from a casual 'one-night-stand.' Luis plays the guitar and says that his music helps him release his frustration. He always "hears music that goes along with my mood." |

11. **The nurse is concerned about the new information received during the initial assessment. What information is the priority?**
    1. Family history.
    2. Trauma history.
    3. History of elated mood.
    4. History of anxiety or worry.

12. **The nurse creates a plan of care based on trauma-informed care. What factors influenced this decision? Select all that apply.**
    1. Sexual abuse by aunt and mother's best friend.
    2. Not completing high school.
    3. Lives with his sister and her daughter.
    4. Selling drugs for the gang.
    5. Sexual abuse by his brother.
    6. Losing his pregnant girlfriend and unborn child.
    7. Not being able to see his child.
    8. Finding out his biological father had abandoned him.

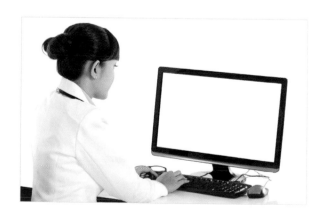

During further conversations, Luis shares that at times he feels like he "can do anything." During these times he is "super focused and feels invincible." Joining the gang is an outlet that allows him to do anything he wants, without limitations. The nurse is concerned that Luis may have bipolar disorder given the recent episode of depression.

13. **The nurse contemplates the differences between bipolar I and II. Mark the box with the appropriate behaviors.**

Behavior	Bipolar I	Bipolar II	Neither
Abnormal or persistently elevated, irritable mood.			
Increased goal-directed activity or energy.			
Inflated self-esteem, grandiosity.			
Excessive anxiety or worry all of the time.			
Decreased need for sleep.			
Distractible.			
History of a depressive episode.			
Suicidal thoughts.			
Causes marked impairment in functioning.			

14. **The nurse is concerned that Luis may have a bipolar disorder and talks to the mental health provider about his current medications. Which medications might be prescribed for Luis in an effort to manage his bipolar disorder? Select all that apply.**
    1. Valproate.
    2. Lamotrigine.
    3. Clozapine.
    4. Risperidone.
    5. Aripiprazole.
    6. Lorazepam.

15. **The mental health care provider is also concerned that Luis may have bipolar disorder and wants to start him on lithium carbonate. Which statement made by the client indicates an understanding of the medication and its side effects?**
    1. "If I have fine hand tremors, I'll just take the benztropine as needed."
    2. "I will have the blood levels tests drawn regularly."
    3. "I will decrease my salt and fluid intake."
    4. "If a skin rash appears, I'll just stop taking my medications."

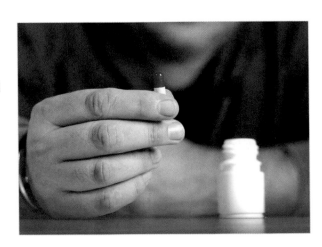

16. **As the nurse is getting ready to administer Luis' morning dose of lithium a coarse hand tremor is noted. What is the nurses' priority action?**

    1. The nurse should administer the morning dose as this is a normal side effect.
    2. The nurse should call the physician immediately as this is a rare and fatal side effect of lithium.
    3. The course hand tremor is a sign of mild toxicity, and the nurse should hold the lithium dose until further assessment.
    4. The nurse will give the lithium, continue to monitor the hand tremor and call the physician when the lithium levels rise to 2.3 mEq/L.

17. **The mental health care provider decided to change Luis's medication to lamotrigine. Which statement made by Luis would require immediate action?**

    1. "I am having difficulty falling asleep at night."
    2. "I noticed a weird rash on my chest that wasn't there before."
    3. "I feel like my thoughts have improved."
    4. "I sure hope I don't get that hand tremor as I had with lithium."

18. **Luis has been stabilized on his medication regimen and discharged from the inpatient unit. The nurse has completed reviewing the discharge instructions with Luis. Which statement(s) require additional follow-up? Select all that apply.**

    1. "When I start to feel better, I can stop taking my medications."
    2. "I will follow-up on my pain management referral so that I can taper off my oxycodone."
    3. "I am glad that my attempt was unsuccessful, I have my children to think about, and so much else to live for."
    4. "I am sure I will be back; these mood issues have been a problem for me for quite some time."
    5. "I need to figure out how to get my GED and start a life without the gang."
    6. "I am worried my prescription for oxycodone won't hold me until my appointment, could you talk to the doctor to get me more?"

---

19. **NurseThink® Prioritization Power!**

    Luis was discharged to a partial hospitalization program. List the **Top 3 Priority** reasons why a partial program would be beneficial for Luis.

    1. _____

    2. _____

    3. _____

---

20. **Luis is concerned about how to get away from the gang and get his life back on track. What suggestions should the nurse make? Select all that apply.**

    1. Change your contact information so they cannot call or text you.
    2. Spend more time with your family.
    3. Find other interests in the community to fill your time.
    4. Let them know that you want out.
    5. Don't be available to them.

Conceptual Debriefing & Case Reflection

1. Compare the emotional responses of Peter Allen and Luis Chaves. How are they the same and how are they different?

   _____

   _____

2. Compare the coping mechanisms of Peter and Luis. How are they the same and how are they different?

   _____

   _____

3. Compare the support systems of Peter and Luis. How are they the same and how are they different?

   _____

   _____

4. In what areas of each case study was therapeutic communication utilized?

   _____

   _____

5. What steps in each case did the nurse take that prevented injury?

   _____

   _____

6. How did the nurse provide culturally sensitive/competent care?

   _____

   _____

7. How will learning about the case of Peter Allen and Luis Chaves impact the care you provide for future clients?

   _____

   _____

Fundamental Quiz

1. The nurse is reviewing clients in the emergency department for inpatient psychiatric unit admission. Which client is the priority?
   1. A toddler with an accidental overdose of psychiatric medication.
   2. A homeless man who is mentally ill, but refuses to take his medications.
   3. A woman with a near-fatal intentional overdose of benzodiazepine medications.
   4. A man with back pain and discloses a suicide attempt at age 30.

2. The client states "I am so worried and anxious about getting discharged." The nurse observes a concerned facial expression. How should the nurse document this interaction?
   1. Flat.
   2. Depressed.
   3. Logical.
   4. Congruent.

3. The nurse is taking care of a client with a history of psychological and physical trauma. What guidelines should be followed?
   1. Limit teaching due to trauma-related alterations in information processing.
   2. Use therapeutic touch to relax the client.
   3. Approach the client in a non-threatening manner.
   4. Don't discuss the trauma in an effort not to re-traumatize the client.

4. The nurse is assessing a child for depression. Which symptoms are most concerning? Select all that apply.
   1. Irritability.
   2. Low self-esteem.
   3. Physical complaints.
   4. Increased concentration.
   5. Negative verbalizations.
   6. Changes in activity level.

5. The nurse is caring for a client who is experiencing an acute panic attack. Which action should the nurse take?
   1. Use distraction techniques to change the focus.
   2. Explore events that led up to the panic attack.
   3. Offer reassurance of safety and security.
   4. Ask open-ended questions to encourage communication.

Advanced Quiz

6. The nurse receives a hand-off report on each of these four clients. Which is displaying the signs and symptoms of a major depressive episode?
   1. The client who has been experiencing a lack of interest in usual activities, excessive guilt, appetite loss, psychomotor slowness, and fatigue for two weeks.
   2. The client who has been experiencing a depressed mood and suicidal ideation with no other symptoms for two weeks.
   3. The client who has been experiencing hopelessness and helplessness, depressed mood, and sleep and appetite disturbance when trying to withdraw from cocaine.
   4. The client who has been experiencing sleep and appetite disturbances, concentration difficulties, feelings of worthlessness, and fatigue for two weeks.

7. The nurse working in an inpatient unit is encouraging a client to attend therapy groups. The client responds, "I don't need to go to group therapy. The medication has helped my anxiety." How can the nurse best respond to this client?
   1. "You will become dependent on the medication if you don't use other strategies such as group therapy."
   2. "All clients are required to attend group therapy. It will help you overcome your anxiety about interacting with others."
   3. "Medication will help the anxious feelings, but it will not address the cause of your anxiety. Group therapy will help you identify some of the causes and enable you to develop strategies to cope with anxious feelings."
   4. "The medication will only continue to help you if you attend group therapy and utilize other supportive treatments."

8. A client with bipolar disorder who is on valproate asks the nurse why the mental health care provider ordered an anticonvulsant when the client has no history of seizures. How should the nurse respond?
   1. "Several anticonvulsant medications, including valproate are used as mood stabilizers."
   2. "Valproate is not an anticonvulsant; it is an antipsychotic medication."
   3. "People with bipolar disorder are at increased risk of having seizures and are treated to prevent them."
   4. "People must be on another medication that lowers the seizure threshold and valproate is protective."

9. A parent of an adolescent being treated in the inpatient unit heard about the black-box warning for antidepressants on a television show and asked the nurse to explain the implications. How should the nurse respond?

    1. "The black-box warning applies to all psychiatric medications."
    2. "The black-box warning emphasizes to providers the importance of maintaining vigilance in monitoring for suicidal thinking and behavior in children, adolescents, and young adults taking antidepressants."
    3. "The black-box warning forbids the use of antidepressants in children and adolescents."
    4. "The black-box warning is based on research demonstrating an increase in suicide completion among those taking antidepressants."

10. The nurse receives a hand-off report on each of these four clients. Which is showing signs and symptoms consistent with a generalized anxiety disorder?

    1. The client who has been experiencing excessive, uncontrolled worry and anxiety most of the time for the last 6 months with restlessness, irritability, and sleep disturbances.
    2. The client who has been experiencing an excessive marked and persistent fear surrounding a specific object for the last 6 months with avoidance of the object that causes the fear.
    3. The client who has had fear and anxiety of social performance or social situations for the last 6 months with social situations avoided.
    4. The client who has had obsessions and compulsions that interfere in daily functioning with repetitive behaviors that are aimed at reducing the anxiety.

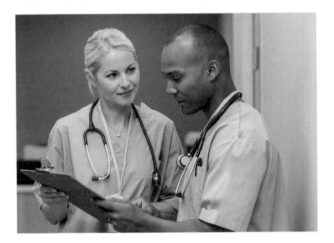

Cognition
Cognitive Functioning

Cognition is the mental action or process of acquiring knowledge and understanding through thought, experience, and the senses. The result of cognitive process is the development of perception, sensation, notion, or intuition about the world at large. The mental processes of cognitive function leads to the acquisition of knowledge and allows for the ability to carry out daily tasks. Cognition is considered a defining characteristic of being human and having a livelihood. For many, their greatest fear is living in a body without adequate cognitive function.

A variety of things impact a person's cognition. Health problems, such as heart disease, diabetes, stroke, depression, and brain injuries; substances like medications, drugs or alcohol; and lifestyle choices, including diet, smoking, sleep patterns, social isolation, and a lack of physical activity, all have an impact. As a person ages, society begins to expect and accept a change in cognition as 'normal.'

The nurse should recognize and teach that this is not as an anticipated event of growing older. Nurses lead the client, family and healthcare team in exploring other etiologies.

Next Gen Clinical Judgment:

> What is the difference between delirium and dementia? Compare and contrast.

> Do you think intellectual disability is considered a cognitive disorder? Why or why not?

> What are the early signs of cognitive disorder?

> List situations that would cause an acute change in cognitive functioning.

_____

_____

_____

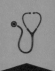

Go To Clinical Case

While caring for this client, be sure to review the concept maps in chapters 3 and 4.

Case 1: Confusion, Dementia, and Loss of Independence

Related Concepts: Nutrition, Mobility, Adaptation
Threaded Topics: Family Dynamics, Medications, Risk for Falls, Home Safety, Restraints, Aspiration Management

Maryann Huston is an 84-year-old female from Chicago, Illinois. She is widowed, has two adult children and seven grandchildren. Maryann is retired from a credit card company, where she spent 40 years in the customer service department. Maryann is 5 foot, 5 inches and weighs 165 pounds (BMI 27.5). Her past medical history includes hypertension, hypercholesterolemia, asthma, chronic obstructive pulmonary disease (COPD), and prediabetes. Maryann lives alone and enjoys cooking and watching game shows on television every night.

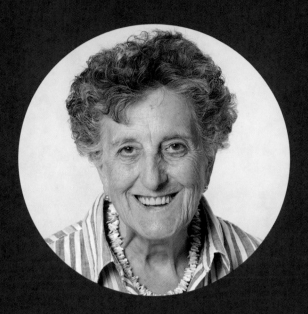

Maryann comes to the clinic today with her daughter, Therese. Therese expresses her concern that her mother might not be as "sharp" as she used to be. She has had very forgetful moments, such as leaving the stove on and forgetting doctor's appointments. Therese shares that Maryann often has a hard time remembering the names of the people that she knows. Richard Spade, a Geriatric Nurse Practitioner, conducts a physical assessment on Maryann.

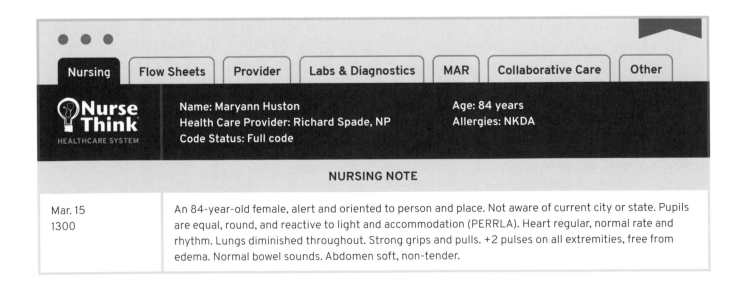

| Nursing | Flow Sheets | Provider | Labs & Diagnostics | MAR | Collaborative Care | Other |

NurseThink HEALTHCARE SYSTEM

Name: Maryann Huston
Health Care Provider: Richard Spade, NP
Code Status: Full code

Age: 84 years
Allergies: NKDA

NURSING NOTE

| Mar. 15 1300 | An 84-year-old female, alert and oriented to person and place. Not aware of current city or state. Pupils are equal, round, and reactive to light and accommodation (PERRLA). Heart regular, normal rate and rhythm. Lungs diminished throughout. Strong grips and pulls. +2 pulses on all extremities, free from edema. Normal bowel sounds. Abdomen soft, non-tender. |

The nurse conducts a mental status exam on Maryann.

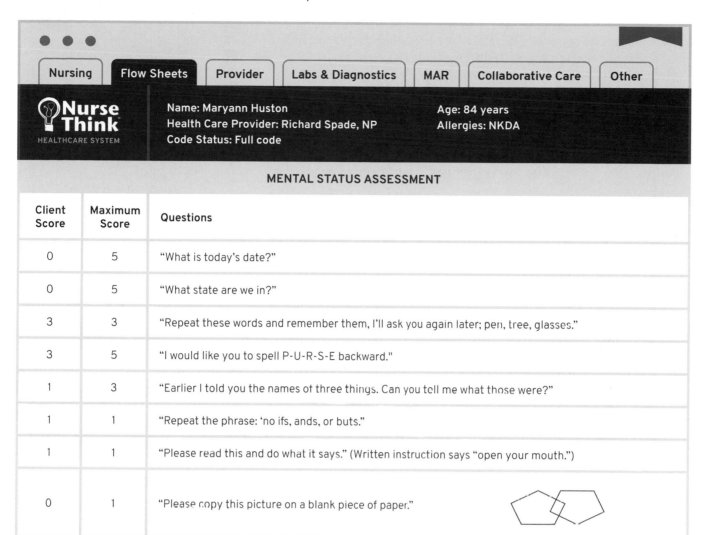

Client Score	Maximum Score	Questions
0	5	"What is today's date?"
0	5	"What state are we in?"
3	3	"Repeat these words and remember them, I'll ask you again later; pen, tree, glasses."
3	5	"I would like you to spell P-U-R-S-E backward."
1	3	"Earlier I told you the names of three things. Can you tell me what those were?"
1	1	"Repeat the phrase: 'no ifs, ands, or buts."
1	1	"Please read this and do what it says." (Written instruction says "open your mouth.")
0	1	"Please copy this picture on a blank piece of paper."
9	24	**Total**

Score	Severity of Disease
19-24	No cognitive impairment
13-18	Mild cognitive impairment
0-12	Severe cognitive impairment

1. **Based on Maryann's mental state exam, how should the nurse interpret the severity of her cognitive impairment?**

2. THIN Thinking Time!

Reflect on the events that have occurred since Maryann came to be evaluated by the nurse and apply **THIN Thinking**.

T – _____

H – _____

I – _____

N – _____

T - Top 3
H - Help Quick
I - Identify Risk to Safety
N - Nursing Process

Scan to access the 10-Minute-Mentor on THIN Thinking. →

NurseThink.com/THINThinking

3. Maryann's daughter Therese begins to cry and says, "How did this happen to my mom? Am I at risk too?" How should the nurse respond? Select all that apply.

1. "We are not sure what ultimately causes Alzheimer's, however it can be genetic."
2. "One can develop Alzheimer's from viruses, deficiencies of neurotransmitters, or autoimmune diseases."
3. "Alzheimer's can be caused by excessive amounts of certain medications, such as thyroid medications."
4. "Yes, you are at risk for developing Alzheimer's disease. You should start medications now as well."
5. "Alzheimer's can be caused by alcohol intake; how much does Maryann drink?"

4. Match the stage of Alzheimer's disease to the description on the right. Each stage may be used more than once.

Stages	Description
A. Stage 1	_____ Major gaps in memory and cognitive defects.
B. Stage 2	_____ Retains names of others but disoriented to place and time.
C. Stage 3	_____ "Mild."
	_____ Loss of ability to speak.
	_____ "Severe."
	_____ Total loss of facial recognition.
	_____ "Moderate."
	_____ Mild cognitive decline.

5. Therese asks what additional diagnostic tests her mother will need to confirm the Alzheimer's diagnosis. Which tests may be ordered on her brain? Select all that apply.

1. Computerized tomography (CT) scan.
2. Magnetic resonance imaging (MRI).
3. X-ray.
4. Positron emission tomography (PET) scan.
5. Angiogram.

6. The nurse practitioner orders additional tests and procedures for Maryann. Complete the chart, identifying if they are appropriate or not appropriate for Maryann's situation.

	Appropriate	Not Appropriate
Complete blood count (CBC)		
Electrocardiography (ECG)		
Lumbar puncture with a collection of cerebrospinal fluid (CSF)		
Electroencephalography (EEG)		
Comprehensive metabolic panel (CMP)		
Nuclear stress test		
Thyroid hormone levels		

7. Maryann's nurse practitioner, Richard, gives Therese a home healthcare referral. What is/are the duty(ies) and responsibility(ies) of a home health nurse? Select all that apply.
   1. Make an individualized plan of care.
   2. Administer medications as needed.
   3. Write prescriptions for medications.
   4. Coordinate care with other health care team members.
   5. Educate clients and families.

8. The healthcare provider prescribes donepezil. Therese asks the nurse how this medication will help Maryann. How should the nurse respond?
   1. "This medication will reverse the progression of Alzheimer's disease."
   2. "Donepezil helps break down the plaques that are found on the brain."
   3. "This medication increases blood flow to the brain, which helps with cognition."
   4. "It helps increase acetylcholine uptake in the brain, which helps maintain memory."

As Maryann's condition deteriorates, she moves in with Therese. Therese and her husband work to sell Maryann's house and move her belongings into their guest room. The nurse visits Therese and Maryann at Therese's home. Therese looks stressed, is short-tempered, and Maryann is screaming.

9. NurseThink® Prioritization Power!
   Evaluate the situation with Maryann and Therese and pick the **Top 3 Priority** actions.

   1. _____

   2. _____

   3. _____

10. When Maryann stops screaming, the nurse plays Maryann's favorite music from her childhood. Therese asks the nurse how listening to music or playing instruments can help Maryann. How should the nurse respond?

_____

11. Therese admits to the nurse that she is having a difficult time caring for Maryann. What resources should the nurse provide?

_____

12. The nurse performs an environmental assessment. Review the image and make an X on the object(s) that could impact Maryann's safety.

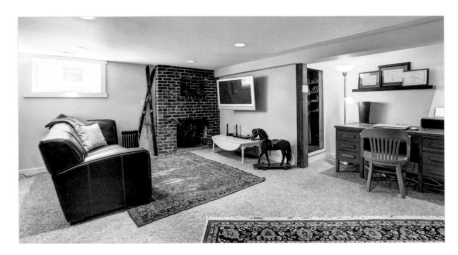

13. The nurse is providing teaching to Maryann and Therese about promoting the independence of self-care for Maryann. The nurse knows teaching has been effective when Therese makes which statement(s)? Select all that apply.
    1. "I will not rush my mom when she is getting ready."
    2. "I will lay out clothes for her to dress herself."
    3. "I will be sure to provide extra time for my mom to get dressed."
    4. "I will help her get dressed to make her feel better."
    5. "I will provide assistive devices such as a button hook to help her."

14. The nurse and Therese discuss Maryann's current environment. For each topic, identify the significance related to Alzheimer's and cognitive function.

    Limited environmental stimuli: _____

    _____

    Scan the QR code on your phone to find more information. →

    www.alz.org

    Regular Routine: _____

    _____

    Familiar environment: _____

    _____

    Calendars and family photos: _____

    _____

15. The nurse is performing a medication reconciliation for Maryann and see's that she has been taking this medication as needed for a hip injury. Mark or circle the statement(s) of why the nurse should question the provider about the use of this medication for Maryann.

Oxycodone
Classification: Opioid pain medication/narcotic
Administration: Take this medication as needed for pain
Side effects: dizziness, lightheadedness, confusion, drowsiness
Precautions: This medication will add to the effects of alcohol and other CNS depressants, such as antihistamines, sedatives, or muscle relaxants. Using narcotics for a long time can cause severe constipation.
Dosage: 10 mg orally every four hours as needed for pain.
Assessment: Monitor pain level, level of consciousness.

16. Therese tells the nurse that she read online that she can restrain Maryann when she needs to get work done around the house. Which instructions are most important to give to Therese? Select all that apply.
    1. Restraints can be used, as long as Maryann is under constant supervision.
    2. Frequent assessments are needed when restraints are used.
    3. Restraints should be avoided as they increase agitation and lead to injury.
    4. Restraints can be used for short periods, such as cleaning a room.
    5. There are legal concerns of restraining a person, and Adult Protective Services can be called.

The nurse evaluates Maryann's dietary needs by performing a 24-hour dietary recall with Therese's assistance.

Maryann's 24-hour Dietary Recall
Breakfast: Sugar-O cereal, orange juice.
Lunch: Ham and cheese sandwich on white bread, apple, hot tea.
Dinner: White pasta with red sauce, garlic bread, a glass of wine.

17. Based on the 24-hour dietary recall, what recommendation(s) should be made by the nurse? Select all that apply.
    1. The diet is nutritionally balanced, but the wine should be eliminated.
    2. More protein is needed in her diet.
    3. An increase in complex carbohydrates is recommended.
    4. Encourage more fruits and vegetables.
    5. Maryann needs more sodium in her diet.
    6. Fluid intake should be increased.

Scan the QR code on your phone to find more information. →

www.choosemyplate.gov

Months pass, and the home health nurse gets a call from Therese saying that Maryann is having trouble swallowing and coughs a lot while eating. The nurse shares that as Alzheimer's progresses, she can develop dysphagia. The nurse suggests adding thickening agents to thin liquids to help prevent aspiration.

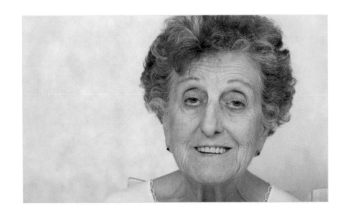

18. **Match the liquid consistency on the left with the definition on the right.**

Consistency	Description
A. Thin liquids	_____ Honey consistency at room temperature.
B. Nectar thick	_____ Watery such as juice, tea, milk, broth.
C. Honey-thick	_____ Too thick to go through a straw.
D. Spoon thick	_____ Slightly thicker liquids, such as thin milkshakes.

During her visit, the home health nurse notices Therese crying at the kitchen table. Therese shares, "I cannot take care of my mom anymore. She doesn't remember a thing, and she cannot do anything herself. I am exhausted."

19. **The home health nurse suggests getting additional help at home or moving Maryann to a skilled nursing facility. Therese asks what services are at a facility. What should the nurse include in the response? Select all that apply.**
    1. Acute medical attention.
    2. Recreational activities.
    3. Physical therapy.
    4. 24-hour supervision.
    5. Administration of IV medications.

20. **The nurse in the skilled nursing facility is performing an admission assessment on Maryann. How will the nurse prevent a client injury? Select all that apply.**
    1. Assigning a room close to the nurse's station.
    2. Keeping the bed in the lowest position.
    3. Using a bed alarm or a chair alarm.
    4. Keeping Maryann in bed at all times.
    5. Thickening all fluids to prevent aspiration.

Visit the Nursing Home Abuse Center and learn 3 new things.

www.nursinghomeabusecenter.com/nursing-home-injuries/prevention/ →

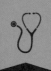

Go To Clinical Case

While caring for this client, be sure to review the concept maps in chapters 3 and 4.

Case 2: Cognitive Impairment from Brain Attack

Related Concepts: Perfusion, Mobility, Nutrition
Threaded Topics: Medication Education, Stroke Protocol, Fall Risk,
Aspiration Risk, Bleeding Risk, Enteral Tubes

Bill Michaelson is a 74-year-old retired computer analyst. His history includes hypertension, hypothyroidism, gout, diabetes type 2, and chronic obstructive pulmonary disease. He smokes one-half pack of cigarettes each day and is moderately overweight (BMI 26.6). Bill was recently diagnosed with atrial fibrillation and was started on warfarin. He and his wife Margie walk their dog 20 minutes each day.

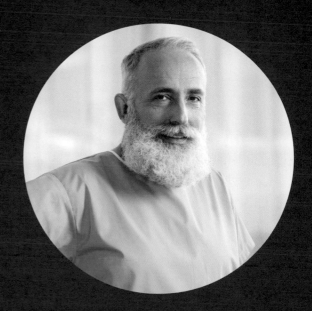

1. **Identify concerns of Bill's health history that are risk factors for stroke.**

Hypertension

____ Gout	____ Overweight (BMI 26.6)	____ Sedentary lifestyle
____ Diabetes type 2	____ Hypothyroidism	____ Chronic obstructive pulmonary disease
____ Current smoker	____ 74-years-old	____ Atrial fibrillation

Bill and Margie present to the emergency department today. Margie says that Bill "isn't himself" and is "acting goofy." The emergency department nurse gathers the health history from Margie.

2. **The emergency department nurse performs a neurological assessment on Bill. Complete the acronym FAST to assess for symptoms of a stroke quickly.**

F -_____

A -_____

S -_____

T -_____

Scan the QR code to learn more about FAST with stroke assessment. →

www.stroke.org/
understand-stroke/recognizing-
stroke/act-fast/

It is determined that Bill is having a stroke and a stroke alert is called. The neurology team comes to the bedside and orders a CT scan of his brain, without contrast, STAT.

3. **How should the nurse prepare Bill for the CT scan?**
   1. Remove all metal from Bill's pockets.
   2. No additional prep is needed.
   3. Place electrodes on Bill's scalp.
   4. Position Bill on his stomach for the scan.

---

4. **THIN Thinking Time!**

   Reflect on the cues and data about Bill and apply **THIN Thinking** to prioritize the concerns.

   T – _____

   H – _____

   I – _____

   N – _____

   T - Top 3
   H - Help Quick
   I - Identify Risk to Safety
   N - Nursing Process

   Scan to access the 10-Minute-Mentor on THIN Thinking. →

   NurseThink.com/THINThinking

The CT scan shows that Bill is experiencing an ischemic stroke caused by a thrombus. The team orders intravenous tissue plasminogen activator (IV-tPA).

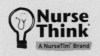

POLICY AND PROCEDURES

Guidelines for administration of Tissue Plasminogen Activator (tPA)

> Confirm no history of gastrointestinal or urinary bleeding within 21 days, no stroke/serious head injury/intracranial surgery within 3 months.

> Do not insert NG tubes, urinary catheter tubes, IV lines, or arterial lines for 24 hours after administration of tPA.

> Monitor coagulation laboratory results during and after tPA administration (PT/INR, platelets, PTT).

> Obtain frequent vital signs and neurologic assessments.

5. NurseThink® Prioritization Power!

Evaluate the guidelines for the administration of tPA and pick the **Top 3 Priority** nursing considerations.

1. _____

2. _____

3. _____

The neurology team decides Bill is an excellent candidate for endovascular therapy. The emergency department places two IVs, both 18 gauges in each antecubital fossa and an indwelling urinary catheter. The stroke team takes Bill to the interventional radiology suite and perform a manual thrombectomy or aspiration and removal of the clot in Bill's brain. The procedure was performed through Bill's right femoral artery. The sheath was removed successfully. The stroke nurse provides hand-off report to the intensive care unit (ICU) nurse.

6. The ICU nurse assesses Bill's right groin and palpates a firm bump above the access site. What would be the best action(s) by the nurse? Select all that apply.

1. Immediately apply manual pressure just above access site.
2. Call the provider.
3. Change the dressing and reassess the site in 15 minutes.
4. Assess and palpate peripheral pulses, bilaterally.
5. Document the findings as normal.

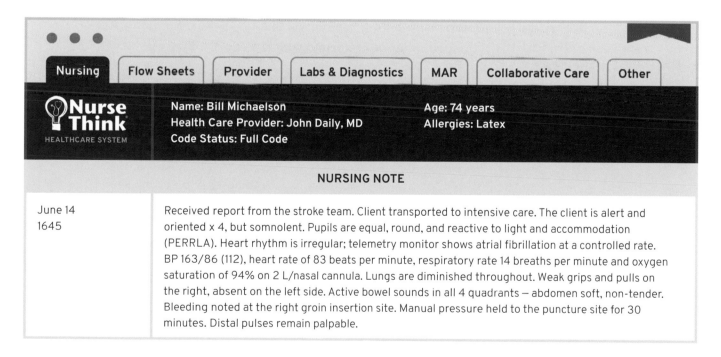

| Nursing | Flow Sheets | Provider | Labs & Diagnostics | MAR | Collaborative Care | Other |

NurseThink HEALTHCARE SYSTEM

Name: Bill Michaelson
Health Care Provider: John Daily, MD
Code Status: Full Code

Age: 74 years
Allergies: Latex

NURSING NOTE

June 14 1645	Received report from the stroke team. Client transported to intensive care. The client is alert and oriented x 4, but somnolent. Pupils are equal, round, and reactive to light and accommodation (PERRLA). Heart rhythm is irregular; telemetry monitor shows atrial fibrillation at a controlled rate. BP 163/86 (112), heart rate of 83 beats per minute, respiratory rate 14 breaths per minute and oxygen saturation of 94% on 2 L/nasal cannula. Lungs are diminished throughout. Weak grips and pulls on the right, absent on the left side. Active bowel sounds in all 4 quadrants – abdomen soft, non-tender. Bleeding noted at the right groin insertion site. Manual pressure held to the puncture site for 30 minutes. Distal pulses remain palpable.

After 30 minutes of manual pressure, the hematoma has resolved. Dorsalis pedis and posterior tibialis pulses are palpable and 2+, bilaterally. Bill is resting comfortably in his bed. Margie is at the bedside and looks distraught.

7. Margie says to the nurse, "This is my entire fault. Bill bruises easily from the warfarin, so we decided to cut the dose in half to help with the bleeding." Which response by the nurse is most appropriate?

1. "It is acceptable to cut medications in half to lessen the side effects."
2. "It is very important to take all medications as prescribed by your provider."
3. "You need to be more careful next time; he could have died from this."
4. "A bleed, not a clot caused Bill's stroke, so it is irrelevant."

The ICU nurse reviews the prescriptions written by the provider.

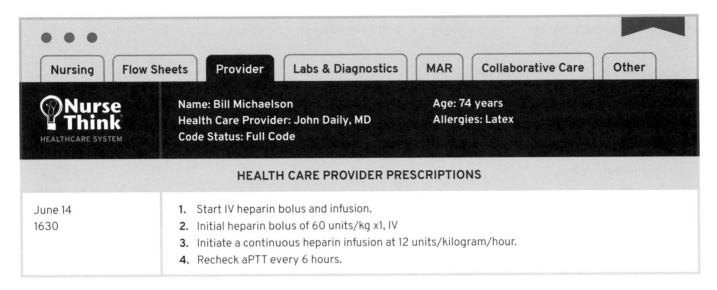

| Nursing | Flow Sheets | Provider | Labs & Diagnostics | MAR | Collaborative Care | Other |

Nurse Think
HEALTHCARE SYSTEM

Name: Bill Michaelson
Health Care Provider: John Daily, MD
Code Status: Full Code

Age: 74 years
Allergies: Latex

HEALTH CARE PROVIDER PRESCRIPTIONS

| June 14 1630 | 1. Start IV heparin bolus and infusion.
2. Initial heparin bolus of 60 units/kg x1, IV
3. Initiate a continuous heparin infusion at 12 units/kilogram/hour.
4. Recheck aPTT every 6 hours. |

8. Bill weighs 175 pounds. How many units of heparin will Bill receive with the initial heparin bolus? How many units of heparin will Bill receive per hour with the continuous infusion? Write out your calculations here.

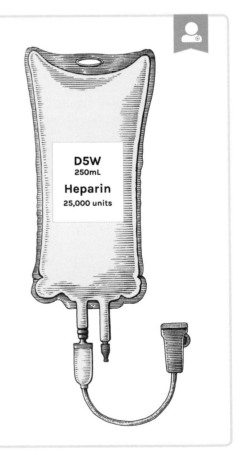

D5W
250mL
Heparin
25,000 units

9. How many mL per hour of heparin will Bill receive with the heparin infusion? Use the image to determine the rate at which the pump should be set. Write out your calculations here.

10. **Margie urgently calls the nurse into the room. Bill starts to mumble, "thirsty very so." Margie looks at the nurse and says, "Why is he talking like that? What is he trying to say?"**

   1. "Bill has receptive aphasia. He does not understand what we are saying to him."
   2. "Bill has expressive aphasia. He can understand us, but he struggles to find the best words."
   3. "Bill has global aphasia. It is a combination of both receptive and expressive aphasia."
   4. "Bill is confused from the medications we gave him."

11. **Because of Bill's aphasia, he has difficulty communicating. How should the nurse respond to Bill?**

   1. Encourage Bill to write when he is having difficulty speaking.
   2. Write everything down on a piece of paper and have Bill read it.
   3. Talk slowly so that Bill can better understand.
   4. Ask Bill to point to what he needs.

12. **Match the neurologic and cognitive deficit on the left to the description on the right.**

Deficit	Description
A. Hemiparesis	_____ Double vision.
B. Hemiplegia	_____ Memory loss.
C. Ataxia	_____ Difficulty in swallowing.
D. Anomia	_____ Misuse of objects because of failure to identify them.
E. Apraxia	_____ Staggering, unsteady gait.
F. Agnosia	_____ Inability to express oneself through speech.
G. Amnesia	_____ Weakness of the face, arm, and leg on the same side.
H. Aphasia	_____ Difficulty in forming words.
I. Diplopia	_____ Inability to remember names of things.
J. Dysphagia	_____ Paralysis of the face, arm, and leg on the same side.
K. Dysarthria	_____ Inability to recognize familiar objects, tastes, sounds and other sensations.

13. **The nurse is rearranging Bill's bedside table. Bill had a left hemispheric stroke; make an X on the image where the nurse should place the bedside table.**

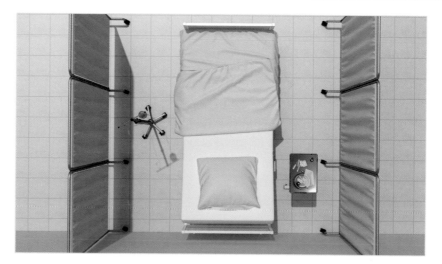

14. **Bill has been working with physical therapy on ambulation and using a walker. Place the steps of using a walker in the correct order. _____, _____, _____, _____.**

    1. Move the walker forward a short distance.
    2. Push up into a standing position.
    3. Step forward with weak leg first, putting weight on palms of the hands.
    4. Place a firm grip on both sides of the walker.

15. **The ICU nurse comes into Bill's room one afternoon and observes Bill flailing his hands in anger and repeating the word "mad." What action(s) is/are best by the nurse? Select all that apply.**

    1. Provide a safe environment.
    2. Support Bill during uncontrollable outbursts.
    3. Give Bill alone time in his room.
    4. Encourage Bill to express his feelings.
    5. Sit and listen to Bill's frustrations.

It has been a few days since Bill's stroke and procedure and Margie hasn't left his side. His condition has stabilized, and he is being transferred to the medical-surgical unit. The indwelling urinary catheter has been removed and Bill has been incontinent of urine. Margie notices that Bill has a difficult time swallowing and coughs a lot. He doesn't eat much of his meals. She voices concern about Bill becoming weak. The nurse reviews the labs and sees that the serum albumin, total protein, and iron levels are low.

16. **Give an SBAR hand-off report from the ICU nurse to the medical-surgical nurse.**

    S – _____

    _____

    B – _____

    _____

    A – _____

    _____

    R – _____

    _____

    Clinical Hint:
    S - Situation
    B - Background
    A - Assessment
    R - Recommendation

17. **Bill is transferred to a new room in the medical-surgical unit. The health care provider prescribed to stop the heparin drip and start Bill on clopidogrel. Fill in the missing pieces of information in the table.**

Medication	Class of Medication	Mechanism of Action	Teaching Points
Clopidogrel 75 mg PO daily			Increases the risk of bruising and bleeding.

The nurse is reviewing additional prescriptions written by the health care provider.

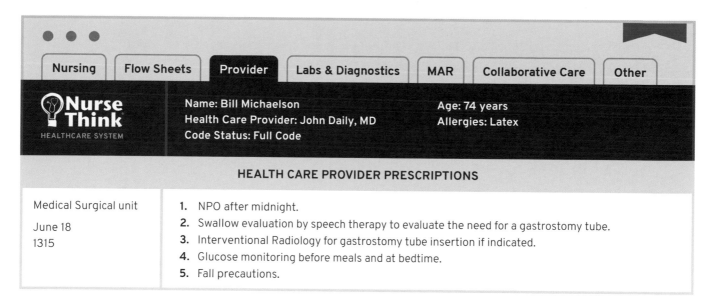

Nurse Think
HEALTHCARE SYSTEM

Name: Bill Michaelson
Health Care Provider: John Daily, MD
Code Status: Full Code

Age: 74 years
Allergies: Latex

HEALTH CARE PROVIDER PRESCRIPTIONS

Medical Surgical unit

June 18

1315

1. NPO after midnight.
2. Swallow evaluation by speech therapy to evaluate the need for a gastrostomy tube.
3. Interventional Radiology for gastrostomy tube insertion if indicated.
4. Glucose monitoring before meals and at bedtime.
5. Fall precautions.

Bill has a swallow evaluation with speech therapy and does not pass. The speech therapist feels that Bill is at high risk for aspiration and recommends a percutaneous gastrostomy tube insertion in interventional radiology. The provider makes Bill NPO.

18. **Margie is concerned and asks the nurse to explain the gastrostomy tube. How should the nurse respond? Select all that apply.**

1. "It is a tube that comes out of the abdomen."
2. "It is used for nutritional feedings since Bill has trouble swallowing."
3. "Bill will need to use this tube for feedings until he gets stronger."
4. "Since Bill cannot swallow, the tube will be permanent."
5. "Liquid nutrition will be administered through the tube."

The charge nurse is making rounds on the clients on the medical-surgical unit and notices this sign on Bill's door.

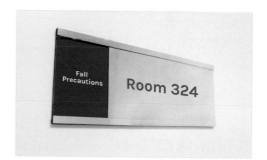

19. **What safety precaution(s) must be in place for fall-risk clients? Select all that apply.**

1. Bed kept in the lowest position at all times.
2. Place the call light and other necessities within reach.
3. Raise the four side rails on the bed.
4. Use bed or chair alarms at all times.
5. Be sure that the clients ambulate with assistance.

After a few days, Bill is discharged from the hospital. The physical therapist suggests Bill be released to a skilled nursing facility for aggressive therapy.

20. **Compare and contrast a skilled nursing facility and nursing home.**

_____

_____

Conceptual Debriefing & Case Reflection

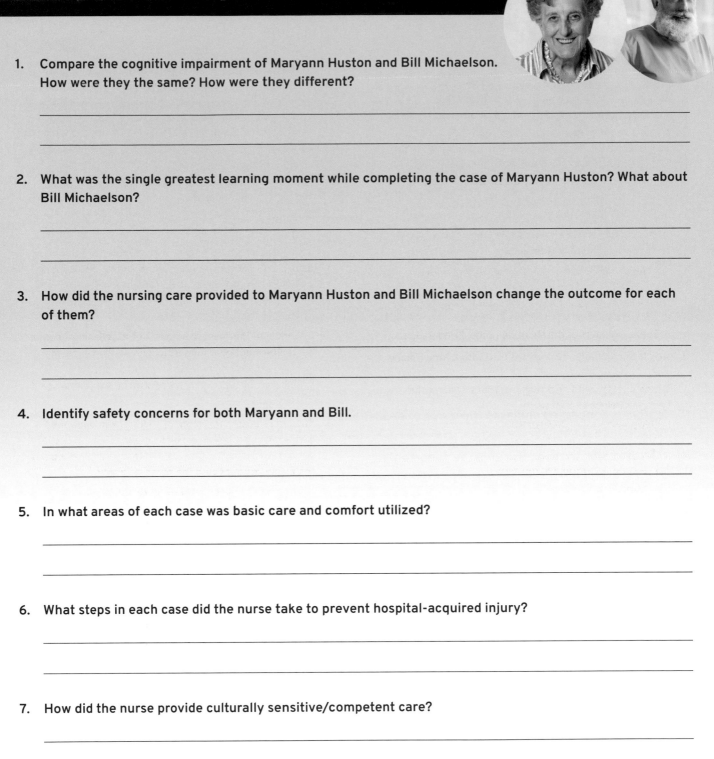

1. Compare the cognitive impairment of Maryann Huston and Bill Michaelson. How were they the same? How were they different?

   _____

   _____

2. What was the single greatest learning moment while completing the case of Maryann Huston? What about Bill Michaelson?

   _____

   _____

3. How did the nursing care provided to Maryann Huston and Bill Michaelson change the outcome for each of them?

   _____

   _____

4. Identify safety concerns for both Maryann and Bill.

   _____

   _____

5. In what areas of each case was basic care and comfort utilized?

   _____

   _____

6. What steps in each case did the nurse take to prevent hospital-acquired injury?

   _____

   _____

7. How did the nurse provide culturally sensitive/competent care?

   _____

   _____

Fundamental Quiz

1. The nurse is caring for a newly admitted older adult in a skilled care facility. Which statement(s) by the client is/are most concerning? Select all that apply.

   1. "I don't remember what I ate for breakfast."
   2. "I don't think I'll enjoy being here."
   3. "My cat 'Mustang' is my baby."
   4. "Did my daughter bring my glasses?"
   5. "I'm in the emergency room."

2. A military veteran is being seen at the clinic for what his wife calls "strange behaviors." Which behavior(s) is/are concerning? Select all that apply.

   1. Panic attacks with an impending sense of doom.
   2. Forgetfulness and leaving food cooking on the stove.
   3. Walking 4-5 times a day throughout the neighborhood.
   4. Hesitation and fear to use the city's public transportation.
   5. Spending hours at the shooting range, firing weapons.

3. An older adult client is hospitalized with a lung infection and has been disoriented and confused since admission. Which cue(s) could be a reason(s) for the cognitive change? Select all that apply.

   1. Oxygen saturation level of 90%
   2. Administration of nephrotoxic antibiotics.
   3. Use of a bedtime sleeping pill.
   4. Temperature of 103.4°F (39.7°C).
   5. Unfamiliar environment.

4. The nurse is planning care for a client with dementia who is disoriented to location, day and time. Physically the client is mobile and has a steady gait. Which priority action should the nurse include?

   1. Reorient the client frequently.
   2. Place suction at the bedside in case of aspiration.
   3. Determine the client's code status with the family.
   4. Place a bed alarm.

5. The nurse is completing a focused assessment to determine the cognitive mental status of an older adult with symptoms of acute hallucinations. Which action is the priority?

   1. Perform the assessment when the client is well-rested.
   2. Reorient the client to time and place during the assessment.
   3. Perform the assessment in a location without distracting stimuli.
   4. Provide a sedative before the assessment to reduce anxiety.

Advanced Quiz

6. An elementary school nurse notices that a child is playing independently and not interacting with others. She gently touches the child on the back, and he jumps away saying "no, don't touch me!" His teacher explains that he has an autistic spectrum disorder. What is the nurse's best action?

   1. Talk gently to the child, keeping a physical distance.
   2. Walk away and leave the child alone.
   3. Encourage the child to play with other children.
   4. Ask the teacher more questions about the child.

7. An adult being treated for attention deficit hyperactivity disorder (ADHD) is brought to the emergency department by paramedics after threatening to injure himself. Which is/are the priority nursing action(s)? Select all that apply.

   1. Provide a quiet, restful environment.
   2. Work with the client to agree to a "no self-harm" contract.
   3. Provide emotional support to increase self-esteem.
   4. Obtain continuous one-on-one observation.
   5. Remove any potentially harmful objects from the environment.

8. The nurse enters the room of a client with advanced dementia to administer routine medications. The client becomes angry and agitated and throws a water cup at the nurse. What should the nurse do next?

   1. Clean up the water spill and leave the room.
   2. Ask why the client is angry.
   3. Call for another healthcare team member to come to the room.
   4. Get another cup of water and try administering the pills again.

9. A client comes to the clinic with her daughter a year after experiencing a stroke. The daughter says she is afraid that her mother has post-stroke dementia. Which symptom(s) support this belief? Select all that apply.

   1. Increased nighttime sleep to 8 hours each night.
   2. Difficulty eating and swallowing with harsh coughing after drinking thin liquids.
   3. A loss of short-term memory and increasing forgetfulness.
   4. The increasing inability to perform simple tasks.
   5. Wandering in the house with a bewildered expression.

10. A client comes to the clinic with a neighbor who reports that the client is often seen wandering in the neighborhood and cannot find the way home. Which question should the nurse ask the client to assess short-term memory?

    1. "Can you tell me your name?"
    2. "Who is the person who brought you in?"
    3. "Where were you were born?"
    4. "What did you eat for breakfast?"

Care of the Multi-Concept Client

Scan QR Code to access the
10-Minute-Mentor
NurseThink.com/casestudy-book

Multi-Concept Client

In this chapter you will find 6-multi-concept cases. These cases are different in that they will combine multiple concepts and exemplars within each case.

Rarely will you care for a client that does not have multiple diseases, issues and concerns. These cases are more realistic to the client that is seen in today's health care system.

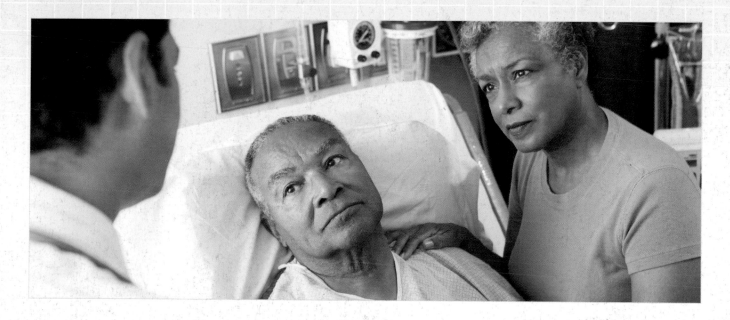

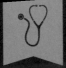

Case 1: Depression, Sexuality, Glucose Regulation, Protection

Related Concepts: Adaptation: Coping and Stress; Communication; Comfort
Threaded Topics: Wellness, Family Dynamics, Self-Management,
Developmental Level, Communication, Documentation

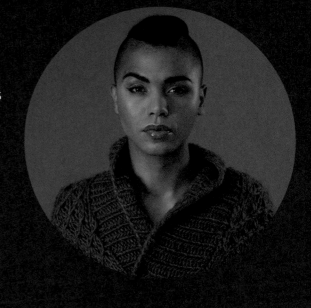

Lucinda Leach is a 16-year-old transgender female who presented to the emergency department with her school counselor after she was observed crying in class at school and making self-injuring statements. She was taken to the school counselor where she revealed that she has been living on the street for 2 days after running away from home because she wanted to kill herself and couldn't "live in that house anymore." This event was followed by a phone conversation with her mother who told her "Do not come home until you can start acting like the boy that our God made you to be!"

Lucinda's medical history includes type I diabetes mellitus since the age of 3 years (maintained on an insulin pump) and Crohn's disease, diagnosed 2 years ago, for which she takes prednisone 2 mg orally each day. She has not had a bowel flare for 6 months.

---

1. **NurseThink® Prioritization Power!**

   Evaluate the information and determine the **Top 3 Priority** concerns or cues.

   1. _____

   2. _____

   3. _____

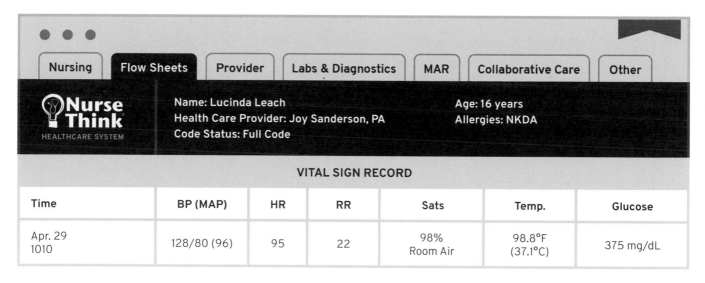

VITAL SIGN RECORD

Time	BP (MAP)	HR	RR	Sats	Temp.	Glucose
Apr. 29 1010	128/80 (96)	95	22	98% Room Air	98.8°F (37.1°C)	375 mg/dL

2. The nurse recognized that Lucinda's insulin pump is not functioning correctly and discontinues it, obtaining a prescription to start her on subcutaneous insulin coverage for glucose > 200 mg/dL. What additional prescriptions should the nurse request? Select all that apply.

   1. Urine for ketones.
   2. Oxygen at 2 L per nasal cannula.
   3. Locked psychiatric unit for suicide precautions.
   4. Glucose monitoring before meals and at bedtime.
   5. Hemoglobin A1C.

3. What statement by Lucinda is most concerning about her current mental state?

   1. "I have nothing to live for; my family doesn't even want me."
   2. "I can't go back home; my mom doesn't agree with my lifestyle."
   3. "I had to run away so that I could feel safe."
   4. "I cry all the time, but my friend has been supportive."

4. Identify the potential stressor(s) impacting Lucinda's life. Select all that apply.

   1. Being transgender.
   2. Being a high school student.
   3. Running away from home.
   4. Not allowed to return home.
   5. Fight with her mom.
   6. Staying on the streets.
   7. Conflict with God.

5. Identify the impact that Lucinda's emotional state has on her physical health risks. Select all that apply.

   1. The risk for hyperglycemia.
   2. The risk of diarrhea.
   3. The risk for bloody stools.
   4. The risk for constipation.
   5. The risk for acidosis.

Lucinda is admitted to the inpatient adolescent psychiatric unit because of her suicidal statements. The nurse works to build a good rapport with Lucinda once she is in the unit. Lucinda reveals that her most recent episode of suicidal thoughts has lasted for 2 weeks. She is experiencing symptoms of hopelessness, overwhelming sadness, inability to function at her previous level, and a decreased appetite with a weight loss of 7 pounds in the last month. She has been thinking of suicide constantly as a means to escape the emotional pain she is

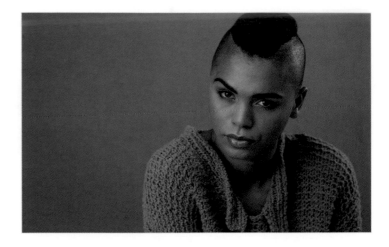

experiencing. She sees no other solution to her problems and feels that suicide is her only option to being "so different from everyone else." She feels she has failed her family and God. At this time, she is verbalizing suicidal thoughts.

6. **Which therapeutic communication technique(s) would help the nurse to build rapport with Lucinda? Select all that apply.**
   1. "I'm concerned about your safety; tell me what's been going on lately."
   2. "Why doesn't your mom want you to dress like a girl?"
   3. "It sounds like you have a lot going on in your life right now."
   4. "It must be tough for you not to have your mom's support."
   5. "All teenagers feel like their parents are against their choices."

7. **The nurse is considering the best approach when interacting with someone who identifies as another gender. Which approach would be best?**
   1. Explain to the client that there will be no judgment as it is not the nurse's right to judge the client's lifestyle choices.
   2. Complete a self-assessment of personal attitudes and preconceived ideas and notions regarding transgender clients.
   3. Approach the nurse manager about the discomfort of having to take care of a transgender client and hand-off care to another nurse.
   4. Explore the client's family history of paraphilias and gender identity disorders to determine the reason for Lucinda's identity.

8. **The nurse wants to find out more information regarding Lucinda's symptoms of depression. Which question would elicit a response indicating other symptoms of depression?**
   1. "Do you worry a lot about what will happen with your life?"
   2. "Do you find that you do not get joy out of doing things you used to like doing?"
   3. "Do you hear or see things that others do not?"
   4. "Do you ever feel like you have so much energy that you don't need as much sleep?"

Lucinda's glucose levels have been consistently between 200-250 mg/dL since admission, and her A1C is 7.6%. She is having intermittent abdominal cramping and 2-3 bloody diarrhea stools each day which has caused her to miss some group therapy sessions.

9. **THIN Thinking!**

   Apply **THIN Thinking** to Lucinda's current situation.

   T – _____

   H – _____

   I – _____

   N – _____

   T - Top 3
   H - Help Quick
   I - Identify Risk to Safety
   N - Nursing Process

   Scan to access the 10-Minute-Mentor on THIN Thinking. →

   NurseThink.com/THINThinking

Lucinda has been living on the street since running away, but she is not sure what to do next. She does not want to return to her mother's home due to the hostile environment, but she is dependent on her mother for medical insurance, medications, and insulin supplies.

10. **The nurse begins to create a plan for the inpatient team to better meet Lucinda's discharge needs. Who should be included in this healthcare team? Select all that apply.**

   1. Diabetic nurse educator.
   2. Medical provider.
   3. Psychological provider.
   4. Occupational therapist.
   5. Chaplain.
   6. Community resource representative.

   Next Gen Clinical Judgment:
   Explore the resources in your local community for a teen in Lucinda's situation.

While Lucinda is in the hospital, she describes the onset of depression as starting in her early childhood. She realized she was in the "wrong body" at the age of 6 and didn't feel comfortable as a male, feeling more like a woman on the inside. She describes hiding her true identity from others for fear of ridicule or bullying. She says that she has always "felt like an outsider" and like she "didn't fit in anywhere." This has limited her from making many friends. She has never had a romantic relationship because she is "unsure of how to approach it." She does feel attracted to men but does not have the energy to seek out a relationship.

11. **The nurse knows that transgender issues and depression are commonly linked. Which symptoms of depression does Lucinda demonstrate? Select all that apply.**

   1. Depressed mood.
   2. Lack of interest in activities that used to be enjoyable.
   3. Change in appetite/weight.
   4. Changes in sleep.
   5. Psychomotor agitation/retardation.
   6. Fatigue or loss of energy.
   7. Feelings of worthlessness.
   8. Inability to concentrate.
   9. Thoughts of death.

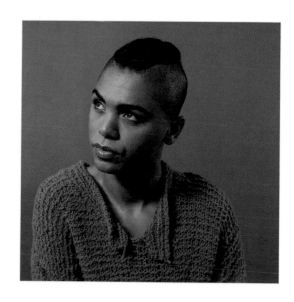

12. **The nurse also considers a diagnosis of gender dysphoria based on the client's presentation. Which of Lucinda's symptoms are congruent with a diagnosis of gender dysphoria?**

    1. An inconsistency of current gender and the need for people to treat them as the other gender.
    2. An intense need to remove primary or secondary sex characteristics.
    3. The need to have the primary or secondary sex characteristics of the other gender.
    4. Inappropriate sexual fantasies and the acting out of these fantasies.

Lucinda begins to feel better with an increased dose of prednisone for Crohn's disease, despite her need to increase her insulin dose. Her diarrhea has subsided, and she can become more engaged with the therapy sessions. Lucinda meets the criteria for both a major depressive episode and gender dysphoria. She begins to make some friends on the unit and continues to open up regarding her childhood, which was filled with domestic abuse and chaos, causing her to feel afraid at home. She witnessed her father abusing her mother, and the police were involved a few times. She expressed relief when her parents separated when she was 10 years old.

13. **The nurse realizes that because of Lucinda's upbringing she continues to work through stages of Erikson's that were not previously met. Which of Erickson's psychosocial levels is she trying to work through?**

    1. Trust vs. mistrust.
    2. Autonomy vs. shame and doubt.
    3. Initiative vs. guilt.
    4. Industry vs. inferiority.

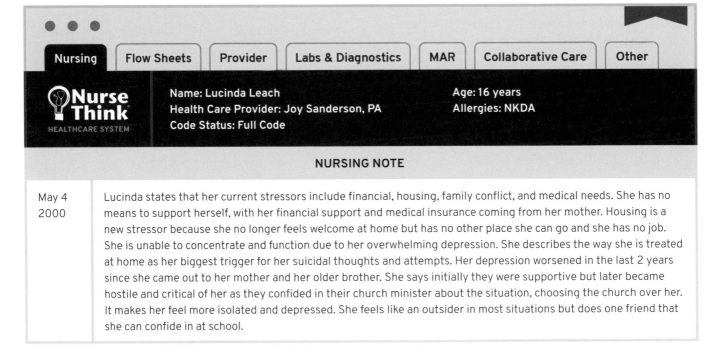

| Nursing | Flow Sheets | Provider | Labs & Diagnostics | MAR | Collaborative Care | Other |

NurseThink HEALTHCARE SYSTEM

Name: Lucinda Leach
Health Care Provider: Joy Sanderson, PA
Code Status: Full Code

Age: 16 years
Allergies: NKDA

NURSING NOTE

| May 4 2000 | Lucinda states that her current stressors include financial, housing, family conflict, and medical needs. She has no means to support herself, with her financial support and medical insurance coming from her mother. Housing is a new stressor because she no longer feels welcome at home but has no other place she can go and she has no job. She is unable to concentrate and function due to her overwhelming depression. She describes the way she is treated at home as her biggest trigger for her suicidal thoughts and attempts. Her depression worsened in the last 2 years since she came out to her mother and her older brother. She says initially they were supportive but later became hostile and critical of her as they confided in their church minister about the situation, choosing the church over her. It makes her feel more isolated and depressed. She feels like an outsider in most situations but does one friend that she can confide in at school. |

14. **The nurse wants to empathize with the client after she has shared this information. Which statement by the nurse is the most empathetic?**

    1. "What does all this mean to you?"
    2. "I can hear how much this must have hurt you."
    3. "I noticed how sad this makes you."
    4. "You feel like you don't fit in."

15. The nurse documents Lucinda's appearance and behavior in the electronic health record. Determine if each statement is adequate and appropriate.

Statement	Adequate and appropriate	Inadequate or inappropriate
Female wearing clean clothes.		
Male who dresses in feminine pajamas with pink nail polish. Has a feminine posture and feature, appears his stated age of 16.		
Unable to see her role in the situation; blames others; unwilling or unable to make significant changes to move forward.		
Has no income but unwilling to obtain a driver's license until she can get an official name change.		
Depressed and hopeless, but willing to open up and talk about issues. She denies hallucinations, delusions, and paranoia. Her speech is slow but coherent.		
Affect and mood congruent. Behavior is guarded. Client is depressed and appears hopeless.		
Client is an underdeveloped transgender female with feminine posture and features. She is wearing hospital pajamas and pink nail polish, appears her stated age of 16.		
Focused on her depression and sees suicide as an option to escape the pain she is in and sees no other way out.		

Lucinda has been in the inpatient psychiatric unit for 3 weeks. She is no longer endorsing suicidal ideation and expresses a desire to live. She is being discharged to her aunt's house. Her aunt is happy to have her, and there have been several family sessions with the aunt included. She will continue on her mother's insurance plan and has been able to replace her insulin pump. Her Crohn's disease is back under control on prednisone 5 mg orally each day.

16. **The mental health care specialist has placed Lucinda on desvenlafaxine 50 mg by mouth daily. What education would the nurse give regarding desvenlafaxine?**

   1. Desvenlafaxine is a serotonin and norepinephrine reuptake inhibitor that works by helping serotonin and norepinephrine get to the synapses where it is needed with fewer side effects.
   2. Desvenlafaxine is a tricyclic antidepressant that works by altering norepinephrine and serotonin levels at the synapse with fewer side effects.
   3. Desvenlafaxine is a heterocyclic that works by inhibiting neuronal uptake of norepinephrine and dopamine with fewer side effects.
   4. Desvenlafaxine is a monoamine oxidase inhibitor that works by blocking the breakdown of tyramine, a precursor to dopamine with fewer side effects.

17. The mental health care specialist refers Lucinda for outpatient psychological treatment. Which would the nurse expect to see as a part of the discharge plan? Select all that apply.

   1. Encourage socialization through the use of group therapy.
   2. Maintain safety of client from self-harm with use of close supervision and monitoring.
   3. Schedule family meeting to obtain collateral information and observe family dynamic in person.
   4. Refer the client to a trans-friendly therapist to assist in raising self-acceptance of identity.
   5. Determine the client's comfort level with a gender identity support group to decrease the sense of aloneness.

Lucinda does well with outpatient therapy and her new life living with her aunt. A few months later, her mother becomes sick with breast cancer and has to undergo chemotherapy. Lucinda decides to return home to help care for her mother. The verbal abuse begins again, the stress builds, and Lucinda returns to her "dark place."

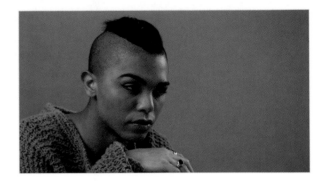

18. What changes would indicate that things have changed for Lucinda? Select all that apply.

   1. Her grades begin to increase at school.
   2. She stops attending her group sessions.
   3. She begins experimenting with drugs and alcohol.
   4. She begins to explore sexual relationships.
   5. She will not respond to her aunt's text messages or phone calls.

19. One day Lucinda's mother enters her room and finds her unconscious and unarousable. In what order should her mother perform these actions?

   _____, _____, _____, _____, _____.

   1. Administer glucagon.
   2. Open the airway.
   3. Call 911.
   4. Obtain a blood glucose level.
   5. Turn off the insulin pump.

20. Lucinda's blood glucose is 29 mg/dL, and she becomes more responsive after the dose of glucagon. Paramedics arrive, begin an intravenous solution with dextrose and transport her to the emergency room. It is determined that she purposely overdosed on insulin after a note to her aunt was found. What are the priority assessments upon admission to the emergency department? Select all that apply.

   1. Level of consciousness.
   2. Blood glucose reading.
   3. Blood pressure.
   4. Suicidal ideations.
   5. Medication dosages.

Go To Clinical Case

While caring for this client, be sure to review the concept maps in chapters 3 and 4.

Case 2: Neurocognitive and Endocrine Disorders

Related Concepts: Adaptation: Coping, Stress, Homeostasis, Comfort, Cognitive Functioning
Threaded Topics: Medications, Depression, GI Bleed, Depression, Dementia

Lola Hamilton is a 72-year-old with a history of fibromyalgia, hypothyroidism, Cushing's disease, diabetes, hypertension, anxiety, and depression. She comes to the emergency department via ambulance after falling at her part-time job. She doesn't recall the events leading up to her hospitalization, but the handoff report from the paramedics said that her coworkers called 911 after she passed out at work. Lola has been having occasional dizziness and forgetfulness for the past year but says these symptoms have worsened over the past several months. She says she often forgets simple things and spends hours trying to recall necessary information.

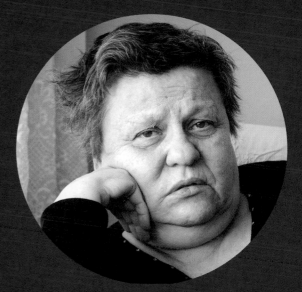

If she doesn't remember something, she will make up a story that "sounds right, to fill in the holes." She also reports severe anxiety at bedtime leading to "almost total insomnia." Lola shares that she averages 6-8 hours of sleep per week. She has been divorced for 30 years and lives alone.

---

1. **NurseThink® Prioritization Power!**

    Evaluate the behaviors that Lola is exhibiting and determine the **Top 3 Priority** assessment findings.

    1. _____

    2. _____

    3. _____

2. **The nurse obtains vital signs, which are all normal other than elevated blood pressure. After speaking to the provider about Lola's symptoms, which diagnostic tests will the nurse anticipate? Select all that apply.**

    1. Complete metabolic panel (CMP).
    2. Thyroid Stimulating Hormone (TSH).
    3. Cardiac enzymes.
    4. Electrocardiogram.
    5. CT scan of the head.
    6. Adrenocorticotropic hormone (ACTH).

3. **The nurse obtains additional information from Lola about her ongoing symptoms. What question(s) are a priority? Select all that apply.**

    1. How often do you feel dizzy?
    2. What does severe anxiety mean to you?
    3. Tell me about other times you have passed out.
    4. Give me an example of something you might forget.
    5. Do you have thoughts of hurting yourself?
    6. Do you have a current support system?
    7. How did you feel about your coworkers calling 911?

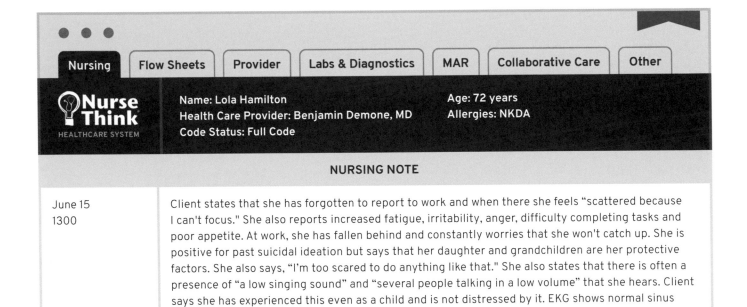

| Nursing | Flow Sheets | Provider | Labs & Diagnostics | MAR | Collaborative Care | Other |

Nurse Think HEALTHCARE SYSTEM

Name: Lola Hamilton
Health Care Provider: Benjamin Demone, MD
Code Status: Full Code

Age: 72 years
Allergies: NKDA

NURSING NOTE

| June 15 1300 | Client states that she has forgotten to report to work and when there she feels "scattered because I can't focus." She also reports increased fatigue, irritability, anger, difficulty completing tasks and poor appetite. At work, she has fallen behind and constantly worries that she won't catch up. She is positive for past suicidal ideation but says that her daughter and grandchildren are her protective factors. She also says, "I'm too scared to do anything like that." She also states that there is often a presence of "a low singing sound" and "several people talking in a low volume" that she hears. Client says she has experienced this even as a child and is not distressed by it. EKG shows normal sinus rhythm — lab report on EHR. |

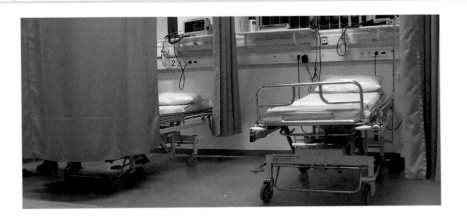

| | Nursing | Flow Sheets | Provider | Labs & Diagnostics | MAR | Collaborative Care | Other |

Nurse Think
HEALTHCARE SYSTEM

Name: Lola Hamilton
Health Care Provider: Benjamin Demone, MD
Code Status: Full Code

Age: 72 years
Allergies: NKDA

LABORATORY REPORT

Lab	Normal	Admit
WBC	4,000 - 10,000 μL	8.9
Hemoglobin	12.0 - 17.0 g/dL	12.0
Hematocrit (%)	36 - 51%	**52 H**
RBC	4.2 - 5.9 cells/L	4.6
Platelets	150,000 to 350,000 μL	200,000
Calcium	9 - 10.5 mg/dL	9.0
Chloride	98 - 106 mEq/L	99
Magnesium	1.5 - 2.4 mEq/L	1.8
Phosphorus	3.0 - 4.5 mg/dL	4.0
Potassium	3.5 - 5.0 mEq/L	**3.4 L**
Sodium	136 - 145 mEq/L	**147 H**
Glucose, fasting	70 – 100 mg/dL	**155 H**
BUN	8 - 20 mg/dL	**43 H**
Creatinine	0.7- 1.3 mg/dL	**1.4 H**
CPK	30 - 170 U/L	55
LDH	60 - 100 U/L	68
AST	0 - 35 U/L	33
ALT	0 - 35 U/L	13
GGT	9-48 U/L	17
Thyroid Stimulating Hormone	0.5 – 5 mU/L	**7 H**

4. **What conclusions can the nurse make based on the lab report?**

   1. The results are consistent with a cardiac event and kidney disease.
   2. The results show liver disease and a neurological disorder.
   3. The results are consistent with adrenal and thyroid disorders.
   4. The results are consistent with an infection and anemia.

The radiology report for Lola's CT scan of the head reveals no abnormalities or bleeds. The 12-lead EKG is not different from a previous reading 1 year ago.

---

5. **THIN Thinking Time!**
   Reflect on the information the nurse has gathered about Lola and apply **THIN Thinking** towards the nurse's actions.

   T – _____

   H – _____

   I – _____

   N – _____

   T - Top 3
   H - Help Quick
   I - Identify Risk to Safety
   N - Nursing Process

   Scan to access the 10-Minute-Mentor → *on THIN Thinking.*

   NurseThink.com/THINThinking

---

6. **The nurse is concerned about Lola's memory loss and forgetfulness. What should the nurse ask to determine if a neurocognitive disorder is present?**
   1. Do you find that you can't recognize close family members?
   2. Do you have angry outbursts that come out of nowhere?
   3. Do you feel like you need to depend on others for your care?
   4. Do you find it harder to learn and remember new things?

The nurse gathers more information regarding Lola's medical history. Lola gives a list of her current medications.

7. **After reviewing the medication list which medication could be causing the dizziness and forgetfulness? Select all that apply.**
   1. Alprazolam.
   2. Duloxetine.
   3. Quetiapine.
   4. Trazodone.
   5. Metformin.

My Medications
Alprazolam 1 mg twice a day as needed
Duloxetine 60 mg daily
Quetiapine 400 mg at bedtime
Trazodone 150 mg twice a day
Metformin 800 mg daily
Metoprolol 50 mg daily
Aldactone 100 mg daily
Levothyroxine 100 mcg daily

8. **The nurse is concerned that some of Lola's physical symptoms could be causing the forgetfulness, and scattered feelings. What could be contributing to these feelings?**
   1. Sleeping 6-8 hours per week.
   2. Past suicidal ideation.
   3. Constant worry.
   4. Being alone.

9. **The nurse assess Lola's mental status. Which assessment(s) best evaluate(s) memory and orientation? Select all that apply.**
   1. What is today's date?
   2. What state are we in now?
   3. Earlier, I told you 3 things, list them for me now.
   4. Repeat the phrase: 'no ifs, ands, or buts'.
   5. Please read this statement and do what it says.

The nurse completes this Mini-Mental Status Exam on Lola.

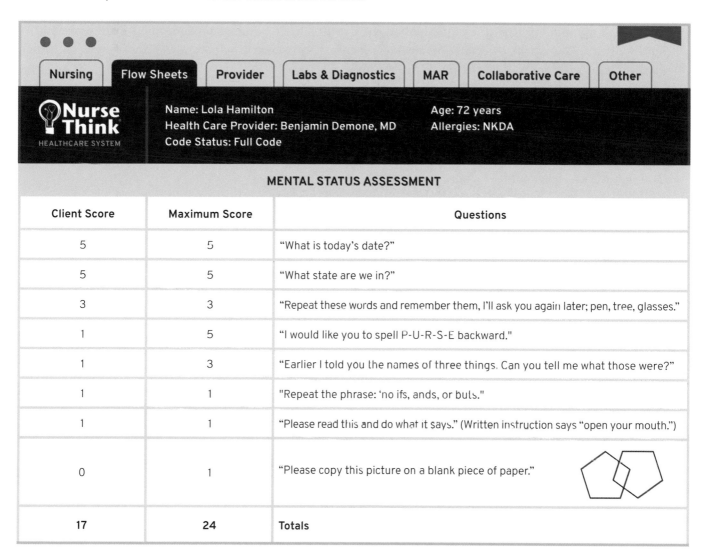

| Nursing | Flow Sheets | Provider | Labs & Diagnostics | MAR | Collaborative Care | Other |

NurseThink HEALTHCARE SYSTEM

Name: Lola Hamilton
Health Care Provider: Benjamin Demone, MD
Code Status: Full Code

Age: 72 years
Allergies: NKDA

MENTAL STATUS ASSESSMENT

Client Score	Maximum Score	Questions
5	5	"What is today's date?"
5	5	"What state are we in?"
3	3	"Repeat these words and remember them, I'll ask you again later; pen, tree, glasses."
1	5	"I would like you to spell P-U-R-S-E backward."
1	3	"Earlier I told you the names of three things. Can you tell me what those were?"
1	1	"Repeat the phrase: 'no ifs, ands, or buts.'"
1	1	"Please read this and do what it says." (Written instruction says "open your mouth.")
0	1	"Please copy this picture on a blank piece of paper."
17	24	Totals

Score	Severity of Disease
19-24	No cognitive impairment
13-18	Mild cognitive impairment
0-12	Severe cognitive impairment

10. **How would the nurse document Lola's perception of the mental status exam based on her presenting symptoms? Select all that apply.**
    1. Client endorses the presence of auditory hallucinations.
    2. Intact. Denies any auditory or visual hallucinations.
    3. Coherent, linear and goal-directed.
    4. No evidence of psychosis noted; the client does not appear to be responding to internal stimuli.
    5. No cognitive impairment.
    6. Mild cognitive impairment.
    7. Severe cognitive impairment.

11. **Lola does not meet criteria for an inpatient physical or psychiatric admission and will be discharged to home with a follow-up visit with her medical and mental health care providers within the next week. Which discharge prescription should the nurse question?**
    1. Alprazolam 1 mg by mouth in the morning and 1 mg by mouth at bedtime for anxiety symptoms.
    2. Duloxetine 60 mg by mouth once per day for increased depressive symptoms and fibromyalgia.
    3. Trazodone 50 mg by mouth at bedtime. Can repeat dose within an hour if unable to sleep.
    4. Levothyroxine 150 mcg daily. Follow up with serum levels in 4 weeks.

The nurse receives a prescription for Lola to wean off of the alprazolam over the next month.

12. **Why would the provider increase the levothyroxine dose?**
    1. Lola is showing signs of depression.
    2. Lola is showing signs of poorly controlled Cushing's disease.
    3. The change is supported by the lab findings.
    4. The medication decreases effectiveness when given with other medicines.

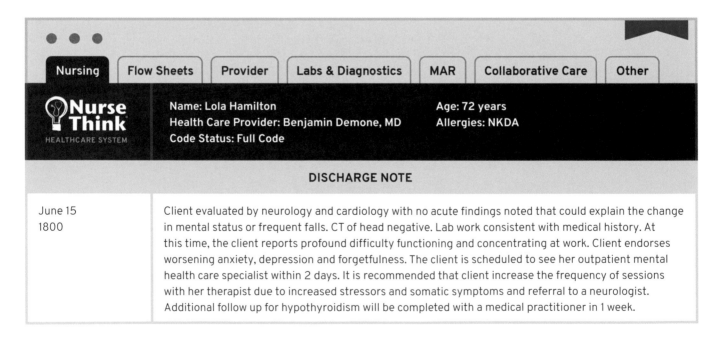

| Nursing | Flow Sheets | Provider | Labs & Diagnostics | MAR | Collaborative Care | Other |

Nurse Think
HEALTHCARE SYSTEM

Name: Lola Hamilton
Health Care Provider: Benjamin Demone, MD
Code Status: Full Code

Age: 72 years
Allergies: NKDA

DISCHARGE NOTE

| June 15 1800 | Client evaluated by neurology and cardiology with no acute findings noted that could explain the change in mental status or frequent falls. CT of head negative. Lab work consistent with medical history. At this time, the client reports profound difficulty functioning and concentrating at work. Client endorses worsening anxiety, depression and forgetfulness. The client is scheduled to see her outpatient mental health care specialist within 2 days. It is recommended that client increase the frequency of sessions with her therapist due to increased stressors and somatic symptoms and referral to a neurologist. Additional follow up for hypothyroidism will be completed with a medical practitioner in 1 week. |

13. NurseThink® Prioritization Power!

Evaluate the discharge note and determine the **Top 3 Priority** teaching needs for Lola.

1. _____

2. _____

3. _____

Lola sees her outpatient mental health care provider who is worried about her memory issues. Lola is currently taking trazodone and duloxetine. She has not taken the quetiapine for 2 days and is only taking half the amount of alprazolam per her discharge instructions. She has an appointment scheduled with a neurologist for a complete work up the following week.

14. The neurologist is concerned that Lola is developing dementia. Which assessment finding supports this diagnosis?

1. Decreased appetite.
2. Feelings of guilt.
3. Sadness and depression.
4. Confabulation.

15. It is important to ensure that Lola is not exhibiting symptoms of depression given her history. Which statement best differentiates between depression and dementia?

1. Dementia develops slowly, while depression may be due to an underlying condition or a recent life change.
2. Attention is intact with both depression and dementia.
3. Clients with both depression and dementia will have a fluctuating or reduced consciousness.
4. Clients with depression will have times where things behaviors are worse in the evening.

16. NurseThink® Prioritization Power!

The nurse knows that when planning care for a client with a neurocognitive disorder that behaviors will slowly deteriorate. List the **Top 3 Priority** educational topics for the caregiver.

1. _____

2. _____

3. _____

As Lola returns to her medical provider for the 4-week follow-up visit, her labs are as follows.

NurseThink
HEALTHCARE SYSTEM

Name: Lola Hamilton
Health Care Provider: Benjamin Demone, MD
Code Status: Full Code

Age: 72 years
Allergies: NKDA

LABORATORY REPORT

Lab	Normal	June 15	July 17
WBC	4,000 - 10,000 µL	8.9	**13.9 H**
Hemoglobin	12.0 - 17.0 g/dL	12.0	**10.0 L**
Hematocrit (%)	36 - 51%	**52 H**	36
RBC	4.2 - 5.9 cells/L	4.6	**3.8 L**
Platelets	150,000 to 350,000 µL	200,000	209,000
Calcium	9 - 10.5 mg/dL	9.0	9.3
Chloride	98 - 106 mEq/L	99	98
Magnesium	1.5 - 2.4 mEq/L	1.8	1.9
Phosphorus	3.0 - 4.5 mg/dL	4.0	4.2
Potassium	3.5 - 5.0 mEq/L	**3.4 L**	3.6
Sodium	136 - 145 mEq/L	**147 H**	**146 H**
Glucose, fasting	70 – 100 mg/dL	**155 H**	**199 H**
BUN	8 - 20 mg/dL	**43 H**	**23 H**
Creatinine	0.7- 1.3 mg/dL	**1.4 H**	**1.6 H**
CPK	30 - 170 U/L	55	67
LDH	60 - 100 U/L	68	88
AST	0 - 35 U/L	33	30
ALT	0 - 35 U/L	13	33
GGT	9-48 U/L	17	20
Thyroid Stimulating Hormone	0.5 – 5 mU/L	**7 H**	5
T3	80-180 ng/dl		155
T4	4.6-12 ug/dl		10

17. **What assumptions can the nurse make about the lab report?**

 1. The hypothyroidism has resolved.
 2. Cushing's disease is better controlled.
 3. Lola's depression has improved.
 4. Lola's infection has resolved.

18. **The nurse notes a decrease in the hemoglobin over the last month and considers possible causes. Which risk is most likely to be the cause?**

 1. A risk for gastrointestinal bleeding from Cushing's disease.
 2. A risk for bone marrow suppression from hypothyroidism.
 3. A risk for poor iron absorption from medications.
 4. A risk for poor nutrition from depression.

19. **Based on this risk, what test should the nurse request?**

 1. Serum protein levels to determine nutritional status.
 2. Hemoccult stool.
 3. Serum iron level.
 4. Bone marrow biopsy.

20. **Lola tells the nurse, "It seems like my body is falling apart. Every time I go to the doctor, they find something new that is wrong with me. Sometimes I feel like I should give up." How should the nurse reply?**

 1. "I'm sure it's difficult for you having many health concerns."
 2. "Tell me what you mean by your statement "I should just give up?"
 3. "I have not ever heard you speak of your family, are they a part of your life?"
 4. "Yes, that is true; your illnesses often cause other illnesses."

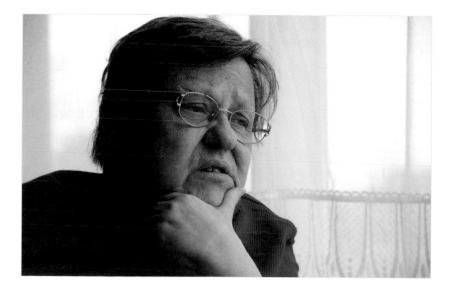

Go To Clinical Case

While caring for this client, be sure to review the concept maps in chapters 3 and 4.

Case 3: Cellular Regulation; Emotion: Grief; Perfusion

Related Concepts: Oxygenation, Elimination
Threaded Topics: Multidisciplinary Healthcare Team,
Blood Transfusion, Delegation, Communication

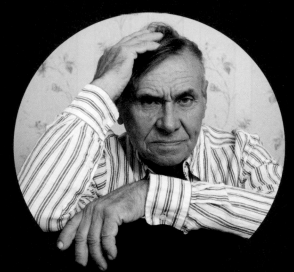

Carl Meyer is a 72-year-old who recently moved to the city from a mining town in Pennsylvania. He is a current smoker, smoking one pack per day since he was 14 years old. Both of his parent's smoked while he was a child. Carl is a retired coal miner and has a familial history of colon cancer. He has been married to his wife Minnie for 50 years, and they have two adult children. He has no known medication allergies.

Carl comes to the clinic today to establish care with a new primary care provider, Michelle Stronge, Family Nurse Practitioner. Michelle completes Carl's past medical history and notes he has hypertension, drinks 2-6 beers a day, and often gets winded while walking around his home. He appears nourished, calm, and well-kept.

1. In reviewing Carl's current state of health and his noted health history, what risk factors does he have for developing cancer and why?

   _____
   _____
   _____
   _____

2. The nurse practitioner completes a thorough physical assessment and finds expiratory wheezes and a dry cough. Carl's blood pressure is 192/102 (132), heart rate of 113 beats per minute, respiratory rate of 28 breaths, and oxygen saturation reading of 89% on room air. What is the priority action by the nurse?

   1. Have Carl take slow pursed-lip breaths.
   2. Assess Carl's level of anxiety and current stressors.
   3. Determine when Carl last took his blood pressure medication.
   4. Place Carl on 2 liters oxygen by nasal cannula.

Michelle asks Carl about his wheezes and dry cough. Carl says that he has had the cough for "about a year now" and it is very dry and he thinks it is allergies. Carl admits to being fatigued and worn down from "getting old." He has lost about 30 pounds this past year without actively trying.

3. **What diagnostic exam should the nurse anticipate will be ordered for Carl?**
    1. Pulmonary function test.
    2. Chest x-ray.
    3. EKG.
    4. Sleep study.

Michelle reviews the chest x-ray with Carl and Minnie and points out a right upper lung nodule. She wants him to have a follow-up lung biopsy. Carl begins to become angry and asks Michelle why he needs a lung biopsy, saying "there's nothing wrong with me!"

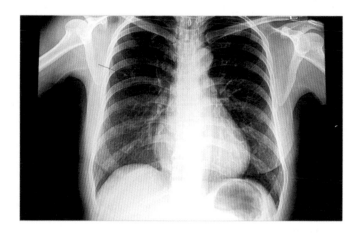

4. **What is the most appropriate response from Michelle?**
    1. "I wouldn't worry about it; this is routine."
    2. "It will be fine. People get lung biopsies all the time."
    3. "Your x-ray showed nodules; it is important to take a biopsy of these nodules to determine if they are benign or malignant."
    4. "The x-ray shows nodules, which shows you have lung cancer. We need to obtain a biopsy to be sure."

5. **Minnie asks about the common risks associated with lung biopsies. What teaching should the nurse provide?**

    _____

    _____

    _____

    _____

Carl's lung biopsy was completed without complication. Michelle refers Carl to Dr. Larry Hewer, a pulmonologist, for consultation and coordination of care. Dr. Hewer tells Carl and Minnie that Carl has non-small cell adenocarcinoma, T2N3M1, and he will need to start a chemotherapy regimen as soon as possible. Dr. Hewer says that because of the stage of Carl's cancer, he is not a surgical candidate and suggests a treatment plan with chemotherapy.

6. **Carl is angry and refuses to talk about the treatment plan. Minnie is crying and asks if he is going to die. Which action is most appropriate at this time?**
    1. Suggest they come back another time to discuss the treatment options.
    2. Offer them both the ability to voice their emotions.
    3. Ask if they can be more appropriate and listen to the options.
    4. Suggest that hospice care may be a nice alternative.

After a few days of working through their anxiety and grief, Carl and Minnie agree that chemotherapy is the best treatment option at this time.

7. **Which are anticipated side effects of chemotherapy?**
   Select all that apply.

   1. Mouth sores.
   2. Peripheral edema.
   3. Increased bruising.
   4. Fatigue.
   5. Hair loss.
   6. Increased heart rate.

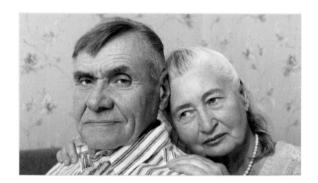

8. **Carl and Minnie are referred to a case manager who develops the multidisciplinary team. Complete the table on the responsibilities of each healthcare team member in the care of Carl and Minnie.**

___Speech Therapist	A. Help alleviate certain treatment-related side effects, such as nausea and vomiting, pain and other common symptoms, such as stress.
___Occupational Therapists	B. Provide hands-on adjustments, massage, stretching, electrical stimulation of the muscles, traction, heat, and ice to reduce the stress of the nervous system.
___Chiropractor	C. Reduce stress, improve mood and energy levels, and decrease perceived pain and anxiety, providing a sense of companionship that combats feelings of isolation.
___Acupuncturist	D. Provide spiritual care before, during, and after treatment.
___Animal-assisted Therapy	E. Provide a plan for the dietary intake that meets the body's caloric needs while minimizing the gastrointestinal side effects of the treatment.
___Nutritionist	F. Provide therapeutic exercises aimed to reduce fatigue and improve physical function, safety and well-being.
___Chaplain	G. Address problems of dry mouth, difficulty swallowing, loss of voice and cognitive changes that may result from cancer treatment.
___ Physical Therapist	H. Assist with daily living activities that are important to routine and quality of life, such as dressing, showering, and eating.
___Care Giver Support	I. Group or individual counseling session to support and provide comfort to the people closest to the client.

Three weeks later, Carl is brought to the emergency department by his wife, Minnie. The triage nurse obtains vital signs: blood pressure 89/50 (63) mmHg, heart rate of 128 beats per minute, a temperature of 102.7°F (39°C), respiratory rate of 34 breaths, and oxygen saturation reading of 82% on room air. The nurse notes that he is pale in color and able to talk in short sentences. Carl reports dizziness and fatigue. Upon palpation of the abdomen, the nurse notes a large lump on the client's right upper quadrant.

9. **NurseThink® Prioritization Power!**
   Evaluate the emergency admission assessment and identify the **Top 3 Priority** assessment concerns.

   1. _____

   2. _____

   3. _____

10. **The triage nurse communicates with the provider to request prescriptions for Carl. Fill out the SBAR from the nurse to the healthcare provider.**

S – _____

B – _____

A – _____

R – _____

> **Clinical Hint:**
> **S** - Situation
> **B** - Background
> **A** - Assessment
> **R** - Recommendation

The healthcare provider provides the following prescriptions.

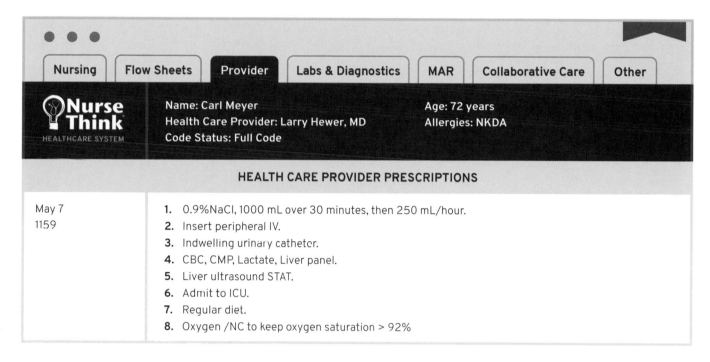

| Nursing | Flow Sheets | Provider | Labs & Diagnostics | MAR | Collaborative Care | Other |

Nurse Think HEALTHCARE SYSTEM

Name: Carl Meyer
Health Care Provider: Larry Hewer, MD
Code Status: Full Code

Age: 72 years
Allergies: NKDA

HEALTH CARE PROVIDER PRESCRIPTIONS

May 7
1159

1. 0.9%NaCl, 1000 mL over 30 minutes, then 250 mL/hour.
2. Insert peripheral IV.
3. Indwelling urinary catheter.
4. CBC, CMP, Lactate, Liver panel.
5. Liver ultrasound STAT.
6. Admit to ICU.
7. Regular diet.
8. Oxygen /NC to keep oxygen saturation > 92%

11. **Which health care prescription(s) should the nurse question? Select all that apply.**
    1. Insert peripheral IV.
    2. Indwelling urinary catheter.
    3. Admit to the ICU.
    4. Regular diet.
    5. 0.9% NaCl, 1000 mL over 30 minutes, then 250 mL/hour.
    6. Liver ultrasound STAT.
    7. CBC, CMP, Lactate, Liver function panel STAT.
    8. Oxygen /NC to keep oxygen saturation > 92%

12. **In which order should the emergency department nurse complete the prescriptions?**

    _____, _____, _____, _____, _____, _____, _____.

    1. Insert peripheral IV.
    2. Indwelling urinary catheter.
    3. Admit to the ICU.
    4. 0.9% NaCl 1000 mL over 30 minutes, then 250 mL/hour.
    5. Liver ultrasound STAT.
    6. CBC, CMP, Lactate, Liver function panel STAT.
    7. Oxygen /NC to keep oxygen saturation > 92%

The emergency department nurse gives a hand-off report to the intensive care nurse.

13. **Complete the following SBAR handoff report.**

    S – _____

    B – _____

    A – _____

    R – _____

Carl arrives at the intensive care via hospital bed with his wife. The ICU arrival team is present, consisting of the primary ICU RN, float, Telemetry RN, and the unlicensed assistive personnel (UAP).

14. **Delegate the following actions to each member of the team. Each member of the team may be used more than once.**

A. Primary ICU RN.	___Complete initial head to toe assessment.
B. Float, Telemetry RN.	___Obtain the initial set of vital signs.
C. Unlicensed assistive personnel (UAP)	___Perform home medication reconciliation.
D. Respiratory Therapist	___Gather toiletries from the clean supply.
	___Obtain additional IV fluids from the med room.
	___Set up oxygen system.

The primary ICU nurse is performing an initial admission assessment, turns Carl to his side to assess his skin, and notices dark red stool with clots of blood. The nurse asks Minnie when this started; Minnie states "This has been going on for three days, we thought it was from the chemotherapy. It happens regularly, and it's hard for me to keep him clean. What does this mean?"

15. **How should the nurse respond to Minnie?**

    1. "This is a normal side effect of chemotherapy."
    2. "Honestly, you should have brought him in sooner."
    3. "He has a gastrointestinal bleed; this is pretty serious."
    4. "It is concerning, as soon as I finish my assessment, I'll speak with the provider."

The nurse continues the assessment, finding clear lung sounds, a rapid, thready pulse, hyperactive bowel sounds, and pale skin with tenting. Another set of vital signs are obtained: blood pressure 92/53 (66) mmHg, heart rate of 123 beats per minute, a temperature of 101.5°F (38.6°C), respiratory rate of 32 breaths, oxygen saturation of 90%.

16. THIN Thinking Time!

Reflect on the nurse's findings and apply **THIN Thinking**.

T – _____

H – _____

I – _____

N – _____

T - Top 3
H - Help Quick
I - Identify Risk to Safety
N - Nursing Process

Scan to access the 10-Minute-Mentor on THIN Thinking.

NurseThink.com/THINThinking

The laboratory results drawn in the emergency department are now available.

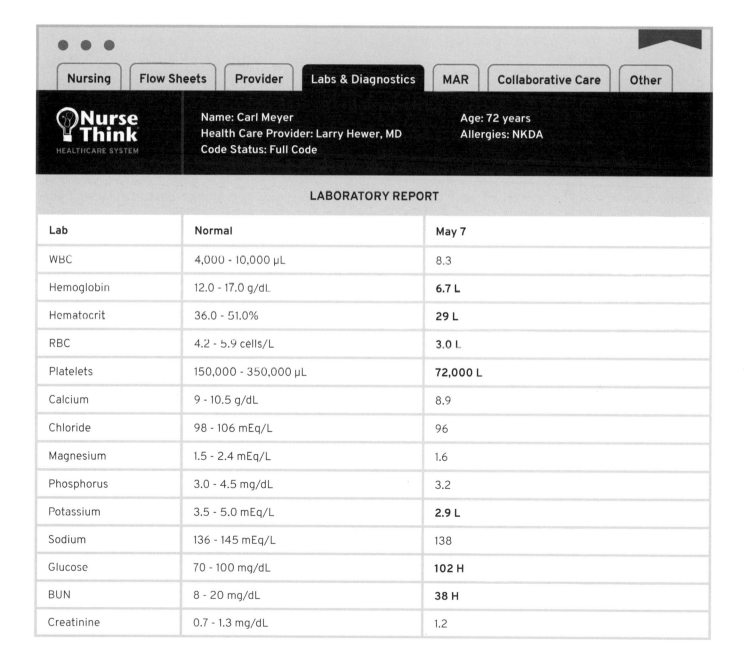

Name: Carl Meyer
Health Care Provider: Larry Hewer, MD
Code Status: Full Code

Age: 72 years
Allergies: NKDA

LABORATORY REPORT

Lab	Normal	May 7
WBC	4,000 - 10,000 µL	8.3
Hemoglobin	12.0 - 17.0 g/dL	**6.7 L**
Hematocrit	36.0 - 51.0%	**29 L**
RBC	4.2 - 5.9 cells/L	**3.0 L**
Platelets	150,000 - 350,000 µL	**72,000 L**
Calcium	9 - 10.5 g/dL	8.9
Chloride	98 - 106 mEq/L	96
Magnesium	1.5 - 2.4 mEq/L	1.6
Phosphorus	3.0 - 4.5 mg/dL	3.2
Potassium	3.5 - 5.0 mEq/L	**2.9 L**
Sodium	136 - 145 mEq/L	138
Glucose	70 - 100 mg/dL	**102 H**
BUN	8 - 20 mg/dL	**38 H**
Creatinine	0.7 - 1.3 mg/dL	1.2

17. **Evaluate the laboratory results and complete the table.**

Abnormal Finding	Risk to Client Safety	Related Assessment Findings	Priority Nursing & Medical Care
Thrombocytopenia			
Anemia			
Hypokalemia			
Elevated BUN			

18. **What prescriptions can the nurse expect to receive after contacting the HCP? Select all that apply.**
    1. Neutropenia precautions.
    2. Packed red blood cell transfusion.
    3. Intravenous hydration.
    4. Bleeding precautions.
    5. Dietary consult.
    6. Contact precautions.

The healthcare provider orders 2 units of packed red blood cells (PRBCs) to be delivered by the nurse.

19. **Which symptom(s) indicate(s) a reason the nurse would stop the blood during the transfusion? Select all that apply.**
    1. Chills.
    2. Sudden back pain.
    3. Fever.
    4. Nausea.
    5. Diarrhea.
    6. Itching.

20. **The nurse evaluates the outcomes from the blood administration. Which assessment finding(s) should the nurse anticipate? Select all that apply.**
    1. Lowering of the blood pressure.
    2. Increase in the hemoglobin count.
    3. Decrease in rectal bleeding.
    4. Pink skin color.
    5. Improvement of the shortness of breath.

The blood transfusion helps Carl and his bleeding stops. Carl begins to strengthen, and he is discharged from the hospital.

Go To Clinical Case

While caring for this client, be sure to review the concept maps in chapters 3 and 4.

Case 4: Fluid and Electrolyte Imbalance; Hormonal Imbalance: Glucose Regulation, Perfusion

Related Concepts: Oxygenation, Homeostasis, Anxiety
Threaded Topics: Medication Reconciliation, Education

Ron Patterson, age 65, is a construction worker in Arizona. His past medical history includes poorly controlled hypertension, diabetes type 2, and he is a current smoker, using 3-4 cigarettes a day. He has mild back pain and has taken ibuprofen several times a week for the past several years. He presents to the emergency department by ambulance for generalized weakness and abdominal pain 4/10. He tells the admission nurse that he was diagnosed with "some kidney problem" a few years ago.

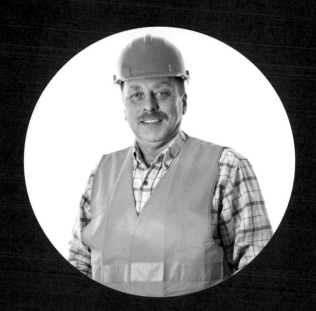

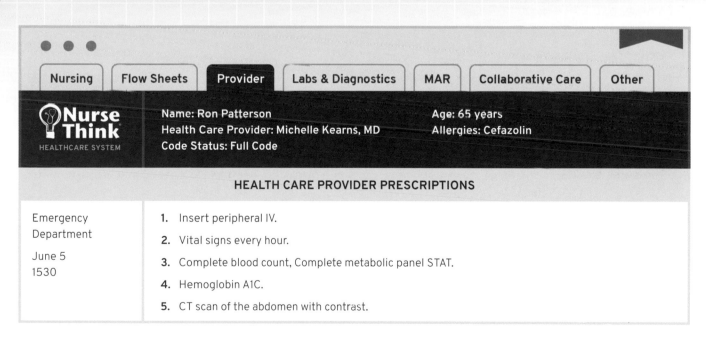

| Nursing | Flow Sheets | Provider | Labs & Diagnostics | MAR | Collaborative Care | Other |

NurseThink HEALTHCARE SYSTEM

Name: Ron Patterson
Health Care Provider: Michelle Kearns, MD
Code Status: Full Code

Age: 65 years
Allergies: Cefazolin

HEALTH CARE PROVIDER PRESCRIPTIONS

Emergency Department

June 5
1530

1. Insert peripheral IV.
2. Vital signs every hour.
3. Complete blood count, Complete metabolic panel STAT.
4. Hemoglobin A1C.
5. CT scan of the abdomen with contrast.

1. **Which health care prescription should the nurse question?**

   1. Insert peripheral IV.
   2. Complete blood count, Complete metabolic panel STAT.
   3. Hemoglobin A1C.
   4. CT scan of the abdomen with contrast.

2. The emergency department nurse is performing an admission medication reconciliation with Ron.

Complete the shaded areas of the table.

Medication	Dose, Route, Frequency	Drug Class	Teaching
Metformin	500 mg, by mouth, every 12 hours	Biguanide	
Dapagliflozin		SGLT2 inhibitors	> Monitor for genital yeast infection; increased urination, or a sore throat and runny or stuffy nose.
Ibuprofen	600 mg, by mouth, every 8 hours as needed for pain		> The maximum dose is 3,200 mg per day. > Can cause stomach or intestinal bleeding > Prolonged use can lead to kidney damage
Lisinopril	20 mg, by mouth, daily	ACE Inhibitor	
Metoprolol	50 mg, by mouth, twice a day	Beta-blocker	

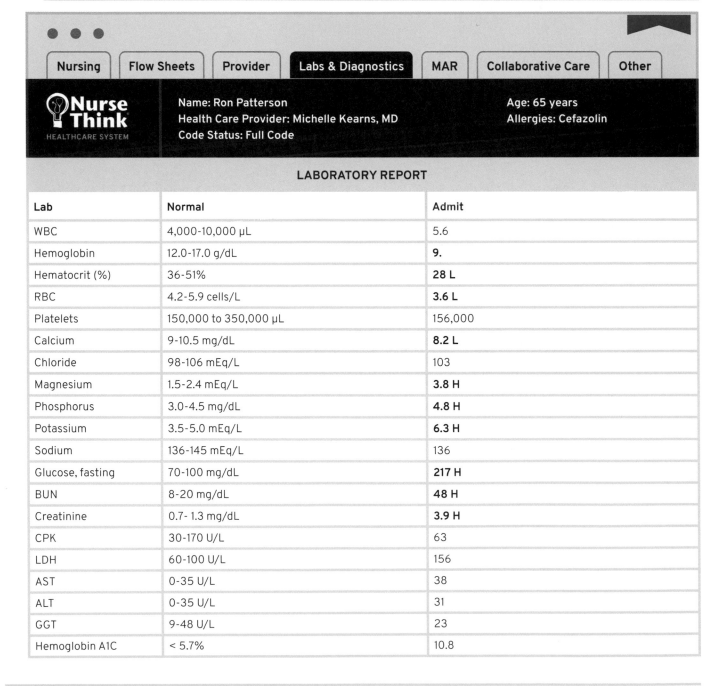

| Nursing | Flow Sheets | Provider | Labs & Diagnostics | MAR | Collaborative Care | Other |

Nurse Think HEALTHCARE SYSTEM

Name: Ron Patterson
Health Care Provider: Michelle Kearns, MD
Code Status: Full Code

Age: 65 years
Allergies: Cefazolin

LABORATORY REPORT

Lab	Normal	Admit
WBC	4,000-10,000 µL	5.6
Hemoglobin	12.0-17.0 g/dL	9.
Hematocrit (%)	36-51%	28 L
RBC	4.2-5.9 cells/L	3.6 L
Platelets	150,000 to 350,000 µL	156,000
Calcium	9-10.5 mg/dL	8.2 L
Chloride	98-106 mEq/L	103
Magnesium	1.5-2.4 mEq/L	3.8 H
Phosphorus	3.0-4.5 mg/dL	4.8 H
Potassium	3.5-5.0 mEq/L	6.3 H
Sodium	136-145 mEq/L	136
Glucose, fasting	70-100 mg/dL	217 H
BUN	8-20 mg/dL	48 H
Creatinine	0.7- 1.3 mg/dL	3.9 H
CPK	30-170 U/L	63
LDH	60-100 U/L	156
AST	0-35 U/L	38
ALT	0-35 U/L	31
GGT	9-48 U/L	23
Hemoglobin A1C	< 5.7%	10.8

3. **Based on the laboratory report, which is/are the priority action(s) by the nurse? Select all that apply.**
    1. Educate the client on bleeding precautions.
    2. Place the client on a cardiac monitor.
    3. Place the client on seizure precautions.
    4. Place a call to the emergency department provider.
    5. Ask the client for a 24-hour dietary recall.

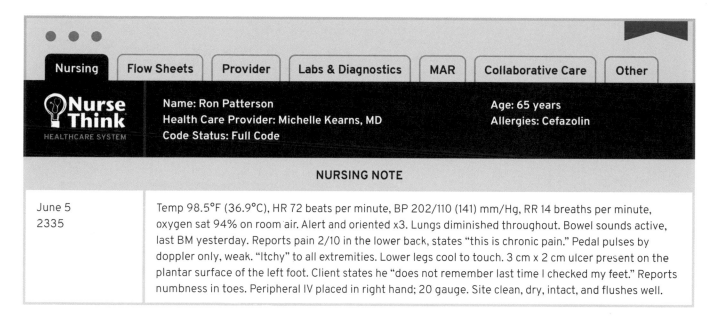

Name: Ron Patterson	**Age:** 65 years
Health Care Provider: Michelle Kearns, MD	**Allergies:** Cefazolin
Code Status: Full Code	

NURSING NOTE

June 5 2335	Temp 98.5°F (36.9°C), HR 72 beats per minute, BP 202/110 (141) mm/Hg, RR 14 breaths per minute, oxygen sat 94% on room air. Alert and oriented x3. Lungs diminished throughout. Bowel sounds active, last BM yesterday. Reports pain 2/10 in the lower back, states "this is chronic pain." Pedal pulses by doppler only, weak. "Itchy" to all extremities. Lower legs cool to touch. 3 cm x 2 cm ulcer present on the plantar surface of the left foot. Client states he "does not remember last time I checked my feet." Reports numbness in toes. Peripheral IV placed in right hand; 20 gauge. Site clean, dry, intact, and flushes well.

4. **The emergency department nurse prepares to teach Ron about the prevention of diabetic foot wounds. Which priority instruction(s) should be given? Select all that apply.**
    1. Check your feet monthly.
    2. Apply lotion to your feet.
    3. Never walk barefoot.
    4. Monitor blood glucose levels.
    5. Wear supportive shoes.

5. **The nurse's note indicates a blood pressure of 202/110 (141) mmHg. What should the nurse do first?**
    1. Ask Ron if he took his blood pressure medicine today.
    2. Retake the blood pressure.
    3. Place a STAT call to the physician.
    4. Document the findings.

The emergency department physician orders a STAT triple lumen dialysis catheter to be inserted in the interventional radiology department. Ron asks the nurse why he needs a dialysis catheter, and the nurse says: "The dialysis catheter will be placed in your arm so that you can go on to a machine and have your blood filtered several times a month because your kidneys have failed."

Critique the nurse's response for accuracy and use of therapeutic communication.

_____

_____

_____

6. **Match the type of dialysis delivery on the left to the client education on the right. The type of dialysis delivery can be used multiple times.**

A. Hemodialysis B. Peritoneal Dialysis	____Risk for developing peritonitis. ____Sterile dextrose dialysate fluid is introduced into the peritoneal cavity through an abdominal catheter at established intervals. ____Requires vascular access. ____Blood removed from the client and filtered through a machine. ____Limit oral fluids and weigh yourself, daily. ____You'll be required to have dialysis several times each week.

7. **The nurse is educating Ron about his dietary changes. The nurse knows teaching has been successful when Ron makes which meal selection?**

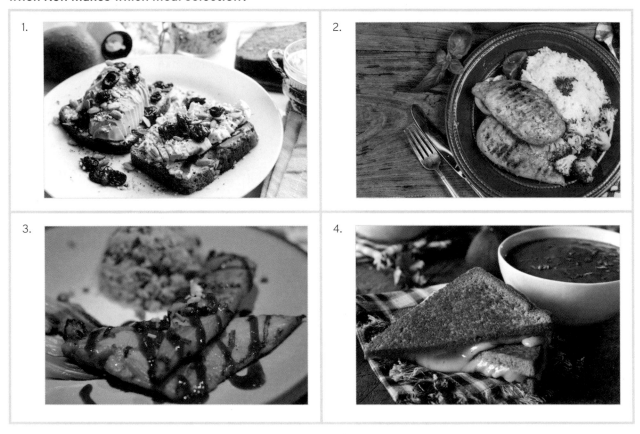

1.

2.

3.

4.

Ron's condition stabilizes after a few dialysis treatments. His temporary dialysis catheter is converted to a tunneled dialysis catheter, and he is discharged from the hospital. The discharge notes instruct Ron to follow up with his health care provider in 7 days. He is scheduled for dialysis three times a week, on Monday, Wednesday, and Friday.

After a couple of weeks, Ron returns to the emergency department with a report of shortness of breath and left-sided weakness. He tells the triage nurse that he goes to dialysis "once or twice" each week.

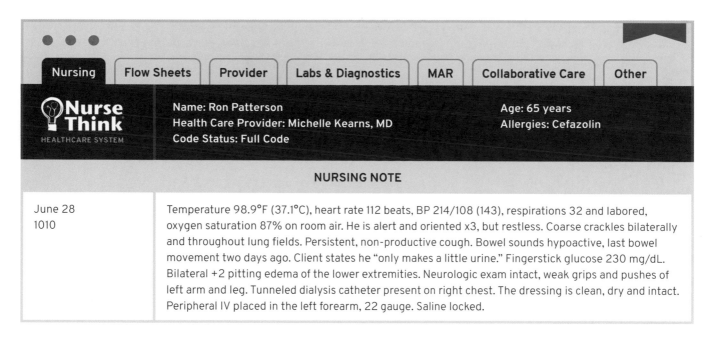

NURSING NOTE

June 28 1010	Temperature 98.9°F (37.1°C), heart rate 112 beats, BP 214/108 (143), respirations 32 and labored, oxygen saturation 87% on room air. He is alert and oriented x3, but restless. Coarse crackles bilaterally and throughout lung fields. Persistent, non-productive cough. Bowel sounds hypoactive, last bowel movement two days ago. Client states he "only makes a little urine." Fingerstick glucose 230 mg/dL. Bilateral +2 pitting edema of the lower extremities. Neurologic exam intact, weak grips and pushes of left arm and leg. Tunneled dialysis catheter present on right chest. The dressing is clean, dry and intact. Peripheral IV placed in the left forearm, 22 gauge. Saline locked.

8. **NurseThink® Prioritization Power!**

   Use the nurse's notes to develop the **Top 3 Priority** cues or concerns.

   1. _____

   2. _____

   3. _____

9. **The health care provider prescribes an echocardiogram and a CT of the head to be completed. Ron asks what an echocardiogram is. What response by the nurse is best?**

   1. "It is a blood test to see if you have too much fluid in your vessels."
   2. "It is an ultrasound done of your heart to check heart function."
   3. "Contrast media is injected into the coronary arteries to assess for blockage."
   4. "Stickers are placed on your chest, and a machine evaluates electrical conduction of your heart."

Ron's tests show that he has an ejection fraction of 30% and he is in heart failure. A brain natriuretic peptide (BNP) is prescribed and returns at 950 pg/mL. His heart rhythm is irregular, and the EKG shows that he is in atrial fibrillation. The CT scan shows an old cerebral vascular accident of the right cerebral hemisphere, explaining his left-sided weakness.

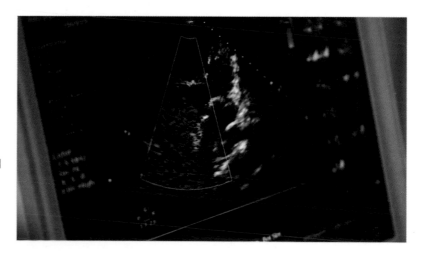

10. Reflect on Ron's medical history and complications. Connect the complications on the left to the contributing factors on the right. Each complication can be associated with more than one contributing factor.

Complications	Contributing Factors
A. Heart Failure B. Renal Failure C. Foot Ulcer D. Stroke	____Poorly controlled hypertension ____Poorly controlled blood glucose levels ____Daily tobacco use ____Excess fluid volume ____Atrial fibrillation

11. Ron is transferred to the telemetry unit. Give a handoff report from the E.D. nurse to the telemetry nurse.

S – _____

B – _____

A – _____

R – _____

Clinical Hint:
S - Situation
B - Background
A - Assessment
R - Recommendation

12. The charge nurse is making bed assignments. In which room should Ron be assigned?

Room 631 ☐

Bed 1: 68-year-old female with an MRSA infection of the urine

Bed 2: open

Room 632 ☐

Bed 1: open

Bed 2: 71-year-old male with influenza receiving breathing treatments every 4 hours

Room 633 ☐

Bed 1: 77-year-old man with a new diagnosis of prostate cancer, anticipating surgery.

Bed 2: open

Room 634 ☐

Bed 1: 82-year-old male with Alzheimer's disease that is confused and agitated.

Bed 2: open

13. The healthcare provider writes prescriptions for medications to treat newly diagnosed heart failure. The nurse prepares to teach Ron about his new medications. Fill in the empty spaces.

Medication	Dose, Route, Frequency	Drug Class	Teaching
	40 mg PO daily	Diuretic	> Monitor potassium levels > Monitor for orthostatic hypotension > Can increase urine output > Monitor blood pressure
Carvedilol	6.25 mg PO daily	Beta-blocker	
Losartan	50 mg PO daily		> Monitor blood pressure > Monitor for orthostatic hypotension

14. **During the morning rounds, the nurse notices that Ron has two bottles of water and three orange juice cups on his bedside table. Which priority instructions should be given?**
    1. "The orange juice is high in potassium; you should drink apple juice instead."
    2. "You are on a fluid restriction; you should know better than that!"
    3. "Because of your heart failure and kidney disease, you should limit your fluid intake."
    4. "It is okay to drink a lot of fluid today as you are getting dialysis this afternoon."

15. **The nurse is teaching Ron about daily care of heart failure. Which statement by Ron is most concerning?**
    1. "It is okay to skip my daily weights if I know I ate bad the night before."
    2. "It is important to take my blood pressure every day and write it down."
    3. "I should call my doctor if I notice increased swelling in my legs or feet."
    4. "I should continue to monitor my dietary choices and fluid intake."

A cardiologist visits Ron and tells him that because of his advanced heart failure, he is at risk for sudden cardiac arrest and may need an implantable cardioverter defibrillator (ICD).

16. **Shortly after the cardiologist's visit, Ron puts on the call light. He is upset and says to the nurse, "Am I going to die? I don't want to die." How should the nurse respond?**
    1. "If you continue to go to dialysis and eat well, you shouldn't need an ICD."
    2. "Your years of self-abuse have taken a toll on your body."
    3. "Listen to the cardiologist; they have your best interest in mind."
    4. "This must be frightening for you to hear. Tell me what you are feeling?"

During the night, Ron begins experiencing some concerning dysrhythmias and is scheduled for the insertion of an ICD. Pre-procedure prescriptions are received.

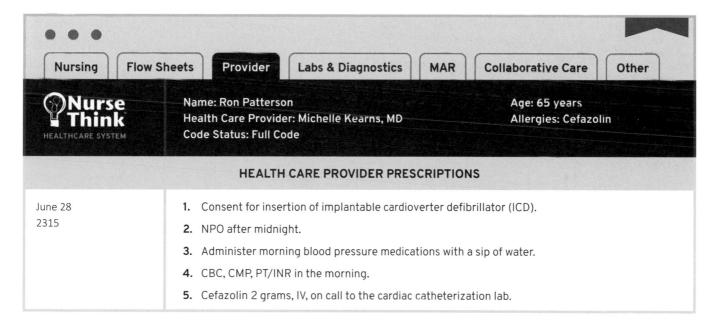

| Nursing | Flow Sheets | Provider | Labs & Diagnostics | MAR | Collaborative Care | Other |

NurseThink
HEALTHCARE SYSTEM

Name: Ron Patterson
Health Care Provider: Michelle Kearns, MD
Code Status: Full Code

Age: 65 years
Allergies: Cefazolin

HEALTH CARE PROVIDER PRESCRIPTIONS

June 28
2315

1. Consent for insertion of implantable cardioverter defibrillator (ICD).
2. NPO after midnight.
3. Administer morning blood pressure medications with a sip of water.
4. CBC, CMP, PT/INR in the morning.
5. Cefazolin 2 grams, IV, on call to the cardiac catheterization lab.

17. **Which prescription should the nurse question?**
    1. NPO after midnight.
    2. Administer morning blood pressure medications with a sip of water.
    3. CBC, CMP, PT/INR in am.
    4. Cefazolin 2 grams, IV, on call to the cardiac catheterization lab.

The next morning, the nurse is checking vital signs and blood glucose and finds that Ron is lethargic and difficult to arouse. His skin is cool and moist.

18. **THIN Thinking Time!**
    Apply **THIN Thinking** to Ron's change in status.

    T – _____

    H – _____

    I – _____

    N – _____

    T - Top 3
    H - Help Quick
    I - Identify Risk to Safety
    N - Nursing Process

    Scan to access the 10-Minute-Mentor on THIN Thinking.

    NurseThink.com/THINThinking

19. **Ron's blood glucose level is 65 mg/dL, and he is unarousable. What should be the nurse's next action?**
    1. Give Ron apple juice, 8 oz and recheck the glucose level in 15 minutes.
    2. Give Ron a half of a sandwich and recheck the glucose level in 15 minutes.
    3. Give Ron D50, ½ amp, IV and recheck the glucose level in 15 minutes.
    4. Call the cardiologist and cancel the procedure.

After Ron's blood glucose is treated, his repeat glucose level is 86 mg/dL. Ron is transported to the catheterization laboratory and has a successful placement of the ICD.

20. **The nurse reviews the post-procedural ICD instructions with Ron. The nurse knows that teaching has been effective when Ron makes which statement? Select all that apply.**
    1. "I will take sponge baths instead of showers for the next few days."
    2. "It is okay to go in a hot tub or swimming pool tomorrow."
    3. "I will not raise my elbow higher than my shoulder for 4 weeks."
    4. "I will not lift anything over 15 pounds for the next month."
    5. "I should stand far from the microwave when it is in use."

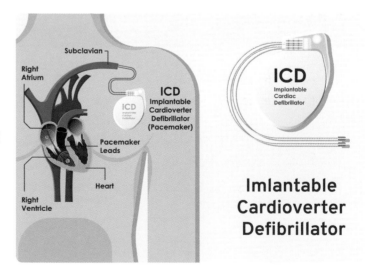

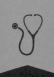

Go To Clinical Case

While caring for this client, be sure to review the concept maps in chapters 3 and 4.

Case 5: Multiple Organ Dysfunction from Trauma and Shock

Related Concepts: Fluid and Electrolytes, Acid-Base Balance, Respiration, Hormonal Regulation, Tissue Integrity, Movement, Comfort, Protection, Homeostasis
Threaded Topics: Ventilator Management, Cardiac Arrest, Critical Care Medications

Gerald Luna is a 45-year-old client with a 15-year history of type 2 diabetes mellitus and a 30-year history of alcoholism. His blood glucose is not well controlled on an oral hypoglycemic agent, and he drinks one six-pack of beer per day. Gerald works at a casino as a slot machine repairman. His wife of 25 years, Andrea, is also employed by the casino in the accounting department. Gerald and Andrea live on a reservation near the casino in a rural setting.

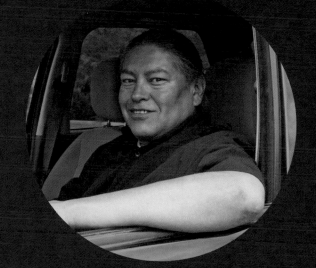

Gerald was involved in a car accident on the way to work. He was not restrained and was thrown from the car into the roadside brush. The crash was witnessed, and bystanders called 911. First responders arrived to find Gerald unconscious with labored breathing and a deformed right lower extremity. A witness stated that Mr. Luna just drove off the road and appeared to be asleep. No other vehicles were involved. The first responders established monitoring equipment, intubated Gerald at the scene, started intravenous fluids with 0.9% normal saline, and splinted his right lower extremity.

1. **NurseThink® Prioritization Power!**
    Evaluate the information in the case and determine the **Top 3 Priority** concerns or cues.

    1. _____

    2. _____

    3. _____

2. **Based on the priority concerns, what action(s) should the nurse perform first as Gerald arrives at the emergency department?**

   1. Obtain a finger sample blood glucose level.
   2. Obtain a oxygen saturation reading.
   3. Take vital signs and place him on the cardiac monitor.
   4. Complete a head to toe assessment.

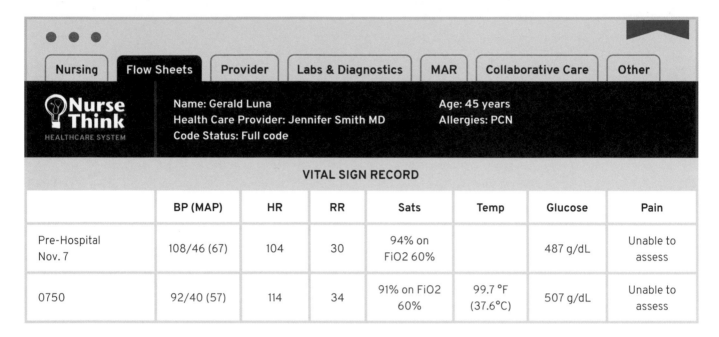

| Nursing | Flow Sheets | Provider | Labs & Diagnostics | MAR | Collaborative Care | Other |

NurseThink
HEALTHCARE SYSTEM

Name: Gerald Luna
Health Care Provider: Jennifer Smith MD
Code Status: Full code

Age: 45 years
Allergies: PCN

VITAL SIGN RECORD

	BP (MAP)	HR	RR	Sats	Temp	Glucose	Pain
Pre-Hospital Nov. 7	108/46 (67)	104	30	94% on FiO2 60%		487 g/dL	Unable to assess
0750	92/40 (57)	114	34	91% on FiO2 60%	99.7 °F (37.6°C)	507 g/dL	Unable to assess

3. **Indicate if the client's condition is improving or declining based on the trends of data?**

   1. Temperature. _____
   2. Pulse. _____
   3. Respirations. _____
   4. Oxygen Saturation. _____
   5. Blood Pressure. _____

Gerald was admitted directly to the intensive care unit for care. The emergency room staff were able to reach Andrea who is having a friend drive her to the hospital.

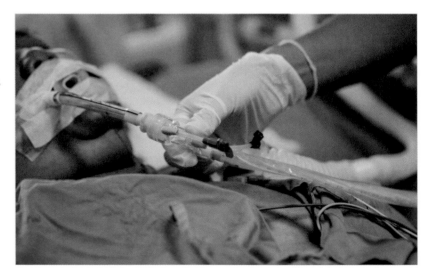

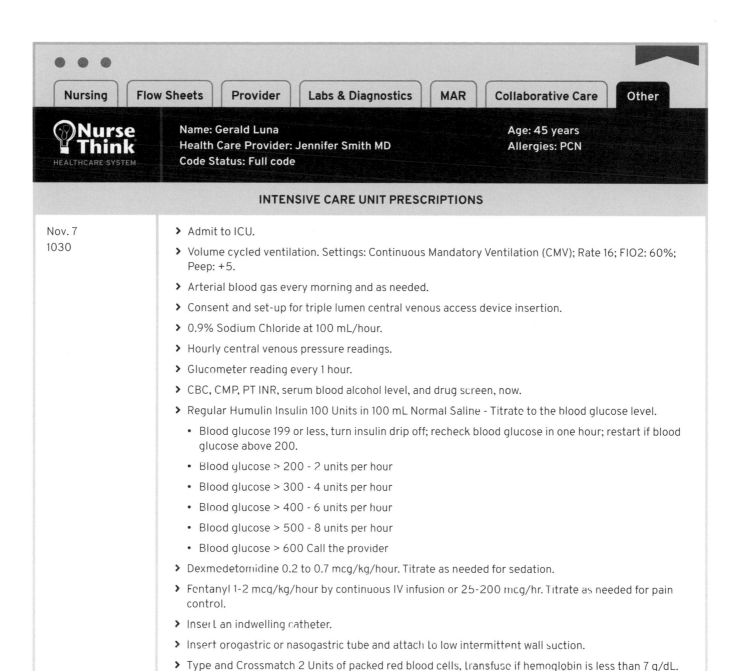

INTENSIVE CARE UNIT PRESCRIPTIONS

Nov. 7 1030	> Admit to ICU.
	> Volume cycled ventilation. Settings: Continuous Mandatory Ventilation (CMV); Rate 16; FIO2: 60%; Peep: +5.
	> Arterial blood gas every morning and as needed.
	> Consent and set-up for triple lumen central venous access device insertion.
	> 0.9% Sodium Chloride at 100 mL/hour.
	> Hourly central venous pressure readings.
	> Glucometer reading every 1 hour.
	> CBC, CMP, PT INR, serum blood alcohol level, and drug screen, now.
	> Regular Humulin Insulin 100 Units in 100 mL Normal Saline - Titrate to the blood glucose level.
	• Blood glucose 199 or less, turn insulin drip off; recheck blood glucose in one hour; restart if blood glucose above 200.
	• Blood glucose > 200 - 2 units per hour
	• Blood glucose > 300 - 4 units per hour
	• Blood glucose > 400 - 6 units per hour
	• Blood glucose > 500 - 8 units per hour
	• Blood glucose > 600 Call the provider
	> Dexmedetomidine 0.2 to 0.7 mcg/kg/hour. Titrate as needed for sedation.
	> Fentanyl 1-2 mcg/kg/hour by continuous IV infusion or 25-200 mcg/hr. Titrate as needed for pain control.
	> Insert an indwelling catheter.
	> Insert orogastric or nasogastric tube and attach to low intermittent wall suction.
	> Type and Crossmatch 2 Units of packed red blood cells, transfuse if hemoglobin is less than 7 g/dL.
	> ICU Standard Emergency Care Protocol.

4. The nurse completes an assessment on Gerald. For each assessment finding, list why it is concerning.

1. Blood glucose. _____

2. Arousable, does not follow commands. _____

3. Lung sounds with crackles bilaterally. _____

4. Blood pressure. _____

5. Respiratory rate. _____

6. Deformity right lower extremity. _____

5. Gerald's blood glucose on arrival to the intensive care unit is 520 mg/dL. What rate will the nurse start the regular insulin drip?

   1. 2 units per hour.
   2. 4 units per hour.
   3. 6 units per hour.
   4. 8 units per hour.

6. The nurse obtains additional information, documented in the chart on the left. Determine if the findings are related or not related to his current trauma situation.

Medical History:
Type 2 diabetes mellitus, alcoholism, smokes tobacco

Vital Signs:
99.7°F (°C); pulse; 114; respiratory rate 34; 88/40 (56)

iStat values:
Hemoglobin 6.2 g/dL, K+ 3.2 mEq/L

Arterial Blood Gas:
pH 7.21
CO_2 65
HCO_3 24
paO_2 58

Finding	Related	Not Related
Cardiac rhythm: Sinus Tachycardia with premature ventricular contractions		
Hyperglycemia		
Respiratory acidosis		
Cool, clammy skin		
Urine output 15 mL/hour		
Jaundice		
Weak pulse right foot		

7. **THIN Thinking Time!**
   Reflect on the nurse's collection of information for Gerald and apply **THIN Thinking.**

   T – _____

   H – _____

   I – _____

   N – _____

   T - Top 3
   H - Help Quick
   I - Identify Risk to Safety
   N - Nursing Process

   Scan to access the 10-Minute-Mentor on THIN Thinking.

   NurseThink.com/THINThinking

8. **Based on the admission assessment and related information provided, what hypothesis can the nurse make?**
   1. Vital signs are stabilizing.
   2. The respiratory condition is improving.
   3. Client's vital signs indicate possible shock.
   4. The client is compensating effectively for loss of volume.

As Gerald's condition is deteriorating, the nurse receives prescriptions from the provider to complete as quickly as possible.

9. **Explain the presenting symptom(s) that support(s) the need for each of the prescriptions.**
   Then describe why the prescription is indicated.

Presenting Symptom	Prescription	Why is it needed?
	Electrolyte replacement protocol.	
	Normal Saline.	
	Blood Transfusion.	
	Norepinephrine drip.	
	Insulin drip.	
	Stat ABG.	
	Insertion of triple lumen central venous access device.	

The nurse begins to complete the prescriptions for Mr. Luna as quickly as possible to help stabilize his condition. The nurse is planning to prepare the norepinephrine. While the nurse is in the medication room, a nurse colleague recommends that it would be essential to consider asking the provider for an order to administer furosemide after the blood transfusion is completed. The nurse consults materials from a drug reference.

Norepinephrine	Furosemide
Classification: Vasopressor. Alpha and Beta-agonist.	**Classification:** Diuretic.
Indications: To restore blood pressure in acute hypotension or severe hypotension during cardiac arrest.	**Indications:** Acute Pulmonary edema, Hypertension.
Dosage: 2-12 mcg/minute by intravenous infusion, average dose is 2-4 mcg/minute.	**Dosage:** 40 to 80 mg intravenous injected slowly over 1-2 minutes. The maximum dose is 200 mg/dose.
Administration: Use a central venous catheter to minimize the risk of extravasation. Use an infusion pump. Monitor blood pressure frequently using arterial line if possible.	**Administration:** For direct infusion, if high dose, dilute with saline, D5W, or lactated ringer solution. Onset is within 5 minutes when administering intravenously. May cause ototoxicity.
Incompatibilities: Alkalis, Iron salts, oxidizers, regular insulin, and thiopental.	**Incompatibilities:** Acidic solutions, amrinone, ciprofloxacin, milrinone.
Side effects: Headache, anxiety, bradycardia, severe hypertension, arrhythmias, ischemic injury, tissue irritation, necrosis and gangrene with extravasation.	**Side effects:** Orthostatic hypotension, weakness, volume depletion and dehydration, hypokalemia, hyponatremia, hyperglycemia.
Precautions: Contraindicated for clients with hypoxia, hypercarbia, and hypotension resulting from blood volume deficit.	**Precautions:** Can cause severe diuresis with water and electrolyte depletion.
Nursing Considerations: The drug is not a substitute for blood or fluid replacement. Gradually slow infusion rate when stopping the medication.	**Nursing Considerations:** Monitor fluid intake and output. Monitor glucose level in diabetic clients. Watch for signs of hypokalemia such as muscle weakness and cramps.

10. **The nurse reviews material for the norepinephrine ordered. Highlight the key information in the reference that the nurse should consider with the administration of norepinephrine. Record the nurse's decisions regarding about administering the medication.**

_____

_____

_____

_____

The nurse colleague recommends that furosemide may be needed since the client is receiving a blood transfusion. Highlight the reasons why the nurse will ask or not ask the provider for a prescription to administer furosemide for this situation.

_____

_____

_____

_____

The nurse prepares the norepinephrine infusion in case it will be needed urgently, but has not started it. An updated assessment for Gerald is documented on the next page.

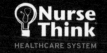

Name: Gerald Luna
Health Care Provider: Jennifer Smith MD
Code Status: Full code

Age: 45 years
Allergies: PCN

INTENSIVE CARE RECORD

Lab	Normal	Nov. 7
Blood Pressure		80/50 (60)
Pulse		115
Respirations		36
Temperature		100.1°F (37.8°C) Temporal
Pain		Unable to assess
Central Venous Pressure	2 – 8 mmHg	**1 mmHg L**
Hemoglobin	12 – 17 g/dl	**5.8 L**
Platelets	150,000 - 350,000 µL	**75 L**
White blood cells	4,000 - 10,000 µ/L	**14.8 H**
Potassium	3.5 - 5.0 mEq/L	**3.0 L**
Sodium	136 - 145 mEq/L	**132 L**
Glucose	70 - 100 mg/dL	**323 H**
Blood urea nitrogen	8 - 20 mg/dL	**85 H**
Creatinine	0.7 - 1.3 mg/dL	**2.8 H**
Albumin	3.5 – 5.0 g/dL	**2.2 L**
Total Protein	6 - 7.8 g/dL	**4.3 L**
Prothrombin	11 - 12.5 sec	**37 H**
INR	0.8 – 1.1	**3.4 H**
AST	0 - 35 U/L	**142 H**
ALT	0 - 35 U/L	**136 H**
Troponin	< 0.10 ng/mL	**0.2 H**
Arterial Blood Gas		
pH	7.35 - 7.45	**7.11 L**
pCO_2	35 - 45 mmHg	**85 H**
HCO_3	22 - 26 mEq/L	**18 L**
paO_2	80-100 mmHg	**59 L**
Respiratory Assessment		Intubated with #8.0 oral endotracheal tube measuring 23 cm at the lip line. Vent settings unchanged since admission.
Cardiac Assessment		Peripheral pulses weak and thready, Capillary refill > 3 seconds, Mean arterial pressure 60.
Neurological Assessment		Arousable, pupils equal and reactive to light, moves upper extremities.
Musculoskeletal Assessment		Right lower extremity with a splint in place, unable to assess movement and sensation, weak pedal pulse.
Chest X-ray		Infiltrates in bilateral lung fields

11. **NurseThink® Prioritization Power!**

    Evaluate the information select the **Top 3 Priority** concerns or cues.

    1. _____

    2. _____

    3. _____

12. **The type and cross-matched blood are available for transfusion. Put in order the steps for administering a blood transfusion.**

    _____, _____, _____, _____, _____.

    1. Start the blood transfusion.
    2. Complete baseline vital signs.
    3. Prime the blood tubing with normal saline.
    4. Identify the client to the blood unit.
    5. Monitor for signs and symptoms of blood transfusion reaction.

13. **As the nurse compares Gerald's current arterial blood gas and respiratory assessment with the one from admission, what change(s) should be anticipated in the ventilator settings? Select all that apply.**

    1. Increase in the peep.
    2. Reduction in FIO2.
    3. Increase in ventilator rate.
    4. Reduction in tidal volume.
    5. No change in ventilator settings.

14. **The nurse is responding to a high-pressure alarm sounding on the ventilator. What are the possible causes of a high-pressure alarm? Select all that apply.**

    1. The lungs are filling with infiltrates.
    2. The ventilator tubing has been disconnected.
    3. The client is biting on the endotracheal tube.
    4. The peep has been increased.
    5. The client has mucus in the airway.

15. **Gerald's wife asks the nurse why he is on life support. What is the nurse's best response?**

    1. "Because he can't breathe without the machine."
    2. "He needs help to breathe since he is bleeding."
    3. "It is too early to know why he can't breathe on his own."
    4. "To help support his breathing effort."

16. **Which findings in the updated assessment make Gerald at risk of bleeding? Select all that apply.**

    1. Platelet level.
    2. Potassium level.
    3. Prothrombin/INR.
    4. Hemoglobin.
    5. Sodium level.

17. **Treatment for Gerald has been in progress for six hours. Which finding(s) would be considered an improvement in his condition? Select all that apply.**

    1. Central venous pressure of 5 mmHg.
    2. MAP of 50 mmHg.
    3. Serum potassium 3.8 mEq/L.
    4. PaO2 80 mmHg.
    5. Following commands.

18. **The nurse enters Gerald's room and sees this rhythm on the cardiac monitor. Mr. Luna is unresponsive. What should the nurse do next?**

    1. Call a code blue.
    2. Start compressions.
    3. Run to get the crash cart.
    4. Remove his wife from the room.

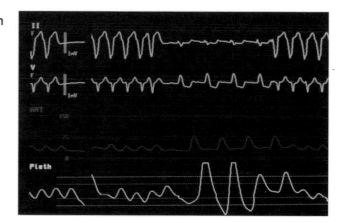

19. **The family approached the nurse to find out if a Native American healer could visit Gerald and perform a ceremony. What is the nurse's best response?**

    1. "He is too ill to have a healer visit right now."
    2. "Could you tell me what the healer would do during the visit?"
    3. "Would there be the use of fire in the ceremony?"
    4. "How long would the ceremony last?"

20. **When reviewing Gerald's case, what evidence is present that confirms multiple organ dysfunction?**

    1. Neurological: _____
    2. Respiratory: _____
    3. Cardiac: _____
    4. Renal: _____
    5. Liver: _____
    6. Other: _____

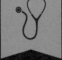
Case 6: Emergency Response Planning

Related Concepts: Perfusion, Respirations, Hormonal Regulation
Threaded Topics: Medication Prioritization, Electronic Medication Error,
Prioritization, Triage

When multiple victims of an accident or disaster are identified at the scene or a care facility, the nurse is faced with the challenge of triage. The goal is to save and care for as many victims as possible by identifying who needs to be cared for first, second, third and so on. Triaging mass emergencies, such as car accidents, is done differently then the process of prioritization that is completed in acute care facilities. When multiple victims are present, the nurse or first responder will identify the victims with the most severe injuries who need care first, or they may not survive. Conversely, those victims who are dead and dying will not be the focus of attention or resources.

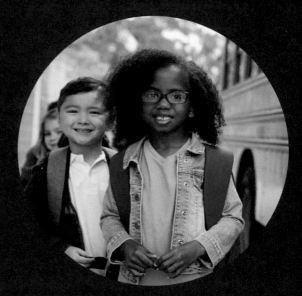

A school bus is headed to a local museum for a 3rd-grade field trip. On the bus are the driver, two teachers, three parents, and 30 students. On the way to the museum, it starts to rain, and the bus driver asks the children to keep the noise down since the weather is worsening. At that moment, an oncoming semitrailer truck starts to slide and hits the school bus head-on. A nurse is driving by and quickly stops to help.

While approaching the vehicles, the truck driver is getting out of the vehicle. The school bus driver's head is down, and visible blood is noted around her. The back door of the bus is opened, and multiple children started jumping out, screaming.

1. **When arriving at the scene of an accident, what is the nurse's most important concern?**
   1. Determining how many people have injuries.
   2. Identifying the location of the accident.
   3. Determine if it is safe to enter the accident scene.
   4. Find the victim that has the most severe injury.

2. **Put in order the triage tagging system listing the most critical to the least critical.**

   _____, _____, _____, _____.

   1. Minor or green tag.
   2. Delayed or yellow tag.
   3. Dead/Dying or black tag.
   4. Emergent/Immediate or red tag.

3. **Which victim should be tagged delayed or yellow?**

   1. Child with a laceration on the right arm.
   2. Adult with a deformed left leg.
   3. Child having pain in the left arm.
   4. Adult with shortness of breath and chest pain.

4. **The nurse is asked to triage victims using triage tags. What triage category is appropriate?**

Triage Tag : No. 3542

Name:_____

Address:_____

Phone #:_____

Major Injuries:

☐ Oriented   ☐ Disoriented   ☐ Unconscious

Time	Pulse	B/P	Respiration

Allergies:

Dead or Dying

No respirations after head tilt

Immediate

Respiratory rate over 30
Capillary refill over 2 seconds
Mental Status – Unable to follow simple commands

Delayed

Otherwise

Minor

Move the walking wounded

1. The semi driver is walking over to the first responders crying and saying that he is so sorry, but his truck lost control, and he had no way to stop.

   Triage Tag:_____

2. The bus driver was carried out and positioned on the ground for triaging. He is unconscious and is not breathing.

   Triage Tag:_____

3. One of the children that was able to climb off the bus and walk to the minor injury care area is now confused and will not follow commands. A large bruise is noted on her forehead.

   Updated Triage Tag:_____

4. An adult on the bus is yelling for help. She is holding her chest. On closer assessment, a large contusion is noted on the left chest with paradoxical chest wall movements. Her respiratory rate is 34 breaths per minute.

   Triage Tag:_____

5. When the first victim arrives at the hospital emergency department, this information is written on Triage Tag No. 5467. The first victim arrives with oxygen at 6 liters by nasal cannula and normal saline 0.9% running wide open. What should be the nurse's first action?

   1. Call a code blue.
   2. Apply a simple mask at 10 liters.
   3. Start a large bore peripheral intravenous line.
   4. Call for a stat chest x-ray at the bedside.

Triage Tag : No. 5467

Name: Rose Wilson

Address: 1234 West Main Street
Chicago, IL 60007

Phone #: (773) 678-1232

Major Injuries: Flail chest, paradoxical chest movements ☐ Oriented ■ Disoriented ☐ Unconscious

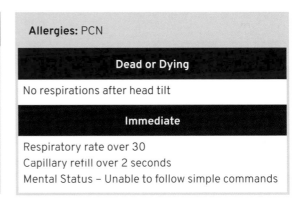

Time	Heart Rate	Blood Pressure	Respiratory Rate	Oxygen Saturation
1000	100	106/50 (69)	32	
1015	112	84/46 (59)	35	89%
On arrival to the Hospital				
1030	115	80/40 (53)	40	85%

Allergies: PCN

Dead or Dying

No respirations after head tilt

Immediate

Respiratory rate over 30
Capillary refill over 2 seconds
Mental Status – Unable to follow simple commands

---

6. **NurseThink® Prioritization Power!**

   Reflect on Rose's assessment findings and identify the **Top 3 Priority** concerns.

   1. _____

   2. _____

   3. _____

---

7. **What critical labs and tests should be ordered for Rose? Select all that apply.**

   1. Chest x-ray.
   2. Complete blood count.
   3. Coagulation labs.
   4. Arterial blood gas.
   5. Venous Doppler study.
   6. Abdominal CT scan.

Review the information given on the following page, which victim should the nurse assess first and why?

_____

_____

_____

Presenting Findings:	Phillip 8-year-old male. Alert, oriented, wheezing bilaterally. He has an inhaler in his pocket	Maria 32-year-old female parent with a chest contusion and chest pain. She is oozing blood from a head laceration	Alison 9-year-old female who is crying and holding her right arm. She has type 1 diabetes who is diaphoretic	Jose 48-year-old male teacher who is diaphoretic, complaining of chest pain and shortness of breath
Allergies	No know allergies	Penicillin	No known allergies	Aspirin
Heart Rate	130	85	112	105
Respiratory Rate	30	30	28	26
Blood Pressure	110/50 (70)	120/80 (93)	100/50 (67)	80/50 (60
Oxygen Saturation	95% on 2 L/NC	85% on 100% non-rebreather mask	95% on room air	92% on 2 L/NC

8. What priority test or information is needed next for each victim? Why?

Phillip: _____ Why? _____

Maria: _____ Why? _____

Alison: _____ Why? _____

Jose: _____ Why? _____

9. **Which medication(s) does the nurse anticipate the provider will order for Phillip? Select all that apply.**
    1. Atropine.
    2. Albuterol.
    3. Oxygen.
    4. Prednisolone.
    5. Furosemide.

10. **The provider ordered Aspirin 160 mg orally stat for Jose. The nurse administered the medication and proceeded to enter the order in the electronic health record. When entering the order, an alert window appeared. What is the nurse's highest priority?**

    Allergy Alert: Aspirin
    Override? Yes   No

    1. Call the provider to report the error.
    2. Monitor Jose for ongoing chest pain.
    3. Assess Jose for signs and symptoms of anaphylaxis.
    4. Delete the order and call the provider.

11. **What signs and symptoms should the nurse anticipate Jose could develop? Select all that apply.**

    1. Hypoxia.
    2. Urticaria.
    3. Phlebitis.
    4. Itching.
    5. Anemia.

12. **Alison has a finger stick glucose reading of 32 mg/dL. What prescription(s) does the nurse anticipate? Select all that apply.**

    1. Administration of magnesium intravenously.
    2. Intravenous administration of insulin.
    3. Laboratory venous blood draw for glucose.
    4. Oral administration of dextrose tablet.
    5. Glucagon administered subcutaneously.

13. **Alison will need surgical intervention to repair her right radius fracture. The surgeon is concerned that the arm is compromised and she needs emergency surgery. What signs and symptoms would the nurse associate with a need for emergency surgery? Select all that apply.**

    1. Mottled right hand.
    2. Right radial pulse absent.
    3. Erythema distal to the injury.
    4. Swelling at the fracture site.
    5. Severe right-hand pain.

14. **The next four victims arrive at the emergency room from the accident. Review the information given, which victim should the nurse assess first and why?**

	Jon	**Marshall**	**Zoe**	**Daniel**
Presenting Findings:	8-year-old male with a history of sickle cell anemia. He is complaining of shortness of breath and joint pain. His mother has been notified of the accident and is on her way to the emergency room.	45-year-old male with a history of anxiety, panic attacks, and Addison's disease. He is hyperventilating and anxious.	2-year-old sister of a student with no known medical problems. Initially, she was crying in her mother's arms but now is not arousable. Her car seat was found 3 rows away from where it was secured.	57-year-old male with a history of coronary artery disease, hypertension, and renal insufficiency. He has a deformed left leg. He is asking for pain medicine now! His pain is 10/10.
Allergies	Morphine	No known allergies	No know allergies	Lisinopril
Heart Rate	125	110	85	52
Respiratory Rate	36	25	16	24
Blood Pressure	92/50 (64)	80/50 (60)	160/40 (80)	186/98 (127)

15. **What test or priority information is needed next for each victim?**

Jon: _____ Why? _____

Marshall: _____ Why? _____

Zoe: _____ Why? _____

Daniel: _____ Why? _____

16. **For Jon, the provider ordered intravenous normal saline 0.9% at 75 mL/hour and morphine sulfate 0.5 mg intravenous push every 15 minutes as needed for pain. What action should the nurse take next?**

_____

17. **For Marshall, the provider ordered intravenous push methylprednisolone 125 mg. What action should the nurse take next?**

_____

18. **For Zoe, the provider ordered a stat CT scan of the head. What action should the nurse take next?**

_____

19. **For Daniel, the provider has ordered hydromorphone 1 mg intravenous push stat. What action should the nurse take next?**

_____

20. **Which victim is showing signs of improvement?**
    1. Jon states he is having shortness of breath with a finger oximeter reading or 85%.
    2. Marshall has a blood pressure of 90/50 and a heart rate of 100 and is asking for water.
    3. Zoe is unresponsive and has started to have a seizure in the radiology department.
    4. Daniel states his pain is 8/10, but his dressing is saturated with bright red blood.

Which victim is showing signs of decline and would be the priority for provider reassessment?
1. Jon states his joint pain is decreasing, and he is breathing easier.
2. Marshall notices that he has abrasions on his legs that are oozing blood.
3. Zoe is no longer having seizures, but one of her pupils is larger than the other.
4. Daniel is complaining of pain 10/10 and needs more pain medicine now!

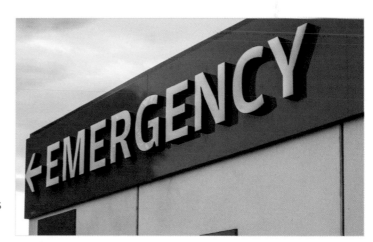

Acute Urinary Retention (2008). Society of Urologic Nurses and Associates.
http://www.suna.org/resources/acuteUrinaryRetention.pdf

American Cancer Society. (Revised 2016). Cancer A-Z. Retrieved from https://www.cancer.org/cancer.html

American Cancer Society. (2018). Guidelines for the early detection of cancer. Retrieved from https://connection.cancer.org/Consumer/PDF/Product/P2070.00.pdf

American College of Obstetrics and Gynecology, www.acog.org.

American Nurses Association. Streamlined Evidence-Based RN Tool: Catheter Associated Urinary Tract Infection (CAUTI) Prevention. Retrieved from: https://www.nursingworld.org

American Pain Society (2008). Principles of analgesic use in the treatment of acute and cancer pain, 6th ed., Glenview, IL.

American Stroke Association. (2015). Complications after stroke. Retrieved from www.strokeassociation.org/letstalkaboutstroke

Center for Disease Control and Prevention. Deaths from Falls Among Persons Aged ≥65 Years — United States, 2007–2016. https://www.cdc.gov.

Center for Disease Control (2018). Urinary Tract Infection: Catheter-Associated Urinary Tract Infection (CAUTI) and Non-Catheter-Associated Urinary Tract Infection, and Other Urinary System Infection [USI]) Events. Retrieved from https://www.cdc.gov/nhsn/pdfs/pscmanual/7psccauticurrent.pdf

Cuellar, E.T. (2017). HESI comprehensive review for the NCLEX-RN® examination. St. Louis, MO: Elsevier.

Folstein M., Folstein S., McHugh P. (1975). Mini-mental state: A practical method for grading the cognitive state of patients for the clinician, Journal of Psychiatric Research, 12 : 189-198.

Giddens, J. (2017). Concepts for Nursing Practice, 2nd ed. Elsevier: St. Louis.

Gould, C., Umscheid, C., et al. (2017). Guideline for prevention of catheter-associated urinary tract infections 2009. Healthcare Infection Control Practices Advisory Committee. Retrieved from https://www.cdc.gov/infectioncontrol/pdf/guidelines/cauti-guidelines.pdf

Gregg, I. (2018). The health care experiences of lesbian women becoming mothers. Nursing for Women's Health, 22(1), 41-50.

Halter, M.J. (2018). Varcarolis' foundations of psychiatric-mental health nursing (8th ed.). St. Louis, MO: Elsevier.

Hayman, B., Wilkes, L., Halcomb, E., & Jackson, D. (2013). Marginalized mothers: Lesbian women negotiating heteronormative healthcare services. Contemporary Nursing, 44(1), 120-127.

Hinkle, J.L., & Cheever, K.H. (2018). Brunner & Suddarth's textbook of medical-surgical nursing (14th ed.).

Philadelphia, PA: Wolters Kluwer.

Hogan, M. (2018). Comprehensive review for NCLEX-RN® (3rd ed.). New York, NY: Pearson.

Holloway, B. & Moredich, C. (2016. OB/GYN Peds Notes: Nurse's Clinical Pocket Guide, 3rd ed. Philadelphia, PA: F.A. Davis Company.

Kaufman, J.S. (2017). Acute exacerbation of COPD: Diagnosis and management. The Nurse Practitioner, 42 (6), 1-7.

Koning, C., Young, L., Bruce, A. (2016). Mind the gap: Women and acute myocardial infarctions: An integrated review of literature. Canadian Journal of Cardiovascular Nursing, 26 (3), 8-14.

Ladewig, P., London, M., & Davidson, M. (2017). Contemporary Maternal-Newborn Nursing, 9th ed. Boston, MA: Pearson.

Lehne, R. (2018). Pharmacology for Nursing Care, 10th ed. St. Louis, MO: Elsevier.

Lewis, S.L., Dirksen, S.R., Heitkemper, M.M., & Bucher, L. (2017). Medical-Surgical Nursing: Assessment and Management of Clinical Problems (10th ed.). St. Louis: Elsevier.

Lilley, L. L., Savoca, D., & Lilley, L. L. (2017) Pharmacology and the nursing process, (8th ed.), Maryland Heights, MO: Mosby.

Lowdemilk, D., Perry, S., Cashion, K., & Alden, K. (2016). Maternity & women's health care, (11th ed). St. Louis, MO: Elsevier.

March of Dimes: Prenatal Tests. https://www.marchofdimes.org/pregnancy/prenatal-tests.aspx

McCuistion, L., Vuljoin-DiMaggio, K., Winton, M.B., & Yeager, J.J. (2018). Pharmacology: A patient-centered nursing process approach (9th ed.). St. Louis, MO: Elsevier.

McKinney, E., James, S., Murray, S. (2018). Maternal-child nursing (5th ed.). Philadelphia, PA: W.B. Saunders.

Metzger, B. (2010). International association of diabetes and pregnancy study groups recommendations on the diagnosis and classification of hyperglycemia in pregnancy, Diabetes Care, 33(3): 676-682.

National Councils of State Boards of Nursing (2018). Substance Use Disorder in Nursing. https://www.ncsbn.org/substance-use-in-nursing.htm

National Council of State Boards of Nursing 2019 NCLEX-RN® Test Plan. Retrieved from www.ncsbn.org.

National Council State Boards of Nursing Next Generation NCLEX® Project. Retrieved from https://www.ncsbn.org/next-generation-nclex.htm

National Institute of Diabetes and Digestive and Kidney Diseases. (2018). Cushing's syndrome. Retrieved from https://www.niddk.nih.gov/health-information/endocrine-diseases/cushings-syndrome

National Institute of Health (2018). Opioid Overdose Crisis. https://www.drugabuse.gov/drugs-abuse/opioids/opioid-overdose-crisis

National Institute of Health and Care Excellence, NICE guideline [NG14]. (2015). Melanoma: Assessment and management. Retrieved from https://www.nice.org.uk/guidance/ng14

Pearson Education. (2019). Nursing: A concept-based approach to learning (Vol. 1-3). Minneapolis, MN: Author.

Pop, V., & Badaut, J. (2011). A neurovascular perspective for long-term changes after brain trauma. Translational Stroke Research, 2(4), 533-545.

Potter, P.A., Perry, A.G., Stockert, P.A., & Hall, A.M. (2017). Fundamentals of nursing (9th ed.). St. Louis, MO: Elsevier.

Ricci, S. (2017). Essentials of maternity, newborn, and women's health nursing (4th ed.). Philadelphia, PA: Wolters Kluwer.

Ricci, S. S., Kyle, T., & Carman, S. (2017). Maternity and pediatric nursing (2nd ed.). Philadelphia, PA: Wolters Kluwer.

Rondal, G., Bruhner, E., & Lindhe, J. (2009). Heteronormative communication with lesbian families in antenatal care, childbirth, and postnatal care. Journal of Advanced Nursing, 65(11), 2337-2344.

Silvestri, L.A. & Silvestri, A. (2017). Saunders comprehensive review for the NCLEX-RN® examination (7th ed.). St. Louis, MO: Elsevier.

Taylor, C., Lillis, C., Lynn, P. & LeMone, P. (2015). Fundamentals of nursing (8th ed.). Philadelphia, PA: Wolters Kluwer.

Texas Nursing Concept-based Curriculum Consortium. Retrieved from http://texasapin.org/faculty/concept-based-curriculum/

Townsend, M. (2015). Psychiatric mental health nursing: Concepts of care in evidence-based practice. Philadelphia, PA: FA Davis.

U.S. Department of Health and Human Services, Centers for Disease Prevention and Control. (2016). The ABCs of hepatitis. Retrieved from https://www.cdc.gov/hepatitis/resources/professionals/pdfs/abctable.pdf

U.S. Department of Health and Human Services, National Institute of Diabetes and Digestive and Kidney Disease. (2018). Adrenal insufficiency and Addison's disease. Retrieved from https://www.niddk.nih.gov/health-information/endocrine-diseases/adrenal-insufficiency-addisons-disease

References

U.S. Department of Health and Human Services, National Institute of Diabetes and Digestive and Kidney Disease. (2018). Cushing's syndrome. Retrieved from https://www.niddk.nih.gov/health-information/endocrinediseases/cushings-syndrome

U.S. Department of Health and Human Services, National Institutes of Health, National Cancer Institute. (2018). Cancer types. Retrieved from https://www.cancer.gov/types

U.S. Department of Health and Human Services, National Institutes of Health, National Heart, Lung, and Blood Institute. (2018). Polycythemia Vera. Retrieved from https://www.nhlbi.nih.gov/health-topics/polycythemia-vera

U.S. Department of Health and Human Services National Institutes of Health, National Institute of Neurological Disorders and Stroke. (2018). Myasthenia gravis fact sheet. Retrieved from https://www.ninds.nih.gov/disorders/patient-caregiver-education/fact-sheets/myasthenia-gravis-fact-sheet

U.S. Department of Health and Human Services National Institutes of Health, National Institute of Neurological Disorders and Stroke. (2018). Peripheral neuropathy fact sheet. Retrieved from https://www.ninds.nih.gov/Disorders/Patient-Caregiver-Education/Fact-Sheets/Peripheral-Neuropathy-Fact-Sheet#3208_1

Vallerand, A. & Sanoski, C. (2019). Davis's drug guide for nurses (16th ed.). Philadelphia, PA: FA Davis.

Vallerand, A.H., Sanoski, C.A, & Deglin, J.H. (2017). Davis's drug guide for nurses (15th ed.). Philadelphia, PA: FA Davis.

Varcarolis, E. M. (2017). Essentials of Psychiatric Mental Health Nursing (3rd ed.). St. Louis: Elsevier.

Ward, S., Hisley, S., & Kennedy, A. (2016). Maternal-Child Nursing Care: Optimizing Outcomes for Mothers, Children and Families 2nd ed. Philadelphia, PA: F. A. Davis Company.

Whelton, P.K, & Carey, R.M. (2017). The 2017 guideline for high blood pressure. JAMA: Journal of the American Medical Association, 318(21). 2073-2074.

Wojnar, D. & Katzenmeyer, A. (2013). Experiences of preconception, pregnancy, and new motherhood for lesbian nonbiological mothers. Journal of Obstetric, Gynecological and Neonatal Nursing, 43, 50-60.

Wolters Kluwer Health, Inc. (2018). In vitro fertilization and embryo transfer. Lippincott Advisor for Education.

Wong, D. L., Hockenberry, M. J., Wilson, D. (2015) Wong's nursing care of infants and children (9th ed.). St. Louis: Elsevier.

Workman, M. & LaCharity, L. (2016). Understanding pharmacology: Essentials for medication safety (2nd ed.). St. Louis, MO: Elsevier.

World Health Organization: Sexual Health. Retrieved from https://www.who.int/topics/sexual_health/en/

Yoder-Wise, P. (2014). Leading and managing in nursing (5th ed.). St. Louis, MO: Elsevier.

Notes

Notes

Notes

NurseThink® Quick Laboratory and Diagnostics

LAB TEST	NORMAL RANGE	CRITICAL CONCERNS	INCREASED	
HEMATOLOGY				
CBC				
*Red Blood Cells / Erythrocytes (RBC)	4.2 - 5.9 cells/L		(Polycythemia), Hemoconcentration	
Reticulocytes	0.5 - 1.5%		Acute Hemorrhage	
*Hemoglobin (Hgb)	12 - 17 g/dL	< 5.0 g/dL or > 20 g/dL		
*Hematocrit (Hct)	36 - 51%	<15% or > 60%		
*White Blood Cells / Leukocytes (WBC)	4,000-10,000 μL or mm³	< 2,500 or > 30,000 μL or mm³	Infections, Inflammation, Stress	
*Neutrophils (polys/segs)	> 75%		Bacterial Infections	
Bands	< 10%	> 10%	Acute Bacterial Infection	
*Absolute Neutrophil Count (ANC)	> 1000 μL or mm³	< 1000 μL or mm³		
*Platelets	150,000-350,000 μL or mm³	< 50,000 or > 1 million μL or mm³	Malignancies	
COAGULATION				
Bleeding time	Less than 10 minutes	> 10 minutes	Low Platelets, DIC, ASA	
Prothrombin Time (PT)	11 - 12.5 seconds	> 20 seconds	Liver dysfunction, Coumadin, Vit K Deficiency	
*International Normalized Ratio (INR)	0.8 - 1.1	> 5.5	Liver dysfunction, Coumadin, Vit K Deficiency	
Activated Partial Thromboplastin Time (aPTT)	25 - 35 seconds	> 70 seconds	Coagulation Deficiencies, Heparin	
Partial Thromboplastin Time (PTT)	60 - 70 seconds	> 100 seconds	Coagulation Deficiencies, Heparin	
D-dimer	< 0.5 mcg/mL		Thrombus	
IMMUNE & INFLAMMATORY				
C-Reactive Protein (CRP)	< 1.0 mg/dL		Bacterial Infection, Inflammation	
Erythrocyte Sedimentation Rate (ESR)	0 - 20 mm/h		Inflammation, Renal Failure, Malignancy	
FLUID, ELECTROLYES & RENAL				
URINE				
*Urine Specific Gravity	1.005 - 1.030		Dehydration, SIADH	
METABOLIC PANEL				
*Blood Urea Nitrogen (BUN)	8 - 20 mg/dL	> 100 mg/dL	Renal Failure, Dehydration, ↑Protein Intake	
*Creatinine	0.7 - 1.3 mg/dL	> 4 mg/dL	Renal Disease	
Electrolytes				
*Potassium (K)	3.5 - 5.0 mEq/L	< 2.5 mEq/L or > 6.5 mEq/L	Acidosis, Renal Failure	
*Sodium (Na)	136 - 145 mEq/L	< 120 mEq/L or > 160 mEq/L	Diabetes Insipidus, Cushing's, HHNK	
*Calcium (Ca)	9 - 10.5 mg/dL	< 6 mg/dL or > 13 mg/dL	Hyperparathyroidism, Renal Failure	
Chloride (Cl)	98 - 106 mEq/L	< 80 mEq/L or > 115 mEq/L	Dehydration, Metabolic Acidosis	
*Magnesium (Mg)	1.5 - 2.4 mEq/L	< 0.5 mEq/L or > 3 mEq/L	Renal Failure	
Phosphorus (Ph)	3.0 - 4.5 mg/dL	<1 mg/dL	Hypoparathyroidism, Renal Failure	
*Glucose	70 - 100 mg/dL	< 50 mg/dL or > 400 mg/dL	Diabetic Ketoacidosis, HHNK	
*Protein - Total	6 - 7.8 g/dL		Hemoconcentration	
*Protein - Albumin	3.5 - 5.0 g/dL		Dehydration	
FLUID STATUS				
* Serum Osmolality	275 - 295 mOsm/kg	< 265 or > 320 mOsm/kg	Diabetes Insipidus, HHNK, Hyperglycemia	
CARDIOPULMONARY				
ABG's				
*pH	7.35 - 7.45	< 7.25 or > 7.55	Alkalosis (resp/metabolic)	
*pO₂	80 - 100 mmHg	< 40 mmHg	Hyperoxygenation	
*pCO₂	35 - 45 mmHg	< 20 mmHg or > 60 mmHg	Hypoventilation	
*HCO₃	22- 26 mEq/L	< 15 mEq/L or > 40 mEq/L	Metabolic alkalosis	
*O₂ saturation	> 94%	< 75%		
Brain natriuretic peptide (BNP)	< 100 pg/mL		Heart failure	
METABOLISM & WASTE				
Ammonia	40 - 80 mcg/dL		Liver dysfunction	
Bilirubin - Total	0.3 - 1.2 mg/dL	Adult: > 12 mg/dL	Liver failure, RBC hemolysis, GB obstruction	
Thyroid Stimulating Hormone (TSH)	0.5 - 5 mU/L		Thyroid dysfunction	
ENZYMES				
Alkaline Phosphatase (ALP.)	36 - 92 U/L	Enzymes will be released and rise with cell damage. Once the damage stops, the enzymes will return to normal.	Liver, Biliary Tract, Bone	
Aminotransferase, Alanine (ALT)	0 - 35 U/L		Liver, (Less in Kidneys, Heart, Muscles)	
Aminotransferase, Aspartate (AST)	0 - 35 U/L		Liver	
Amylase	0 - 130 U/L		Pancreas	
Creatine Kinase (CPK)	30 - 170 U/L		Heart, Brain, Muscle	
Lactic Dehydrogenase (LDH)	60 - 100 U/L		Heart, Liver, Kidneys, Muscles, Brain, Lungs	
Lipase	< 95 U/L		Pancreas	
Troponin I & T	< 0.5ng/mL & < 0.10 ng/mL		Cardiac	
THERAPUETIC DRUG LEVELS				
Peak and Trough				
Digoxin	0.8-2.0 ng/mL	> 2.4 ng/mL = toxic level		
Lithium	0.6- 1.2 mEq/L	> 1.5 mEq/L = toxic level	Renal Failure, ↓consciousness, ECG changes	

* Know APPROXIMATE Normal for NCLEX® Exam   References: American College of Physicians & Mosby's Diagnostic and Laboratory Test Reference, 10th ed.

Do not memorize specific lab numbers - they vary greatly.
It is more important to know **approximate** normal and recognize **critical concerns** - this is when a nursing action is required.

DECREASED	SPECIAL NOTES	PRIORITY LABS
		Infection, Inflammation & Immunity
		WBCs, Segs, Bands, ANC, CRP, ESR
(Anemia), Blood Loss, Hemodilution	↑ with Epoetin; Too High = Clot formation; Too Low = O₂ Transport	**Liver Disorders**
Bone Marrow Failure	Immature RBCs	Liver Enzymes; PT/PTT/INR; Albumin; Ammonia, Bilirubin
		Na, K, Glucose
	Oxygen Carrying Capacity; PRBC < 7 g/dL	**Renal Disorders**
	Hydration Dependent	BUN; Creatinine; Osmolality, K, Na, Ca, Ph, RBCs, Urine SG
Chemo, Bone Marrow Failure	↑ with Filgrastim	**Cardiac Disorders**
Chemo, Bone Marrow Failure	Poly/Segs are Mature WBCs	Cardiac Enzymes, BNP, ABGs, Digoxin Level
Bone Marrow Failure	Increase = Left Shift	**Pancreas Disorders**
(Neutropenia)	ANC = WBC x (% Neutrophils + % Bands); < 1000 = Isolation	Amylase, Lipase, Ca, Glucose
ITP, Leukemia, Chemo	< 20,000: = Spontaneous Bleed; ↑ with Oprelvekin	**Hemorrhage - DIC**
		RBCs, Reticulocytes, Hgb, Hct, Platelets, Coagulation Studies
		Fluid Imbalance
	Therapeutic is > 1.5 - 2 times control with warfarin therapy	Protein, Albumin, Na, Urine SG, Osmolality, RBCs, Hgb,
		Hct, BUN
	Therapeutic is 1.5 to 4 with warfarin therapy	
	Therapeutic is 1.5-2.5 times the control with heparin therapy	
	Cardiac marker but not specific to myocardium	
Sickle Cell Anemia, Polycythemia Vera		
Excessive Diuresis, Diabetes Insipidus	Fluctuates Fluid Status	
Hepatic Failure, Overhydration	End By-Product of Protein Breakdown	
Decreased Muscle Mass	Doubling of level indicates 50% reduction in the GFR	
Diuretics, Gastrointestinal Loss	Abnormal level leads to arrhythmias, muscle cramps	
SIADH, Addison's	↓ = Lethargy, Stupor, Coma, Seizures; ↑ = Agitation, Seizures	
Hypoparathyroidism, Pancreatitis, Low Protein	↓ = Tetany; ↑ = Osteomalacia, Dehydration	
Gastrointestinal Loss, Low Na Diet	↓ = Hyperexcitability; ↑ = Weakness, Lethargy	
Alcoholism; Renal Disease	Abnormal level leads to arrhythmias, muscle irritability	
Hyperparathyroidism, Vit D Deficiency	↓ = Osteomalacia; ↑ Hypocalcemia (tetany)	
↓ Glucose intake or absorption, Exercise		
Malnutrition, Burns, Blood Loss	Needed for wound healing	
Liver Dysfunction, Nephrotic Syndrome	Impacts fluid shift in and out of the vascular space	
SIADH, Overhydration	Measures concentration of dissolved particles in blood	
Acidosis(resp/metabolic)	pH is inversely proportional to H+ concentration	
Hypoxemia (pneumonia, etc.)	Indirect measure of O₂ concentration in arterial blood	
Hyperventilation	Measurement of ventilation	
Metabolic acidosis	Measures metabolic component of acid-base balance	
Hypoxemia/Anemia	Indication of the % of Hgb saturated with oxygen	
	The higher the number the weaker the left ventricular contractions	
	Product of protein breakdown; Neurotoxic; Treated with Lactulose	
	Neurotoxic to newborns	
Pituitary dysfunction, Hyperthyroidism	T3, T4, T7 often needed to rule out thyroid dysfunction	
	Biochemical Markers for Cardiac Disease	
	Monitors therapeutic drug levels of nephrotoxic medications	
Subtherapeutic	Cardiac Glycoside	
Subtherapeutic: symptoms poorly controlled	Lithium clearance from the body is increased during pregnancy	

Chapter Exemplars

Chapter 5: Sexuality: Reproduction / Sexuality

Case 1: Infertility; Conception; Miscarriage; Domestic Violence

Case 2: Pregnancy; Gestational Diabetes; Vaginal Delivery; Newborn Care; Maternal Health

Chapter 6: Circulation: Perfusion / Clotting

Case 1: Acute Myocardial Infarction

Case 2: Hypertension; Heart Failure;

Chapter 7: Protection: Immunity / Inflammation / Infection

Case 1: Hip Fracture; Perioperative; Catheter Associated Urinary Tract Infection

Case 2: Severe Allergic Reaction; Appendicitis; Pediatric

Chapter 8: Homeostasis: Fluid and Electrolyte Balance / Acid-Base Balance

Case 1: Aspirin Toxicity; Blood Gases; Older Adult

Case 2: Diabetes; Renal Failure;

Chapter 9: Respiration: Oxygenation / Gas Exchange

Case 1: Emphysema; Blood Gases

Case 2: Pneumonia; Pleural Effusion; Chest Tube; Pediatric

Chapter 10: Regulation: Cellular / Intracranial / Thermo

Case 1: Melanoma; Central Line; Death and Dying

Case 2: Brain Injury; Ventilator; Seizure

Chapter 11: Nutrition: Digestion / Elimination

Case 1: Diverticular Disease; Intestinal Obstruction; Nasogastric Tube

Case 2: Hepatitis; Liver Failure; Pediatric

Chapter 12: Hormonal: Neuroendocrine / Glucose Regulation / Metabolism

Case 1: Metabolic Syndrome; Type 2 Diabetes; Insulin Dependence

Case 2: Pituitary Tumor Removal; Perioperative

Chapter 13: Movement: Mobility / Sensory / Nerve Conduction

Case 1: Parkinson's Disease; Fall Risk; Fracture

Case 2: Paraplegia from Fracture

Chapter 14: Comfort: Pain / Tissue Integrity / Fatigue

Case 1: Pressure Ulcers; Confusion; Older Adult

Case 2: Burns; Pain Management; Perioperative

Chapter 15: Adaptation: Stress / Violence / Coping / Addiction

Case 1: Obsessive Compulsive; Ineffective Coping; Mental Health

Case 2: Opioid Addiction; Professional Role; Mental Health

Chapter 16: Emotion: Mood / Anxiety / Grief

Case 1: Anxiety; Loss; Mental Health

Case 2: Bipolar; Depression; Suicide; Mental Health

Chapter 17: Cognition: Cognitive Functioning

Case 1: Confusion; Dementia; Older Adult

Case 2: Brain Attack

Chapter 18: Multi-Concept Clients

Case 1: Depression; Sexual Identity; Diabetes; Crohns; Pediatric

Case 2: Fibromyalgia; Hypothyroidism; Cushing's Disease; Diabetes; Hypertension; Anxiety; Depression

Case 3: Lung Cancer; Liver Metastasis; GI Bleed; Transfusion

Case 4: Hypertension; Diabetes; Acute Kidney Injury; Heart Failure; Implantable Cardioverter Defibrillator

Case 5: Trauma; Ventilator; Blood Transfusion; Cardiac Arrest; Multi-Organ Failure

Case 6: Triage of Mass Victim Event; Pediatric